'A deep read, rich with valuable information that will ...... the understanding of every yoga therapist. Rarely have I encountered such a generous offering of scientific information contextualised specifically for those in the field of yoga therapy. This book will definitely be a required read for my yoga therapy training programme going forward!'

– Robin Rothenberg, C-IAYT yoga therapist, author of *Restoring Prana: A Therapeutic Guide to Pranayama and Healing Through the Breath for Yoga Therapists, Yoga Teachers and Healthcare Practitioners*

'Charlotte reviews a unique tapestry of concepts not found elsewhere, providing the reader with a broad overview of the self from the inside out. Weaving together a description of the mind, the immune system, fascia and the respiratory and nervous systems, she connects the dots in ways not done before and buttresses this with practical tools and tips for the profound development of wellbeing.'

– Heather Mason, Founder of The Minded Institute

'This book is an enjoyable blend of scientific information and mindful practice. It is a resource for yoga teachers and serious practitioners who are ready to bring their curiosity to the inner world of movement and breath. Charlotte balances the complex subject matter with scholarly clarity while also encouraging the exploration of awareness. A welcome contribution to the study of yoga!'

– Dr Kristen MacPherson, DPhil (Oxon), MSc (Oxon), BA, E-RYT, YACEP

'Charlotte's knowledge is born out of deep, sustained curiosity to understand the interrelated systems of the human biome and our shared environment. This book is the result of Charlotte's determination to truly understand the respiratory system spurred on by the COVID pandemic, and the desire to help others through it. It is the body owner's manual we all need to understand how our vital systems work, and how to work with them.'

– Lisa Kaley-Isley, clinical psychologist, yoga teacher, IAYT certified yoga therapist and yoga educator

YOGA AND SOMATICS FOR IMMUNE AND RESPIRATORY HEALTH

YOGA AND SOMATICS FOR IMMUNE AND RESPIRATORY HEALTH

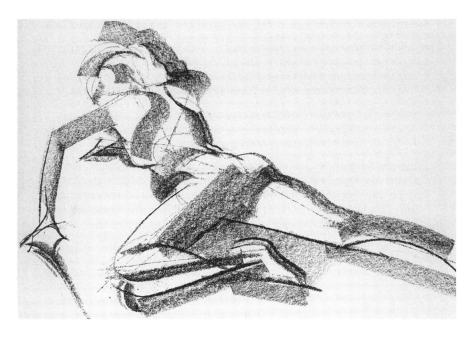

CHARLOTTE WATTS *with* Leonie Taylor

Foreword by Joanne Avison

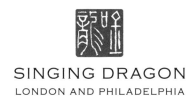

SINGING DRAGON

LONDON AND PHILADELPHIA

First published in Great Britain in 2023 by Singing Dragon,
an imprint of Jessica Kingsley Publishers
An imprint of Hodder & Stoughton Ltd
An Hachette Company

I

A CIP catalogue record for this title is available from the
British Library and the Library of Congress

ISBN 978 1 83997 087 0
eISBN 978 1 83997 088 7

Printed and bound in Great Britain by TJ Books Ltd

Jessica Kingsley Publishers' policy is to use papers that are natural, renewable and recyclable
products and made from wood grown in sustainable forests. The logging and manufacturing
processes are expected to conform to the environmental regulations of the country of origin.

Jessica Kingsley Publishers
Carmelite House
50 Victoria Embankment
London EC4Y 0DZ

www.singingdragon.com

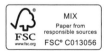

For lovely Maisie, Sam, Peter, Nancy, Sandy, Alan and Oscar
– my constellation

CONTENTS

FOREWORD

Yoga and Somatics for Immune and Respiratory Health is for anyone studying or teaching the human body/being. The emphasis is on 'health', using the lens of yogic wisdom, to visualise and embody many deep and subtle practices that are described and beautifully illustrated throughout the text. Each practice is relevant to the topic and each topic is woven together to make sense of the person practising or teaching. That's a feat – and it's a brave achievement.

Why brave? Because we are in the new era of a new age! So much has gone online, so much has shifted our 'normal', and so many of us are looking to make sense of what has changed and what longs to be the same. Beyond that, there is a deeper need to make sense of the impact we are navigating together – upon ourselves as individuals and as a collective. Yoga stands the test of time, and with a work like this, students and teachers of its art and science are equipped with an updated, invaluable and relevant guide to traverse these new landscapes. Charlotte has managed to distinguish the fears and concerns that we have experienced (personally and professionally) around the globe over recent years, and to demonstrate how they can be managed and changed, and improved through knowledge and thoughtful practice and exploration. Whether you are a teacher, therapist or simply interested, you will find gold in this enquiry and the guidance threaded compassionately through it.

In our modern, technology-driven society, there is a minefield of misinformation, Instagram anatomy and marketing-speak readily available at the touch of a social media button. Charlotte takes them all on – explaining these complex, interrelated health issues clearly and practically – and then gets you *moving* to put the resolutions into practice, through her knowledge of yoga and deep understanding of the intelligent logic and variety it provides. That way, her explanations can make sense and make a difference to your work directly – because you can apply the information immediately. Every part explains, highlights (including references and quotes where needed to support an idea or consideration) and then illustrates movements, postures and iterations that will allow you to implement and experiment with what you have just learned. That's why it's brave; it is workable.

When you meet Charlotte, you quickly pick up the energy of a bright mind, an open heart, and a hunger to learn and teach, with a passion for making sense of what can really make a difference in practice. Charlotte insists on *making* that difference to those her work is aimed at, to educate and encourage. Charlotte's way, in a professional, personal and family field, bears the hallmark of enthusiasm and integrity *in action*. It is no different with this book. Charlotte has managed to weave her intense and disciplined knowledge into a practical, useful, useable treasure that is so current, it is an essential for anyone practising today. It helps all of us to make a bigger difference.

What you have in your hands, as a yoga teacher, yoga therapist or practitioner of any stripe, is a gift of clear references to complex subjects and issues that have (had to) become a part of *everyone's* repertoire. Big subjects such as 'stress', 'inflammation', 'mindfulness', 'fluid adaptation', 'embodied awareness' and the subtleties of resonance can be difficult to grasp and even harder to digest when they are analysed and regurgitated in dense academic language – that Charlotte manages to keep to an essential minimum. Using plain English and speaking from experience, her book encourages and enlightens our sense of safety and creates a safe and sacred environment, for ourselves and for our students to appreciate. Indeed, we can flourish with this approach in the everyday world of real-time yoga practice.

Here are some aspects, among many, that this work takes on and elaborates beautifully:

- Optimising health through fluidity in movement and breath. We are guided to feel into what we need rather than being told the form we should be in. Consider that, if we are stressed, a prescribed postural set can be more (rather than less) imposing. With the value of appreciating the fascial matrix and naturally fluid motion of our internal structure, the practice becomes more about curiosity than calculated shapes.
- Classical reductionist viewpoints of 'condition X = solution Y' are sacrificed to promote more self-aware and non-judgemental inquiries that honour the beginner's mindset (page 72) and deeply encourage a state of presence. Charlotte demonstrates the value of nurturing that approach and its profound impact on the immune system and somatic balance and adaptability. The practices with every part invite you to

experience the difference. When you have the 'why', it is so much easier to find the 'how', and to take it away to explore on the mat.

- The book really demonstrates how yoga can offer a philosophy and model to support our everyday resilience and self-care, if we select appropriately from both the subtle and the strong practices. Recognising the connections between structure, system signalling and sensory awareness (with diagrams to make sense of how systems correspond and communicate), we can translate the work into practical application with confidence.

- A highlight of this work is how certain kinds of appropriate movement (recognising the innate properties of the fascial matrix) can enhance our embodied awareness. This spontaneously connects us with our own breath, which naturally brings multiple benefits to our health, wellbeing and self-confidence on or off the mat.

As we navigate our way, collectively, from the 'double dead anatomy' of the 20th century and into the new world of fascia and its implications for immunity and respiration in the 21st, we need these careful descriptions of how our fluid bodies move and breathe and self-sense their way into form. Beyond that, Charlotte takes us through the subtle advantages of building on these explorations to improve our resilience.

Charlotte is not the kind of author who lays out her ideas, lists a pile of references to demonstrate her intellectual organisational skills and leaves you, the reader, wondering exactly how to take that detail from chapter to classroom. Charlotte is the kind of author who has (obviously in this case) taken a carefully considered practice *from experience of teaching in live classes to live people* and teased open all the assets for you, as participant, practitioner or experienced teacher or therapist. It has been written with her wit, wisdom and compassion, and there is no doubt you will be as delighted as I am to have it in your library.

Wishing you so well my dear, in gratitude for this work that you crafted with Leonie.

Joanne Avison, MSS, ERYT500, C-IAYT
Brighton, England

ACKNOWLEDGEMENTS

Firstly, large heartfelt thanks to my lovely friend Leonie Taylor. Leo is included as a co-author of this work to crucially acknowledge the instrumental part she played gathering the written, spoken and taught content of my 'Yoga for Immune and Respiratory Health' course. She skilfully played a vital part in shaping the content, research and viewpoint that is this book.

Many thanks to all of the teachers who have inspired this content in so many different and fascinating ways, in particular the lovely Tias Little, whose teaching and wisdom is woven through this work, not just where quoted directly, but also so inspirationally through his SATYA (Sensory Awareness Training for Yoga Attunement) somatic training, run with Surya Little. This course took many threads that I had explored before, forming them in his compassionate and playful way.

Gratitude to the lovely Joanne Avison for her generous Foreword (thank you for capturing my intention so eloquently!) and for all the reasons I asked her to write it – her incredible depth of knowledge of form, movement, expression and what it is to be alive within this thing we call body. Her anatomy teaching and writing is a true, deep resource and guide.

Much thanks go to Jim Feil for his incredible guidance in Stanley Keleman's body psychotherapy work as Formative Embodiment. The journey was one of the most deeply inspirational for my experiential understanding of what embodying actually means, what it is to be human and to express.

Also gratitude to Daniel Simpson, whose work on yoga history and *pranayama* was invaluable for that content within the book; also his time and advice.

Great thanks go to Laurie Booth for his illuminating teaching and constant playful enquiry within our movement sessions, and how he brings my anatomical connection to life. His quotes in this book truly meet the spirit of the work.

Heartfelt thanks to my original teacher Jim Tarran of the Vajrasati school of yoga; his sensitive voice and beautiful turn of phrase can be found throughout these pages as a huge influence on my relationship with guiding inwards towards awareness.

Much gratitude to Karin Gurtner for her course 'Anatomy Trains in Motion', which was such a turning point for me to be able to bring the lines in bodies I could see and sense into such a real and living form. Also to Steve Haines for his trauma-informed training within TRE (tension- and trauma-releasing exercises), which led me in many directions to understand the depth and nature of how we embed trauma and the possibilities of growth beyond. Thanks to Judith Hanson Lasater for her teachings on bringing yoga philosophy to life within practice and Cathy-Mae Karelse for illuminating my understanding and language around mindfulness. Also Donna Farhi for her depth in bringing curious, somatic work into yoga practice for me.

A special thank you goes to my co-teacher at Yogacampus Leah Barnett – working together on the 'Teaching Yoga for Stress, Burnout and Fatigue' course has been a deep influence, and Leah's subtle and sensitive relationship with sounding and *mantra* within yoga is a large influence in Part 6.

This work has also been influenced and inspired by many teachers, writers and speakers who are both fascinating and excited by embodiment, and what it is to relate from our phenomenological experience to the outside world and back again. Gary Carter, Simon Low, Mimi-Kuo Deemer, Kate Ellis and Aki Omori are all such teachers who even in short exposures tapped into some true fundamentals of exploration of all it is to be human through movement. Much gratitude also to the other various yoga, somatics, Feldenkrais, qi gong, nei gong and primal movement teachers I have explored with along the way, who resonate with this need to draw together an understanding of our somatic or body psychotherapy – and simply move in ways that express our needs, feel our boundaries, help us treat ourselves kindly and support compassionate relating with others.

The subject matter for this book is also hugely influenced by my study and work as a nutritional therapist, and the research within that field and the systemic viewpoint that offers, as well as the agency for human health. A great source of much of the immune-based research in this book has been via the *Integrative Healthcare & Applied Nutrition* magazine (IHCAN), and thanks are due to the writers and esteemed editor Simon Martin. Other notable sources of information are from Dr Leo Pruimboom and his teachings on psycho-neuro-immunology, Dr Jeffrey Bland and his Functional Medicine model and Dr Robert Verkerk of the Alliance for Natural Health. I would also like to thank the wonderful naturopath Marion Kirkham for setting me on the path around 20 years ago to understanding what stress means for the modern human, which was a huge influence on everything that I have studied since.

I also need to acknowledge the trauma work of people such as Drs Stephen Porges, Gabor Maté and Bessel van der Kolk, to name a few. Their illumination of the collective needs of the modern human is invaluable to those with the courage to listen.

Large thanks to Yogacampus (particularly Elizabeth Stanley and Lisa Kaley-Isley) and The Minded Institute (and Heather Mason; thanks also to Heather for her reading and advice on this work) for the opportunity to teach on their esteemed Yoga Therapy courses. It is in the research, preparation and teaching of lecture and course content where I find the seeds that grow into larger works such as these. Being part of something larger and within such valuable work has been of such huge support for the confidence to take my voice out of my head (and off the paper!) into the world. In this context, gratitude must also go to the esteemed yoga teacher Fiona Agombar for trusting and recommending me to these members of our community – much love.

Much thanks to all the students I have had the amazing pleasure of guiding through therapeutic and somatic lenses within yoga – the conversations, communal practice and reflections we have are always so insightful, inspired, intimate, courageous and real. These have been some of my most profound learning moments.

Lastly, a big thank you to Claire, Masooma and Carys (and anyone else involved I didn't have direct contact with!) at Singing Dragon for their support in bringing this piece of work to fruition.

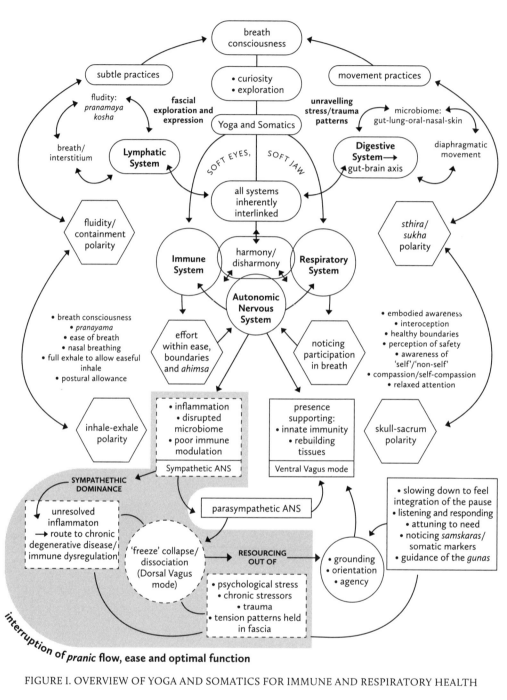

FIGURE 1. OVERVIEW OF YOGA AND SOMATICS FOR IMMUNE AND RESPIRATORY HEALTH

INTRODUCTION

I am very pleased to bring you the fruition of this work that began its journey when the UK went into its first lockdown period in March 2020 as a result of COVID-19. With people separated and restricted from social contact, for many yoga teachers and those who made a living meeting and connecting with people face to face, this was a time of great uncertainty. For me this also presented the irony of knowing how crucial social engagement and the free flow of movement are to our basic health, and in particular, the very immune and respiratory function that was feeling so tremulous for many.

As someone who has supported people with immune and respiratory conditions for two decades, my first thought was to put together a course to help yoga teachers work with students in ways that supported their sense of self-care, specific to the needs that the COVID-19 virus was highlighting. This was a way to disseminate information that I have always thought that everybody would benefit from knowing – offering us involvement and agency within our own body-mind states and processes. To know how stress, trauma, breath, movement and posture (to name just a few) affect the capacity of our body systems is crucial to truly feeling what we need to support our own health. Engaging with our vitality through the movement we were designed to express is to be able to meet what comes our way with the best chance of elegance and coping.

I contacted the wonderful Elizabeth Stanley at Yogacampus (I have taught for this London-based educational body for many years) and offered her a proposal for a six-week online course. Given the current national and worldwide situation, she deemed this a good idea, and so I set about gathering together the content from across the many fields I am interested in and that naturally feed into modern yoga teaching.

That course was (and still is!) called 'Teaching Yoga for Immune and Respiratory Health', and gave me a wonderful opportunity to pull together what I had learned and practised over the last 20 years as a nutritional therapist, to weave into my ongoing work as a therapeutically based yoga teacher.

This book is laid out along the same six themes within the course it evolved from: healthy defences, stress and inflammation, fluid adaptation, mindful boundaries, embodied awareness and good vibrations. This follows an arc to correlate with the practices for each part, that together build up a complete cycle – from the ground up to standing and back down again, to bring in sound at the end, a final resonance. I wanted to write the book because the initial material for the course only brought up areas of enquiry for me. I both wanted to expand on areas I knew more about in a nutritional therapy capacity and research their place within a yoga context, and to know more about areas that are clearly so important in linking our immunity and respiratory functions. So in many ways this book has become the manual for the course.

You'll find that throughout, although some disease states are discussed, there is no list of conditions and specific protocols for each. This is a step away from the more medical model of 'What is wrong?' and 'How do we fix it?' – within both systemic models of yoga and Ayurveda, and nutritional therapy and functional medicine (the model behind much modern nutrition practices), there is a focus on exploring how systems function and how to support their optimal capacity. They are always coming from the perspective that we are whole (not a collection of separate parts), and that orchestration within its entirety (including our emotional landscape and psychological story) is always relevant. We differentiate – that is, look at different components – only to integrate, to come back to whole, to healing.

As well as my teaching and consulting work, my personal health journey has been one of peeling back the layers. Delving beneath the surface expressions of dis-ease (in yoga and Ayurveda, this concept of ease, *sukha*, is the route to health on all levels), we can peel back the layers to reveal the effects that factors such as chronic stress and childhood trauma are running in the background. I came to both nutrition and yoga through long-term ill health, much of it related to the stress-related inflammation discussed throughout the book, which breath consciousness and embodied physical practices can so profoundly help to alleviate.

In the light of these times of COVID-19, there has been much (often heated!) discussion around the part we can play in our own protection against this or other viruses and the post-viral load that can ensue, such as long COVID more recently. As someone who had post-viral long-term chronic fatigue, understanding factors that predispose us to these chronic conditions has long been of interest and deep research. We live in times where exciting ways of viewing how our experiences affect our health are being researched and brought into therapeutic yoga – neuroscience, epigenetics, psycho-neuro-immunology, polyvagal theory and more. If you haven't come across these terms, worry not – we delve into them in the following pages, and maybe more importantly, we observe how they might correlate with facets within yoga models and their influences: *koshas*, *samskaras*, *kleshas* and *gunas*, to name a few. This can particularly guide how we bring such theory into reality, via meditative, mindful and somatic practice.

With so much emphasis on acquired immunity to disease (antibodies to specific pathogens or invaders – see Part 1) as the main route to protection, the (well-researched and increasingly understood) ways that we can engage with and support our innate immune function are often undervalued and even dismissed as less important or even ineffective. The reality is very different, as we will explore. Our innate immunity is where we can not only support our acquired immune function, but is also actually necessary to enable its function. This is a rich area that allows us agency within our own health, where we can interface with our internal processes and play a part in how we feel.

Exploring how immunity resides in, communicates with and is influenced by other body systems is to enter into the story of what it is to be human. As the immune system can seem such an amorphous, abstract entity, we see its defensive and survival actions turn up in symptoms rippling through other parts – heat and inflammation through the autonomic nervous system, upset through the digestive tract, and, linking to our other focus here, the respiratory system – changes in breath and its self-regulatory qualities. To support immune health, we can facilitate how it can most optimally operate – not too little where we struggle to deal with invaders or too much where we get stuck in inflammation. Rather, we are looking for modulation, an appropriate response that seeds the potential for recovery throughout all systems.

So health here (and particularly how it is bound up in the way we move) is to support all the facets of our bodily existence – which includes and is always interrelated with our psyche and emotional landscapes. A key example that is more understood in recent years is how free flowing and responsive, organised fascia allows the same qualities in immune response. Back to the breath, and we weave in how autonomic responses (how 'safe' or 'unsafe' we perceive ourselves to be at any given time) are constantly being shown in the quality and tone of each cycle of inhale–exhale. We can tune into these communications to understand our responses and needs.

To talk 'health' in a modern context is to recognise the need to be 'trauma-informed' – not to identify or diagnose trauma (we don't even need to use the word in teaching), but to be aware of the conditionings and drivers that can surface in a survival response to a time or event from the past. Allowing these to be present – with compassion and without reaction or judgement – can offer a route back towards post-traumatic growth and the regulation within body systems that gets lost. This dysregulation can show up as symptoms such as inflammatory disorders, autoimmune conditions, respiratory conditions and related digestive issues, the latter, as you will see, play such a large part in immunity and are so affected by the breath (explored in greater depth in my book *Yoga Therapy for Digestive Health*).[1]

The practices

The engaged and embodied movement practices within this book are not based around flexibility, acrobatics or athleticism – they all work within a natural range of movement and, as such, offer more functional movement or primal shapes than 'traditional' yoga *asana* (posture) alone. As many of these poses (now taught and practised within modern postural yoga) were taken from influences such as the British Army's rule,[2] the shift in physical practice has been long part of its 'Westernisation', but when including such change under the umbrella of yoga practice, we need to acknowledge its lineage.

We refer back to the wisdom of the foundational yoga, *Vedanta* and Tantric texts as a guide to continually dropping beneath the physical practices as only surface movement. As Daniel Simpson, author of *The Truth of Yoga*, states:

> There has never been any such thing as "One True Yoga". The practice and the theories behind it have evolved, becoming combined in a variety of ways. None of these is "truer" than others. Each makes sense in context, but there is no obligation to pick one text, or one form of yoga, and uncritically follow whatever it says. We are free to ignore what might not seem relevant. But that makes it important to know what traditional teachings say, and to distinguish this from how we interpret them.[3]

Within this context, the practices are not in the category of 'gentle', which so often these days seems to imply less, or for those who cannot do the 'real stuff'. They may not be extreme for the body, but they are deeper and richer in so

---

1   Watts (2018).
2   Shearer (2020).
3   Simpson (2021).

many ways – they ask us to be with space, to meet the voices coming up from our deeper unconscious patterns, and to have a relationship with vulnerability.

Somatic practices, such as those from Thomas Hanna and the Feldenkrais system, are becoming more commonly incorporated into yoga teachings as the need to move in more fluid and explorative forms within our sedentary and stressed culture becomes clear. These movements can be specific and pre-scribed, or more free-form – to follow all of the various patterns that we evolve with from babies learning to move and strengthen. More fluid movements invite us to feel the experience, without attachment to 'the form'. This can help us unravel patterns imprinted in adulthood born more of tension or habit, which can become more robotic and stuck.

I would like to give the floor here to one of my favourite yoga teachers, Tias Little, with whom I have studied for many years and whose SATYA (Sensory Awareness Training for Yoga Attunement) training has particularly influenced my inclusion of somatics within a yoga framework:

> In subtle body training, we move through layers of membrane, connective tissue, bone and fluid into the depth of our being. Always the aim is to have a fluid presence and to sense and feel a kind of submersion. Gliding, undulating, and pulsating, we move with little effort, sensing how movement emerges from within. As we penetrate layer by layer into our interior, we experience not only physical but psychic absorption. This soaking inward is profoundly healing for both body and mind. It is like being in the amniotic sea of embryological development. The experience of soaking inward is akin to states of *samadhi* celebrated in the teachings of yoga.[4]

In many ways, the context of the immune and respiratory systems lends itself to more fluid, nuanced practices, as this is not the stuff of the more obvious struc-tural body. As you'll see throughout the book, everything is body-wide – both the immune and respiratory body systems animate us and create our boundaries and sense of edge within the structure, so we can explore our body psychology through these fluid and breath bodies (*pranamaya kosha*; page 151).

In any practice with a physical component, so much focus can hone in on the musculoskeletal system as driving the whole show; to drop back into the softer, more pulsatory and fluid realms of the breath, fascia, interstitium and lymphatics is to meet our softer animal body rather than viewing ourselves as

---

4   Little and Little (no date).

mechanical beings. Here we can tune into the quality of movement as gesture, expression, emotional body – spiralling, reaching out, drawing in, organisation around the midline, noticing continual introspection and extraversion. This can meet our true needs as an antidote to the often-damaging driver to do more, do it faster and even beyond our own boundaries, that can be given so much credit in our goal-oriented world.

As the practices in the book often incorporate small, subtle movements to refine awareness and listen in to the quieter voices, this can begin to allow us to drop beneath the louder voices of the mind. Creating this room for kind attention, movement from self-compassion and respect for our own boundaries can begin to foster the safety that can resolve heightened responses that show up in the immune and respiratory systems.

This can also involve moving into patterns held in body tissues and triggers (*samskaras*, somatic markers) to move out and unravel old stories laid down as present experience. Movement can feel it offers us the vehicle for adaptation and shifting perspective when it is guided from nervous system and emotional body cues, rather than purely musculoskeletal physicality, connecting with fascial, fluid, breath and organ bodies via the skin to bring mental, emotional, wisdom, spiritual bodies to consciousness.

Self-reflective practice

For each of the six parts in the book, five self-enquiry questions are set as self-study (*svadyaya*) for you to consider alongside the practices. They are designed to help bring the theory into the embodied, and to guide you to a living, breathing connection with the whole body-mind effects of the immune and respiratory systems.

The questions are best answered from an experiential point of view, bringing the poetic, descriptive, felt sense into any analysing or describing from an anatomical or biomechanical standpoint. Find out how this enquiry can help you translate the theory of body systems into the real, individual experience felt by yourself and your students.

If the questions relate to practices, come back to them over and over again, so you can see that there are no definitive answers. Notice which of these help you to most tune inwards. It is these that can be used moving forwards as ways to continual insight through practice that might feed into guiding others within teaching.

Remember, there are no right or wrong answers – reflections are not about seeking improvement or identifying what is 'wrong' and must be 'fixed'. Enquiry formed from curiosity and exploration can open up paths and insights that are easily quashed when we view ourselves as a collection of issues, rather than a systemic whole. In the words of Steve Haines, 'You're an organic garden, not a broken machine.'[5]

Resources at the end of each part

The subjects explored within this book are vast, and so we have provided further resources for reading and learning on subjects throughout each of the six parts. These include books that were influential to the content, and that can offer you deeper insight into parts that were not possible to fully expound within these pages.

We have included what can be most helpfully applied within the context here, for deepening practice to guide body systems back into equilibrium. We can so often want to understand 'why' to connect and be motivated to engage in a practice – feeling this ourselves, if we are teachers, we can empathise with which words and phrases draw others into presence and embodiment. How we sow this understanding of the links between breath, movement and health within guidance for others – to talk directly to body tissues – can enrich the experience for both student and teacher.

The resources are all their own starting points, and I humbly suggest that you follow what truly speaks to you, rather than feeling you need to know it all. The modern 'yoga world' is benefiting from more and more knowledge in a myriad of directions, and while this can be illuminating, it runs the risk of adding to current common overwhelm. Simply knowing more can also never take the place of the deeper wisdom gained from an attuned and curious practice.

We all need to be mindful that we are not grasping at more knowledge as a distraction from the trickier and more vulnerable business of tuning inwardly – I know that I can be pulled down that particular rabbit hole!

Sanskrit terms and spelling

Throughout the text, the Sanskrit terms used have been written in the anglicised form, in italics. The decision not to use the diacritical marks (or to cite the Nagari or Devanagari script used for Classical Sanskrit) was chosen carefully,

---

5   Haines (2021).

from respectfully not wishing to make errors – neither of the book's contributors are Sanskrit scholars, but deeply respect that work. There is, however, a Glossary at the end of the book to show the commonly used words with their diacritics and any spelling changes from the Latin alphabet they bring.

References

Haines, S. (2021) 'You're an organic garden, not a broken machine.' Body College, 4 November. Available at: https://bodycollege.net/youre-an-organic-garden-not-a-broken-machine

Little, T. and Little, S. (no date) SATYA (Sensory Awareness Training for Yoga Attunement) [course training manual]. Accessed 2019.

Shearer, A. (2020) *The Story of Yoga: From Ancient India to the Modern West*. London: C. Hurst & Co Publishers Ltd.

Simpson, D. (2021) *The Truth of Yoga: A Comprehensive Guide to Yoga's History, Texts, Philosophy, and Practices*. New York: North Point Press.

Watts, C. (2018) *Yoga Therapy for Digestive Health*. London and Philadelphia, PA: Singing Dragon.

PART 1

HEALTHY DEFENCES

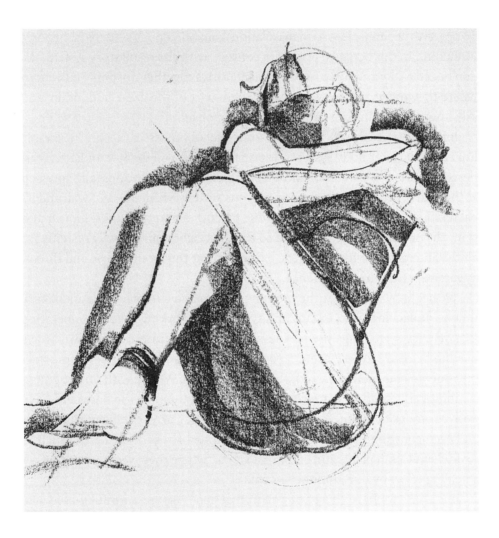

Exploring the territory that the immune and respiratory systems occupy and their intertwining roles within the whole organism. Using the contexts of breath, movement, awareness and enquiry, we can connect with these continual processes as part of a whole orchestration.

In this first part, we will look at what the 'health of our defences and breathing' mean, in terms of the whole territory, organisation and interplay. We look specifically at the immune and respiratory systems, the anatomy and physiology of how they work together, and how they interact, particularly with the autonomic nervous system.

Supporting our boundaries and breath – the territory

To observe the immune system in isolation from other body systems is a myopic viewpoint. In this book we place it in context, with the respiratory system. We don't need to try and force two separate entities together or simply talk about where they meet; rather, we consider them part of the great hum of life and ask, how are they in constant reciprocal response?

Immunity is a complex and orchestrated set of processes that are inexorably linked to all other body systems, especially, as we will explore in Part 2, our nervous system and states of energy, being, safety and emotions (all expressed at the heart), including the enteric nervous system within our gut wall and its bacterial colony or microbiome. These extend out to the lungs, mouth and skin, all communicating back, and so the dance goes on. All body systems are always interacting with all others, particularly at the mouth, nose and throat, as gateways for immune defence.

We begin by looking at the immune system as a complex network of very unique molecules, cells, organs and systems, all working together, operating as a defence system against invaders, under the assumption that we always need to be ready to assess and respond to factors entering from the outside: microorganisms such as bacteria, fungi and viruses. We live with some of these symbiotically, such as gut bacteria – we expect them in the body and have evolved alongside them. Others may not be particularly pathogenic (harmful) and even contribute to hormesis (adaptation to a stress or challenge) such as toxic chemicals in plants and herbs that we eat, where these very toxins provoke a healing effect by our immune system.

It is when we have those coming in that can be more harmful (or we perceive them to be) that we mount the defences. We also defend against some chemicals (more and more of which are manmade or industrial), as well as natural pathogens where nature is defending itself against *us*, such as pollen, Poison Ivy or venom.

To live is to be constantly interacting with (and often defending ourselves against) compounds that occur in nature, or cells within ourselves. When our own cells go through ageing or dying off processes, and in the face of malignant cells or those that would be more cancer producing, an immune response is needed to clean these up. Immunity is a hugely complicated system, counteracting a very, very broad range of situations and threats.

The immune territory

Our immune system includes many interacting processes, such as inflammation (covered in much detail in Part 2), phagocytosis (the eating of other cells), antibody synthesis (mounting for specific attack), and many more. The immune system is body-wide and produced by different systems, such as the lymphatic system and bone marrow, the thymus and spleen (Figure 1a). All of these different localities and effects combine to be able to protect the whole being that is us, to respond immediately, and hopefully appropriately, as needed.

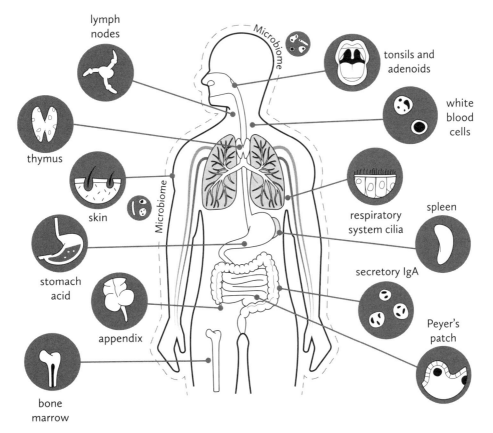

FIGURE 1A. BODY-WIDE IMMUNE SITES

In this book we will also look at situations where response is not appropriate, such as in autoimmune disorders or being caught in inflammatory conditions. What we're particularly interested in (within the scope of yoga teaching and yoga therapy) is developing ways to stimulate appropriate immune response or immune modulation, that is, not reacting more than necessary, allowing ourselves to consciously regulate how we respond to threat or danger coming into the body (and why the word 'boost' is not just inaccurate, but even problematic). Equally, ensuring that defences are not underreacting to something coming in that warrants a specific attack.

While the immune system is distributed body-wide, it's important to remember that 70 per cent is located in the gut. The gut wall contains 'associated lymphoid tissue' and antibodies – one of the reasons why there has been more and more interest in recent years in the immune system's microbiome cellular components. Our gut is continually assessing whether something is beneficial or pathogenic; in autoimmunity, this discernment is confused. The confusion is seeing our own cells as pathogenic (something to be attacked) – an inappropriate response. To function properly, our immune system must detect a huge variety of agents and pathogens, from viruses to parasitic worms, and distinguish them from our own healthy tissue. This identification between matter is a massive part of immune signalling.

This is a simplistic overview of the immune system in order for us to understand as teachers and therapists the main branches of the immune system.

The two branches of the immune system

Immunity is described as having two distinct parts – the more generalised and non-specific responses of our innate immune system and the more targeted strategies of the acquired immune system – towards specific invading organisms and substances. The implication of this is often seen within the context of germ theory – the idea that we are under constant attack from natural forces, and if we could only dominate and suppress them through sterilisation and sanitisation, we would 'win' and not succumb to disease (pages 34 and 220).

As we will explore in Part 4, looking at the whole terrain allows us more interaction and regulation throughout our complete body system.

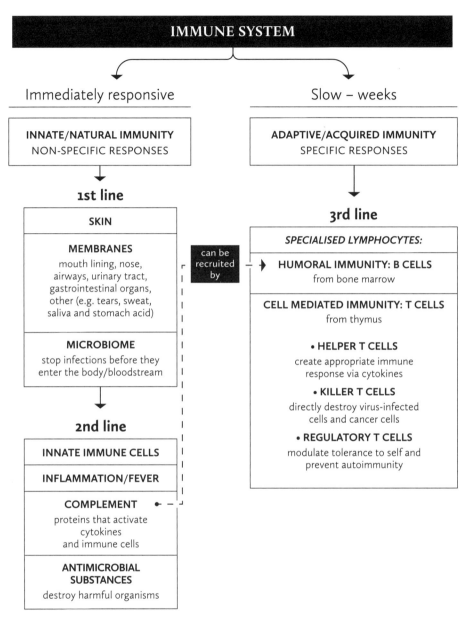

FIGURE 1B. THE IMMUNE SYSTEM

Innate immunity

Our innate immune system is ancient and primal. Although we build up our acquired immunity over time (which is why children tend to get ill more often than teens or adults), we are born with a certain level of defence, as well as some borrowed from our mother as passive immunity, through the placenta and then breast milk.

This is our innate immunity, our first-line, non-specific response to any breach of our body and its boundaries, and it has a profound part to play in our health and longevity.[1,2] This includes inflammation but is also our physical barriers: the skin, mucous membranes, saliva, stomach acid, the flushing action of urine, tears and the cilia in the lungs. The respiratory system has an important part to play, as does the blood – bringing the breath and the heart (that moves the blood) into the picture.

(Acquired immunity is more specific and involves memory – such as acquiring immunity to a specific disease or via vaccination. It's something that becomes specific to a certain organism coming in, such as a virus or bacteria, and the remembering of it so that we can mount a similar and more efficient attack next time. We discuss this further on page 33.)

Immune responses kick in a few seconds after an antigen enters our body in a way that is designed for adaptation and protection; for example, the proteins on a virus are recognised by human cells to take it in and create protection and memory of it. Most viruses don't need a response as we don't view them as harmful, but rather as providing key genetic material – how we take in information from the world around us so we can respond appropriately.[3]

As the adaptive immune system doesn't produce antibodies until weeks after the first exposure and symptoms of a disease (innate system responses), it is the innate immunity that responds to any new antigen immediately. This is how we stay in relation to the 10^{15} (add 15 zeros after the 10!) viruses estimated to be in our bloodstreams at any given time, not to mention the 10^{31} in the air that we breathe. These are not figures that should alarm us; rather, they offer an amazing view of the constant interrelating we have with the milieu of organisms on Earth. We are part of nature, and the less we come from a stance of 'them against us', the more we can support the sophisticated ways our innate immune system supports health.

If we simply run the narrative that it is the acquired, adaptive immune system that will save us from the perceived threat of disease, we dismiss and neglect the agency and vitality that makes up the innate relationship to the organisms we live with – internally in our microbiome and in the larger world around us.

Much of what we're talking about here (and what we can meet through our practices) is in support of our innate immunity, which actually helps activate

---

1   Candore *et al.* (2006).
2   Moskalev, Stambler and Caruso (2020).
3   Liang and Bushman (2021).

and regulate, and gives more potency to, acquired immunity. Innate immunity is always active, always ready to respond in a healthy system, ready to recognise any active microbial agents entering in the lungs or other tissues.

Our innate immunity also includes our microbiome, or supportive beneficial bacteria, often referred to as probiotic bacteria. Supportive bacteria, which are not just in the gut but all across our skin, in our lungs, our mouth or throat, or any other orifices, are our first line of defence against anything from the outside world. This also includes the barrier of the gut because essentially that is outside until something moves across the gut barrier into the bloodstream.

Throughout this book we explore how we can meet, understand and interface with these defences as real, living, responsive and expressive companions to our autonomic nervous system, and how the respiratory system intertwines the two. The regulation of these systems relies on our parasympathetic nervous system, the healing of tissues and building back up of innate compounds. Healthy functioning of our innate immune system requires us to have really good quality sleep, conscious rest and dropping down from the constant reactivity and doing that mobilises our sympathetic nervous system. This means spending the time needed to truly bring down active states, so we can gather back up vital resources. This is clearly the realm of restorative, mindful and meditative yoga practices, and why they can be of such benefit to our immune and respiratory health.

INNATE IMMUNITY CHARACTERISTICS

Our innate immunity has some crucial characteristics that influence how we can practise movement, breath and compassionate attention – how to support our immune capacity to offer us constant and appropriate protection. We can remember that it:

- Is always active and immediately responsive.
- Is ready to recognise and inactivate microbial products entering the lungs and other tissues.
- Includes the microbiome (supportive organisms such as beneficial bacteria and viruses) throughout the body, including on the skin, gut and lungs that make up a large part of our entire cellular organism.
- Relies on parasympathetic tone for regulation.

The four actions of innate immunity

Essentially, innate immunity is orchestrated by four processes: mechanical barriers, chemical barriers, inflammation and fever. These can be put within two categories: structural and functional components.

STRUCTURAL COMPONENTS

- *Mechanical barriers* (endothelial system) include the skin and membranes that line our mouths, nose, airways, urinary tracts and gastrointestinal organs. When these are intact, with a healthy microbiome, they provide a physical barrier against the entry of toxins and harmful organisms (see Part 4).

FUNCTIONAL COMPONENTS

Zach Bush[4] describes the remaining three: '[they] involve a multitude of cells and biochemical cascades. The functional actions of the innate immune system are often overlooked and over simplified. In reality, it's a complex and dynamic set of actions that has a life of its own – literally.'[5]

- *Chemical barriers* include sweat, tears, saliva, stomach acids, mucus and other fluids secreted by the body (see Part 3).
- *Inflammation* occurs when the mechanical and chemical barriers to foreign invaders have failed (see Part 2).
- *Fever* is a healthy reaction to bacteria and viruses that are sensitive to extremes in temperature, excreting substances that trigger a temperature increase. This symptom that we might see as unwanted is crucial because invading organisms cannot tolerate elevated temperatures for an extended period of time.[6] Overuse of medication that brings down uncomplicated fever (anti-pyretic) is a common practice that may be linked to harmful effects.[7,8]

---

4   Zach Bush MD is a physician specialising in internal medicine, endocrinology and hospice care with a focus on the microbiome as it relates to health, disease and food systems. Internal medicine is the medical speciality dealing with the prevention, diagnosis and treatment of internal diseases, and practitioners are skilled in the management of patients with undifferentiated or multisystem disease processes.
5   Bush (2021).
6   Gardner (2012).
7   De Ronne (2010).
8   Purssell (2007).

THE INNATE SYSTEM PARTY OF PLAYERS

The various innate actions listed above are carried out by three different types of response:

- *Cell response* (following page).
- The *biochemical or complement cascade*, which is composed of several proteins produced by the liver that circulate in our blood. They attach to any foreign material they find, targeting it for attack by the other cells in the immune response.
- *Genomic editing* is how the innate immune system addresses viral genomic material coming in, and is of much interest at the moment with the development of RNA 'vaccines' that do not inoculate, but rather genetically modify our responses to RNA viruses. RNA and DNA viruses generate genetic fragments inside our cells (in the cytoplasm) that are called pathogen-associated molecular patterns (PAMPs – these are what PCR tests measure).

According to Zach Bush and Peter Cummings[9], it was previously assumed that the genetic information in viruses was integrated into the human genome for the survival and replication of the virus. But it can be argued that this integration of viral code into our genome in fact increases our biodiversity and is allowed in by our innate immune system. The adaptations brought about by viral genes are actually responsible for many metabolic and physiological functions and the origins of over half of our genome can be traced back to viral sources.

---

9   Bush and Cummings (2021).

The cells of the immune system

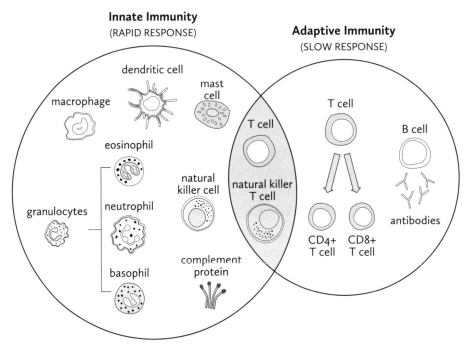

FIGURE 1C. INNATE AND ADAPTIVE IMMUNITY
Source: Adapted from Dranoff (2004)

The following cells have specialised roles in innate and adaptive immune responses:

- Granulocytes are white blood cells that fight pathogens and recycle damaged cells. There are four different types:
  - Neutrophils may leave blood for the tissues to attack organisms such as bacteria and fungi.
  - Basophils initiate an inflammatory response to environmental antigens.
  - Eosinophils defend against parasites; they are prolific in allergic diseases and asthma.
  - Mast cells are most abundant in mucous membranes. They secrete chemicals including histamine. Chronic mast cell activation – high levels of histamine – is associated with allergic diseases and asthma (page 148).
- Macrophages, a type of phagocyte ('cell eater'; page 41), that digest pathogens, secreting cytokines (page 88) to signal to T lymphocytes that other immune cells are needed.

- Dendritic cells communicate between the innate and acquired immune systems.
- Natural killer cells destroy infected cells.
- T cells are lymphocytes (following page) that evolve in bone marrow and mature in the thymus gland (page 106). Sub-types of T cells are CD4+ T cells, 'helper' cells, which distinguish what is and what is not 'self', while CD8+ T cells directly kill virus-infected cells.
- B cells also develop in bone marrow and bind to specific antigens to produce an immune response.

Acquired or adaptive immunity

When we think of the immune system as 'fighting off invaders', this is the action of the acquired or adaptive branch. It is a learned response to a specific foreign agent, that is, something coming in from the outside that we deem harmful. These invaders are referred to as antigens, which are basically any substance that, when introduced into the body, stimulate the production of an antibody (aka an immunoglobulin) by the immune system.

Antibodies are large Y-shaped proteins that identify and deactivate unwanted visitors such as pathogenic (harmful) bacteria and viruses. Antigens can also include toxins, such as environmental and chemical agents, foreign blood cells and the cells of transplanted organs:

Many of the cells in the innate immune system (such as dendritic cells, macrophages, mast cells, neutrophils, basophils and eosinophils) produce cytokines or interact with other cells directly in order to activate the adaptive immune system. The innate immune response has an important role in controlling infections during the first seven days after an infection.[10]

Our acquired immunity learns what we have previously reacted to and created antibodies for. This means that when it is exposed to the same antigen years later, it remembers and can launch a quicker attack, often with less severity of symptoms. With exposure to different diseases over time (or via vaccination), we accumulate a library of antibodies – an immunological memory bank. While innate responses occur in seconds, adaptive immune responses occur much more slowly – in days (or even weeks for full antibody memory) after exposure.[11]

10 ASTRO (no date).
11 Owen *et al.* (2018).

There are two main parts to acquired immunity, and the action of both is carried out by lymphatic cells or lymphocytes (page 40). These are white blood cells that make up about one-third of those circulating around our bodies, moving around in the blood, but also living in tissues, essentially roving freely in the body, primed for action. There are two types: T lymphocytes or T cells and B lymphocytes or B cells. Some B lymphocytes become plasma cells, which, in response to a particular antigen, can remember an invader at a future exposure and produce specific antibodies.

Cell-mediated immunity

Cell-mediated or T cell immunity (confusingly, T cells also work within so-called B cell immunity) uses T lymphocytes as its main weapon, although the interaction between T lymphocytes and B lymphocytes often occurs. After a foreign invader is digested by a macrophage, it presents details about the antigens on the surface of that microorganism to T lymphocytes.

One type of T lymphocyte, the helper T cell, will bring that information to other T lymphocytes (so they will recognise the invader), natural killer cells (that will seek out and kill the organism) and B lymphocytes (that initiate the humoral immune response).

Another type of T lymphocyte, the cytotoxic T cell, uses a more direct approach and kills cells that it recognises as non-self or as potentially harmful.

Humoral immunity

Humoral or B cell immunity involves the production of antibodies, or immunoglobulins, proteins produced by B lymphocyte plasma cells in response to the recognition of a specific antigen. Antibodies can prevent viruses from entering healthy cells, neutralise the invader's toxins, or break down the microorganism and leave them for the scavenger phagocytic cells to eliminate.

Two halves of a whole

The interplay of the immune system means that hard-and-fast rules are tricky to pin down; hence research and understanding is ongoing and 'the science' is only ever a phrase that can approximate a current opinion – of which there are many.

The relationship between the acquired and innate immune systems is often described as the innate having efficacy in the short term, with the acquired providing more long-term and continued protection. This is where germ theory (and recent science around COVID-19) focuses, the vast majority towards acquired 'germ-fighting' rhetoric as our only saviour and 'fighting the virus' the only public health message, beyond a cursory nod to the part we play within our self-care. This downplays the extremely important part the innate immunity has to play in our defences, especially when we view our relationship with viruses via genomic editing, and that acquired actions are way downstream to innate actions in the timescale of defences.

If we see health solely as the territory of the medical, pharmaceutical and chemical industries, rather than a correlate or reflection of nature, we can actually dampen down its defences and leave ourselves reliant only on antibody protection. Whether it's too much washing (especially with harsh chemicals) destroying our protective microbiome, dampening a fever or inflammation with regular pharmaceuticals or poor nutrition that doesn't allow full healing of the lungs, gut, skin or other barriers, these all wear down the potential of our first-line defences. The symphony of the innate immune system components is what allows us to relate to the organisms coming into the body (and the important information they bring in with them about the outside world) without being overwhelmed by them.

Holistic immunity

It is important to have an overview of both innate and acquired immunity as a whole, but it is our innate defences that we relate to within therapeutic movement, breath and awareness practices – that which we can tune into through breath, touch, the states of our nervous system, sound and the ways in which we find ourselves able to move at any given time. The relationship between our immunity and how safe or unsafe we feel is tied in to our breath, which becomes faster and shallower when we enter protective nervous system states. Healing becomes compromised when we become stuck in heightened stress responses; we cannot be in survival and growth at the same time (more on this in Part 2). According to Donna Farhi:

> It begins when we are still in the womb – an expanding, condensing rhythm, threaded together by moments of pause. It is the pulse of the universe, and from the moment of conception we are that. While we are in our mother's body, the breath is an interior movement, a process of shimmering cellular respiration. At the moment of birth, when we first breathe into the lungs, we are initiated into the family of things. Suddenly the world is in us and we are in the world. We draw the breath inside the body, for a moment it becomes us, and we exhale

a part of what has become us back into the world. While we are young we tend to breathe with the kind of complete freedom and ease that is an expression of our innocence and fearlessness. As we age and lose some of that innocence, rubbing up against life's challenges, we unconsciously shut down, and we do this first and foremost by constricting our breath.[12]

Understanding how our immune system shapes our boundaries between the outside world and our internal landscape is key to supporting it, so it can respond to perceived threat and danger. Our respiratory system has a similar response to the internal and external, constantly taking in nourishment through the inhalation and releasing what does not serve us through the exhalation.

These two systems are intrinsically linked in our functional health and how we relate to the world around us. We explore how the immune and respiratory systems relate to movement, embodied awareness and self-compassion throughout the book to develop a sound understanding of how to structure effective sequences.

The respiratory system

The respiratory system includes the upper respiratory tract of the mouth and throat as well as the lungs, an intricate, tree-like structure. All of these cavities allow the passage of air and need to be open and responsive, with all of their linings healthy. Well-functioning barriers are healthy places of life that support colonies of bacteria. The mucosal quality of those linings as boundaries is key to the health of the respiratory and immune systems as a whole.

The cilia are very fine, hair-like projections that line the airways of the respiratory system, moving mucus and contaminants upwards and outwards. These add a vital extra surface area for beneficial bacteria and immune components, lining the barrier to the territory between the outside world, the air coming in and the interior of our bodies – what is allowed into the bloodstream.

During respiration, oxygen is inhaled and carbon dioxide exhaled, mirrored at the micro level within every cell of the body, where the lungs meet the cardiovascular system for oxygen delivery. All blood in the body is filtered through the lungs every minute, taking its carbon dioxide back for breathing out and picking up new oxygen to take around the body, pumped by the heart. Optimally, we take in about ½ litre of air roughly 12–15 times each minute.

---

12   Donna Farhi, quoted in Gardiner (2013).

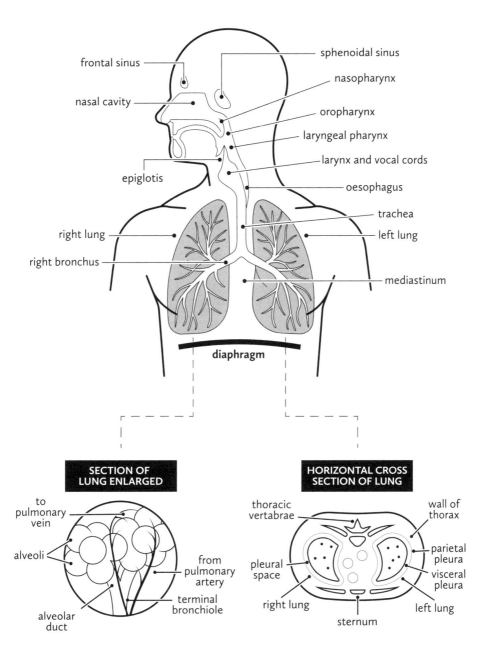

FIGURE 1D. THE RESPIRATORY SYSTEM

The lungs

IN RELATION TO THE HEART

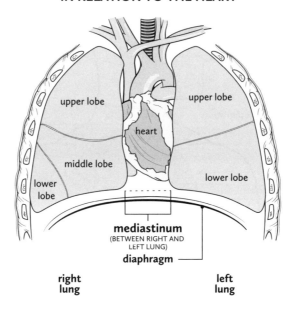

IN RELATION TO THE STOMACH AND LIVER

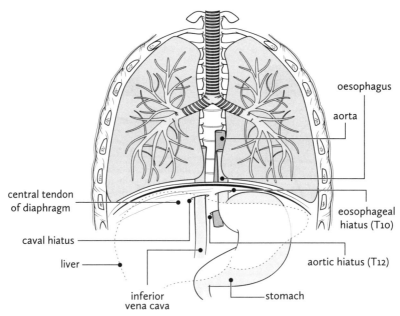

FIGURE 1E. THE LUNGS AND DIAPHRAGM

The lungs are incredibly beautiful, butterfly-like structures rather than the 'bags opening and closing like bellows' that we may have heard cued in yoga teaching.

They are rather more porous, more like elastic sea sponges in texture, and respiration is the act of rinsing gases in and out. We draw in oxygen, fuelling all cells. Within that respiration, a chemical reaction occurs within each and every cell, the exhaust fume of which is carbon dioxide. We essentially breathe that out of every cell, which is then transported through the bloodstream, back out into the lungs.

Jonathan Parsons MD, at the Ohio State University Asthma Center, states: 'In healthy people without chronic lung disease, even at maximum exercise intensity, we only use 70 percent of the possible lung capacity.'[13] Lung capacity is the maximum amount of air that your lungs can hold. It predicts health and longevity, begins to decline at 30 years old and is as much as 50 per cent lower by the age of 50.[14] There are lung/breath capacity tests that measure how much we're able to take in and release. Often, lack of lung capacity is because of focus on the breath either at the top of the chest or down into the belly rather than inclusive patterning of the chest, diaphragm and the belly (we'll look at this more in Part 2).

The moving and somatic practices that we explore in this section rely on the movement of the whole body, fluidity in the spine and throughout the whole of the fascia – opening us from the inside out. All are involved in the breathing in a fluid, rather than a mechanistic, way – 'mechanism' is not a word with which we should describe the body as it implies that we are robotic and articulated, rather than the pulsating, responsive and rhythmic beings that we are!

Joanne Avison writes compellingly on the incredible fluidity of the breath, supporting the shift away from mechanical language: 'This "opening and closing" of a closed, kinematic chain mechanism that is whole and complete (in the round) will be referred to here as the "expansion and in-drawing" motions of breathing. It is an important distinction that deliberately avoids "contraction and relaxation" of muscles.'[15]

A more tidal, pulsing rhythm is a more accurate description for the breath. We need fluidity within its expression, which comes from opening the front of the spine as we inhale, opening the back of the spine as we exhale; movements such as spine undulations (explored in Part 2's practices) help to free the quality of the breath throughout the whole body. We can combine this with core stabilisation – this doesn't mean 'tight abs', but rather awareness of how the ribs relate to the pelvis and so offer support around the lower back. This supports

---

13   Quoted in Centers for Respiratory Health (2021).
14   Schünemann *et al.* (2000).
15   Avison (2021).

the movement of breath into the upper body, and we will explore this through the physical practices in this book.[16]

The lymphatic system

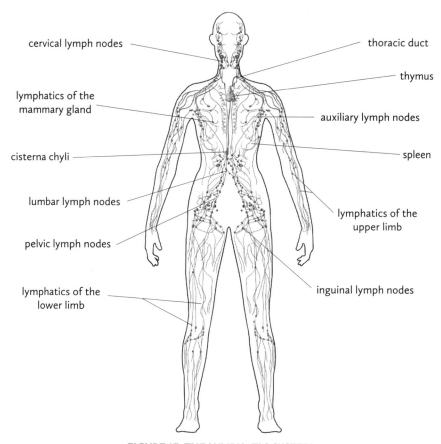

cervical lymph nodes

thoracic duct

thymus

lymphatics of the mammary gland

auxiliary lymph nodes

cisterna chyli

spleen

lumbar lymph nodes

lymphatics of the upper limb

pelvic lymph nodes

lymphatics of the lower limb

inguinal lymph nodes

FIGURE 1F. THE LYMPHATIC SYSTEM
Source: This illustration first appeared in Yoga Therapy for Digestive Health *by Charlotte Watts*

The lymphatic system is a very important part of the immune system, sitting closely with the respiratory system, moving up to it, coming into contact with it and taking away anything that is harmful. It defends the body against infection by supplying disease-fighting cells, lymphocytes. It appears as a beautiful, silvery web that extends throughout the whole of the body. Key sites are into the throat, which drains out to the collarbone, down into the groin, the solar plexus and under the armpits. All of these nodes rely on muscle movement and

16   Bradley and Esformes (2014).

raising the heart rate, and are vital for lymphatic drainage and the removal of toxins from the body.

White blood cells (leukocytes)

White blood cells are key immune players; they are part of the lymphatic system and produced in bone marrow, from where they travel body-wide. They are on constant patrol, looking for pathogens; when they find a target, they multiply and send signals out to other cell types to do the same.

They are stored in different places in the body, referred to as lymphoid organs, including the following:

- Thymus, a gland between the lungs and just below the neck.
- Spleen, which sits in the upper left of the abdomen, filters blood.
- Bone marrow, found in the centre of the bones; it also produces red blood cells.
- Lymph nodes, small glands positioned throughout the body, linked by lymphatic vessels.

There are two main types:

- Phagocytes: these cells surround and absorb pathogens and break them down, effectively eating them. There are several types, including:
  - Neutrophils, the most common, which tend to attack bacteria.
  - Monocytes, the largest, with several roles.
  - Macrophages, that patrol for pathogens and also remove dead and dying cells.
  - Mast cells, multitaskers, helping to heal wounds and defend against pathogens.
- Lymphocytes: these help the body to remember previous invaders and recognise them if they recur. Lymphocytes begin their life in bone marrow. Some stay there and develop into B lymphocytes (B cells); others become T lymphocytes (T cells) in the thymus. In the gut lining these are called Peyer's patches, constituting 70 per cent of the immune system here as GALT, gut-associated lymphoid tissue.

The throat – back of the oral cavity

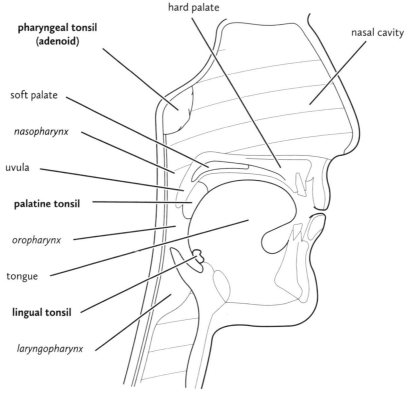

FIGURE 1G. THE TONSILS AND THROAT

The uvula hangs down from the top of the throat from the soft palate. To the side of the
tongue three sets of adenoids between the back of the nose and throat supply and drain out
via many more lymphatic nodes and ducts in the throat, the neck and the collarbone.

The oral cavity and throat is another important aspect of the immune system that
is also connected to the lymphatic system. We might often see swellings in the
base of the throat or up underneath the ears or around any of these areas as they
respond to pathogens. Until recently, people often had their tonsils or adenoids
removed, but it is now understood how integral to the immune system they are.

What makes this a particularly complicated and important site is that we
take food and air in here – the things of nourishment, *prana*. The quality of
how we take in breath and food has a huge part to play in both immune and
respiratory health. This is where we can be conscious through breath and the
quality of our nourishment – not just what, but also how we eat or breathe.
This is where practices such as *anapanasati* (mindfulness of breathing; page 69)
or mindful eating and conscious diet all have a huge impact on our ability to
respond to the world where it meets our body.

Protective fluids in the mouth and stomach

We have many protective fluids in the mouth and stomach. Saliva is a key part of our first immune defence, particularly in relation to what's coming in from the outside world – the amount we chew and how mindfully we eat has a huge effect. Chewing has been shown to inhibit stress-induced neuronal responses in the brain. In a trial studying the effects of chewing gum on post-operative patients and those with a tendency to heart arrhythmia, it was ascertained that 'chewing may contribute to maintaining visceral autonomic balance and gastrointestinal homeostasis' and that 'chewing suppresses an excessive sympathetic response'.[17] So when we chew, we are activating parasympathetic tone, the body's ability to rest and digest. When we don't chew thoroughly, we don't produce enough saliva, we might gulp stuff down, or we might drink more water, over-diluting digestive fluids.

When things from the outside make their way down that are too pernicious to be killed off by saliva, the high pH of stomach acid kills pathogens, but this also relies on the parasympathetic tone to be produced. Further down in the gut, immune capacity relies on calm eating and calm states, being able to come down to conscious, inactive relaxation for full functionality.

In his book *Breath*, James Nestor explores the shifts in our chewing habits post-industrially and the link to poor breathing. Combined with 'morphological changes to the human head…that lowering of the larynx that clogged our throats, the expansion of our brains that lengthened our faces', rapid industrialisation of farmed foods has meant that, 'within just a few generations of eating this stuff, modern humans became the worst breathers in Homo history, the worst breathers in the animal kingdom'.[18]

Breath as the conductor of respiratory and immune systems

With these post-industrial and evolutionary shifts in our breathing patterns, it is common to have respiratory problems linked to difficulty with nasal breathing. Difficulties in breathing might also be postural (which we will explore in Part 3) or it might be habit, possibly from repeated stress responses. The benefits of nasal breathing are numerous, as are the health issues associated with mouth breathing.

The tone of our breathing can allow us to drop into calm, relaxed states, as well as protecting the health of tissues in the mouth and the nose and immunity

---

17   Koizumi *et al.* (2011).
18   Nestor (2020).

through the whole of the body. This is encouraged in yoga practices. At the very least, focusing on breathing in through the nose, even if breathing out through the mouth, is advised, and will vastly improve the tone of the nervous system and subsequently our immune response.

Nasal breathing

Yogic breathing or *pranayama* (page 307) 'extends life force' by bringing attention to both the inhale and the exhale in different patterns, as a means of calming mental states. The majority of practices are nasal and encourage expansion of the whole respiratory system to support mental and physical vitality.

Air is warmed as it comes in through the nose, which opens lung cells more for optimal oxygen absorption. Taking air in through the nose routes it past tiny filtering hairs and mucus linings with immune components that prevent and even destroy impurities entering the body. Cold air coming into the nose cools down the frontal lobe of the brain, which calms its activity.

Through nasal breathing, we also produce the chemical Nitric Oxide, which opens the cells of the lungs to receive oxygen, supporting bronchial tone by regulating how well the airways in the respiratory tract are able to contract and relax with the breath. This creates homeostasis, a coming into balance that works body wide and signals (through the autonomic nervous system) to relax inner muscles of the blood vessels. This increases natural blood flow, allowing dilation where appropriate and lowers blood pressure where it tends to be high, which is more constrictive. This has a protective effect on the immune system. In balance, Nitric Oxide is an important component within the immune system, controlling and destroying invaders, but it can be damaging within the context of high inflammation in the body.[19]

Mouth breathing

According to James Nestor's research into the breath, we lose 40 per cent more water at night by mouth breathing, also losing our first defence against oral bacteria. Mouth breathing and the resultant drying out of mucosal linings in the airways can lead to malocclusion (misalignment between the upper and lower teeth)[20] and oral hygiene problems as well as long-term systemic issues such as asthma, snoring and sleep apnoea, and gastrointestinal disorders.[21] When we don't sleep deeply because we are disrupted by our own breathing

19   Sharma, Al-Omran and Parvathy (2007).
20   Paolantonio *et al.* (2019).
21   Flutter (2006).

patterns, hormones are unbalanced, and we don't receive enough oxygen to the brain, so even growth and intelligence can be affected as well as our energy levels in general, leading to associated issues such as 'attention deficit disorder (ADHD), diabetes, high blood pressure, cancer and so on...'[22]

Patiently retraining our *samskaras*, or habits, through *pranayama* practices (conscious breathing), we can, over time, help to overcome patterned mouth breathing (page 168).

The diaphragm

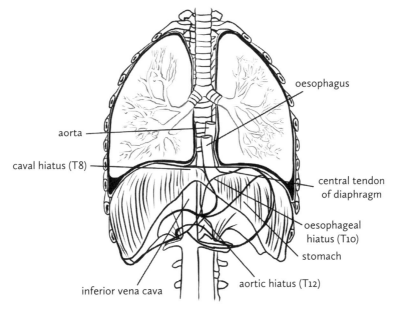

FIGURE 1H. THE DIAPHRAGM
Source: This illustration first appeared in Yoga Therapy for Digestive Health *by Charlotte Watts*

Lungs are not muscles, but rely on the movement of the diaphragm, a key part of our breathing mechanism and an integral part of the movement of everything above and below, interconnected and symbiotic. This upside-down, bowl-shaped muscle at the bottom of the ribs separates the abdominal from the thoracic cavities. Above, we have the lungs and the heart; below, we have the liver nestling up in the right-hand side and the stomach in the left.

Functional movement of the diaphragm is also paramount for digestive health and for immunity of the digestive wall. Moving into the cave of the rib cage, the diaphragm ideally works in a really beautiful, pulsing motion

---

22   Nestor (2020).

in symbiosis with the intercostal muscles between the ribs. Diaphragmatic movement moves fluids through the fascia, making space for and hydrating the organs and abdomen.

If we can visualise the movement of the diaphragm, not in mechanical terms but rather as a fluid movement comparable to that of a jellyfish, gracefully expanding as we inhale, releasing as we exhale, we better appreciate its poetic nature. This also gives us a more accurate idea of it as multidimensional, moving to the sides and out to the back, not just focusing on the front, as we see in two-dimensional drawings.

THE INHALATION

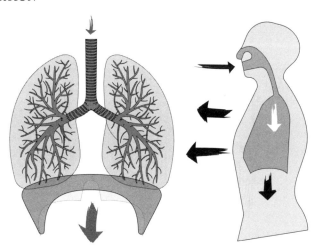

FIGURE 11. INHALATION

On the inhalation, the diaphragm contracts and moves downwards towards the belly to increase the volume of the thoracic cavity, creating a partial vacuum, drawing air into the lungs.

The inhalation is the action of the diaphragm drawing in, related to the 'doing' sympathetic tone of the autonomic nervous system. When everything orchestrates together, the muscular action of the diaphragm moves in and downwards towards the belly and increases the volume of the thoracic cavity, pushing the belly move outwards, creating a partial vacuum by drawing air into the lungs.

We can feel this in our yoga practice as we often activate expansive, more dynamic movements on an inhalation, feeling its opening nature, the sense of motion. We may visualise and connect to the inhale bringing in nourishment to every cell of the body, the circulation of energy, vitality:

Much like the original cell (of us) and the planet upon which we breathe, the breath occurs naturally in 360 degrees of roundness. However we describe it, it somehow helps to remember this in practice. It is important in understanding the biotensegrity of the breath. Lengthy descriptions of the anatomy and biomechanics of breathing function may provide useful information. However, lest we forget in our hunger for naming parts, the breath is round, and we survive because the air surrounding us is alchemised into something we call Life Force. Yoga calls it Prana. Martial Arts call it Chi or Qi or Ki. Whatever it is, it animates our form and functions.[23]

THE EXHALATION

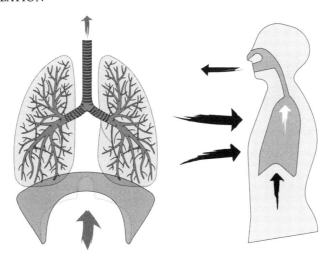

FIGURE 1J. EXHALATION
On the exhale, the diaphragm is drawn upwards, ribs inwards, and carbon dioxide is expelled.

The exhalation, in its most relaxed state, doesn't require any action. It is simply the diaphragm releasing back up, an elastic recoil up into the chest. It is a relaxed tone – we simply allow it to happen, which is why we often practise diaphragmatic breathing on the back so that we don't require any postural muscle action to stand or even sit. Where we can be as relaxed in the whole body as possible, an easeful exhalation is the result of allowing a complete inhalation to come to its full conclusion, or peak, and then allowing the exhalation to spontaneously flow. This is the breath we can feel just below the nostrils, but not to the level of the chin.

We often release movements in our *asana* practice on the exhalation, embodying the sense of letting go, not 'doing' but 'being', becoming more

23   Avison (2021).

spacious. This is the parasympathetic domain, where the body restores, rests, digests and processes the action of the inhale.

The intercostals

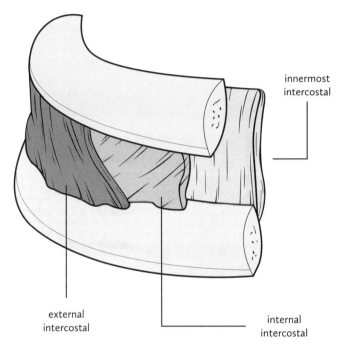

innermost
intercostal

external
intercostal

internal
intercostal

FIGURE 1K. THE INTERCOSTALS
On the inhalation, external intercostals contract to allow the inside space to expand. The internal intercostals only contract in the forced out-breath of stress response.

The intercostals are the muscles between the ribs. The external intercostals are more involved in the inhalation; it might sound counterintuitive, but these contract on the inhale as the ribs are actually expanding. Picture the opening of the ribs out to the side, the back and the front to allow the inside space to open up so that the innermost intercostals can expand.

The exhalation only involves contraction of the internal intercostals when there's a forced out-breath, which may happen if we go into the stress response, exertion or panic mode. This can also happen in particular yoga practices where we consciously force the out-breath, such as *kapalabathi pranayama* (skull shining breath), where the breath is pumped out in short, sharp bursts. Ideally, most of the time we want the tone of our exhalation to be fluid and relaxed.

The cycle of the breath

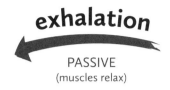

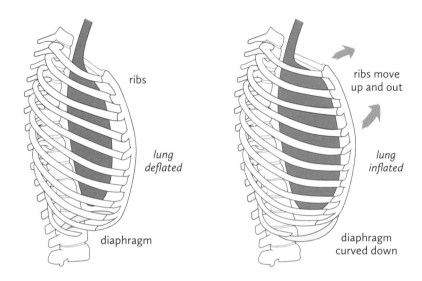

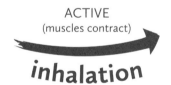

FIGURE 1L. EXHALATION AND INHALATION

The breath is a cycle, a continuum, fluid and felt through the tissues of the whole body, moving seamlessly through passive and active phases, regulating nervous system tone. As John Stirk says: 'Waiting at the end of an exhale invites respiratory intelligence to attract an inhalation at the precise moment it is needed, something we cannot know in advance. The slightest anticipation disturbs the breath's natural creativity. We can stand back to the extent that it hardly feels like the breath, just a sliver of understated sensory activity passing through spatial consciousness.'[24]

---

24 Stirk (2021).

The *four continuous stages of the breath* (see more on page 309) are:

1. *Puraka* (inhalation), the process of drawing in air. This should be smooth and continuous, drawing in *prana*, life. Imagine the inhale as if it is coming up a hill; it needs energy and action, but not more than enough.
2. *Abhyantara kumbhaka* ('full pause' or 'full pot' after inhaling), cessation of the flow of air at the top of the inhale, the suspension of the air in the lungs. This is practised with *ahimsa*, a lack of force. Here we get to the top of the hill and there's that peak holding-in space. The retention of air in the lungs allows the oxygen to be taken across the barrier and into the circulation.
3. *Rechaka* (exhalation), the smooth and continuous release of the breath. This is like the falling over the other side of the hill that follows the pause. Reducing the tendency to add force to the exhale is beneficial to parasympathetic tone. The language of *pranayama* (yogic breathing practices; page 307) is very much around ease and release rather than 'full' or 'deep' (which can become grasping and lose subtlety), rather looking to calm the mind fluctuations through *isvara pranidhana* (surrender).
4. *Bahya kumbhaka* ('empty pause' or 'empty pot' after exhaling) completes the cycle that terminates as the pause ends and a new inhalation begins. In *pranayama*, this moment is the 'perfectly peaceful pause'. Here, everything has potential, and if we look at the exhalation as expiration, it can also be seen as a 'little death'.

We have the polarity of life coming in with the inspiration and going out with the expiration, a continual cycle that mirrors life itself. Each breath has its story, its own unique point in time, its own particular potential and context within our embodied state. We can let go of each breath, the old, in the pause, at the still point of every single cycle. *Anapanasati* (mindfulness of breathing; page 69) is being completely in the moment, not grasping at something to come or holding on to what has been.

Bringing awareness of these stages of breath into any nature of physical practice can help both bring it to life – as it responds to nervous system states and shifts – and provide a guide for our attunement to our need for space, release and, so very often, slowing down.

PHYSICAL PRACTICE: SOMATIC AND LOOSENING SEQUENCE

In this first part, we arrive into the territory of our whole being, close to the ground. Lifting ourselves minimally against the forces of gravity, we offer the room to open out, to broaden into our tissues. We might settle into a sense of the whole, with less imperative to 'do', to 'get going'.

As our focus, our context of immune and respiratory health represents our self-protective and vital capacities, we can meet these realms arriving into our meditative space. This is a fostering of embodied awareness, with the home of our body offering us a route into the very real act of grounding. This is acknowledging our physicality, as it is (the size and shape it is) in the here and now – presence – allowing our body systems to find their way back to equilibrium.

Somatics encompasses movement practices such as those here, which meet this presence through interoception (internal physical perception and experience). They often remove a sense of form and allow us to feel a more fluid, fascial identity, rather than moving from muscle and strength. They work by helping retrain neural pathways out into the somatic nervous system that may have lost their communication routes, remembering that this communication comes from the brain (page 81). As Moshé Feldenkrais said: 'What I'm after isn't flexible bodies, but flexible brains. What I'm after is to restore each person to their human dignity.'[25]

In allowing an opening of space, we are inviting the space for expression and function to find the path of least resistance, where dropping back into equilibrium is most available. Rather than what can we do, how does it feel? How do we listen and respond with curiosity, rather than imposing our will on our physical being?

As well as providing a guide for exploration, through pulsing or rocking movement around and awareness of the diaphragm, we also encourage free movement through the lymphatics into the belly and all the way up into the collarbone and throat. We free the tissues around and between the ribs, and fascial movement through all of the organs. This supports the health of the mucosa and the microbiome in all of our tissues, and frees up our movement patterns from the centre outwards.

---

25   Moshé Feldenkrais, quoted in Leutenegger (no date).

These movements can be easier on the ground – where we don't have to hold the shoulders up, we can have more ease to release the jaw. Softening the jaw and throat is crucial for oral health, as the front line of immune health. Lying down also reduces possible issues that our postural habits bring into the breath and the holding of the body when we sit or stand. Priming from the ground in this way, as we come further up from it, we support both respiration and immunity. Where we can find self-support relies least on tension and more on easeful calibration up through our bipedal design.

In terms of our innate defences, these practices also allow us to sense our own boundaries, where 'enough' is found at any point. Freed from the rigidity of prescribed form, we can creatively explore where tension resides or arises in the tissues, moment to moment, and make space, allowing release.

> Resistance in the tissues is ideally soft, pliant, and can be dispersed by the slightest suggestion from the mind. It takes time to reveal this quality which is dependent on the quality of consciousness.
>
> **John Stirk**[26]

In any of the positions offered here, you always have the agency and autonomy to feel movement emerge and evolve as your body informs you where it wants to go. When we are listening in to these inner voices of intuition, we can foster a deeper connection with attending to our true needs, beneath the constant vigilance of the front brain.

Adding in any rolling, rocking, pulsing, wriggling, shimmying and free-form moving that feels natural throughout the practice hands over trust that this is your body and you know what it needs more than any imposition on it. This playfulness is like meditation – it needs no purpose. As Donna Farhi states:

As we come up against the discomfort of tight muscles or challenging positions, we learn to soften and breathe into our tightness or breathe through our difficulty. When an upsetting emotion arises during meditation, we learn to give this feeling room by allowing our breath to rise and fall. This teaches us

26   Stirk (2021).

that while we cannot control what is going to happen to us, we can control our response. We can choose to open up or to shut down, to soften or to harden.[27]

Sensory motor amnesia

Sensory motor amnesia (SMA) is a term coined by Thomas Hanna to describe when muscular activation has become switched off or is inefficient.[28] These are so deeply habitual that we cannot even sense, let alone control, them, and they can easily create chronic issues within breath and immune responses.

A common, modern postural pattern is to lose the signals to relax the neck, lower back or shoulders, keeping us stuck in secondary breathing modes (page 85). Moving into areas where the 'new normal' is tension or they have forgotten to let go isn't simply about pushing in a new form or looking for a 'fix' to this issue. We need to recognise that these are patterns of self-protection, and as such, they need gratitude. Like many such tissue habits – they get locked into a shape or place that is no longer appropriate to the moment. Somatic practices can help us move into patterns to evolve out of them, exploring areas as we are invited in and not crashing against our own boundaries – to write new stories.

Much of this stuckness (*granthis*; page 153) is a direct result of modern living – a mixture of sedentary behaviours, chronic psycho-social stress and societal traumas such as isolation and fear all play their part, as do any other trauma states. These modes that have wandered far away from our original, primal beings shut down parts of us that then become over- or under-used. We can signal both soothing and a 'waking up' through all of our tissues by attending to some key areas that are affected via modern habits:

- Observing where our faces get caught into 'masks' from social norms or presenting a 'persona' to the world – move into all of the muscles in the face, opening the mouth wide, sticking out the tongue and making faces.
- Noticing when we are clenching our jaw from chronic stress – slacken the lower jaw and move it from side to side.
- Chronically tight diaphragm, psoas, throat – practices in this book.
- Recognising habitual tension held in our hands from technology use – move fingers and wrists, interlink the fingers and make 'figure-of-eight' motions with the wrists.

---

27 Donna Farhi, quoted in Gardiner (2013).
28 Hanna (2004).

- Over-focusing with the eyes towards screens and tightening the muscles around them – softening and massaging the forehead, sinuses and temples.

Continually bringing ease and kind attention to these areas within our practice can help free the tension that is also an inherent part of the stress response that we will explore in Part 2.

THE INNATE WISDOM OF THE BODY

1. Environmental stressors and physiological or emotional threats provoke reactivity in the body, where it will manifest as muscle tension, granthis (knots) or the development of unhealthy habits.
2. All experience in the body is impermanent.
3. Traumatic experiences held in the body can be triggered and re-experienced as feelings, sensations and memories.
4. The body, as the mind, has plasticity, constantly changing and remoulding.
5. Healing and self-repair is possible at any point.
6. Practising non-judgemental awareness, compassion and patience create the perfect environment in which the body's innate wisdom can arise.
7. The body is the route to deep healing and transformation of emotional trauma.

The wisdom of the pause

Interspersing the directed movements here with spaces of simply lying down and exploring what feels congruent in the body fosters a felt sense of autonomy and trust. This is taking time and space to simply be, to allow the previous moments to be received, processed and assimilated. Like a conversation, information from movement needs time to settle in, shift and become integrated.

We can notice in the pauses offered here (in positions such as constructive rest, *apanasana* (wind-relieving pose), *balasana* (child's pose) and *savasana* (corpse pose)) that it is part of our nature to anticipate (an important protective trait), but this can provoke conditioned responses that we rush towards.

Noticing these pulls of the mind and dropping beneath to listen to the nuances of our inner experience offers us an insight into the rhythms beneath the noise of constantly doing. This is tuning into the symphony of our body processes and goes a long way to allowing them to function in easeful harmony.

Constructive rest position

First, come to the ground in constructive rest position (CRP), to connect into the breath, to tune into our nervous system (or energetic) state. We are setting the scene for practice here, stepping away from habits of 'doing' or 'fixing', simply noticing your body as it is, without adjustment. In this way you can allow the space to arrive – a process. Notice the very real physical movement of your breath in your body, inviting you into the here and now.

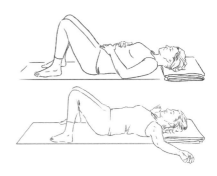

- A place to arrive, to tune into needs and move into somatic or other practices.
- Neutral positioning for the psoas – potential for release before moving into pliability there. Knees bent for the lower back to move with the motions of the breath, to talk to the psoas. Allows breath to drop away from the chest and shoulders, down into the belly and diaphragm.
- Alternate meditation position when fatigued or when sitting upright may create tension.

1. Start with a neatly folded towel or blanket under your skull so that there is a softness in the throat and at the root of your tongue. Your feet should be about hip-width apart, not too close to the buttocks, so that it is easeful; the back muscles are passive (not anticipating action). If there is any pinching at the lumbar or the feet, or it feels as if the legs are dropping out, turn the feet inwards and drop the knees together for support. If arms are out to the side, elbows bent to whatever degree allows them to soften and release – where your wrists, and, therefore, shoulders, can drop.
2. Notice the jaw and temples. Lightly draw the chin towards the throat, as this can ease the passage of breath through the nose. Allow the

lower jaw to slacken away from the top teeth, then move the lower jaw gently to release, attending to any tension around the skull with gentle rolling of the head, side to side. Invite an 'aah' sound with the exhalation, creating space between the back of the teeth, feeling the vibration around the jaw and throat.

3. Sense around the ears (another site of immune defence, where mucosal immune responses in the middle ear and Eustachian tube generally respond efficiently to pathogens).

4. Peacefulness in the nervous system is represented by softness of the inhale through the nose. Try not to 'do' or 'fix' here, but rather simply notice the body as it is, without adjustment, in this way, sensing the difference between left and right, top and bottom body, and where the body meets the ground. Notice the very real physical movement of the breath in the body.

5. Softly position the hands on the abdomen. Tune into the rise on the inhalation, the fall on the exhalation. This positions the psoas neutrally so we can better notice breath into the belly.

6. Slide the hands up to the diaphragm, feeling the easeful movement of the lungs and ribs – a tidal rhythm, each breath unique.

7. Come back to this position between movements to let them integrate and assimilate through body tissues, moments of 'pause' and letting things settle in. CRP is a reset for our natural spinal curves and a place to allow space and cultivate internal awareness of unconscious, habitual instincts.

8. After 10–15 minutes observing the breath, move the jaw and face, wriggle the shoulders and take the arms out to the side at shoulder height.

9. Exhale the head to roll it to one side, without pushing or forcing. Inhale it back to centre and exhale to the left. As the neck softens, as the head turns to one side, reach the opposite arm out from the centre to make space in that shoulder. Inhale back to centre and move that side to side, feeling out into the space around you.

Pandiculation

Although the term 'pandiculation' is often used to refer to the act of a combined yawn and stretch, our automatic pandicular response can be performed as conscious movement, as a fundamental part of our neuromuscular functioning (for more on pandiculation, see page 290). According to Heidi Hadley:

What we do in a pandiculation is threefold: Pandiculation sends biofeedback to our nervous system regarding the level of contraction in our muscles, thereby helping to prevent the build-up of chronic muscular tension. This is an extremely important function of the pandicular response. A pandiculation contracts and releases muscles in such a way that the gamma loop, a feedback loop in our nervous system that regulates the level of tension in our muscles, is naturally reset. This resetting reduces muscular tension and restores conscious, voluntary control over our muscles.[29]

Pandiculation prepares us for normal sensing and moving, readying the voluntary cortex for efficient functioning. Beginning by contracting and releasing small groups of muscles, we can reroute brain wiring to involuntary muscle tension (held as sensory motor amnesia, SMA; page 53) by resetting the alpha–gamma feedback loop in the brain. We can take natural pandiculating movement into larger movements that integrate muscular releases into natural, efficient full-body movement patterns.

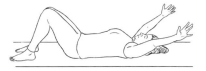

- A nervous system reset, into parts where gathering tension to experience release feels intuitively helpful – limbs, jaw, whole body...
- Allowing exploration to unfold from here.
- We can punctuate a practice with moments of reaching, yawning and spontaneous noise.

1. From CRP (or any other position) with arms bent, lift the arms a little off the ground and move the ribs and shoulders in an exploratory way, letting that open out into a reach in any direction as that evolves.
2. Through that reach, feel any part of you that tenses to evoke an accompanying yawn and then consciously release with a sigh.
3. Let this tension–release cycle move into any part of you that naturally joins in, for example one or two legs at a time, reaching across the diagonals, etc.

---

29 Hadley (2019).

Lying spine undulations

We explore spine undulations further in Part 2, but come here to this lying version to attune to the animating, physical motions of the breath, to the central axis and belly, and to offer ease into all connections into the spine and therefore radiating out – the potential of space and release.

- Can differ from ventral–dorsal undulations on other planes as there is a counter-movement between the lower back and the neck – a lymphatic pump.
- On the inhale as the chest rises and the chin draws in to meet it, a gentle *jalandhara bandha* is formed (page 336).
- As the chin rocks up to the ceiling on the exhale, a little compression in the base of the skull occurs – this floods this area with fluids on the release of the inhalation to come. Between is a wave-like motion up the spine.

1. Lying comfortably on the back, tune into the natural rhythm of the breath.
2. To ease into the side of the spine before the forward–back motion, move the tailbone side to side, as if wagging the tail – this may mean that there is also motion in the knees; allow this spontaneously. Even the head may move side to side so that the whole body may join in; this is a very primal, reptilian or fish-like movement, freeing up the ribs, diaphragm, organs and lymphatics.
3. Gradually reduce this movement, eventually settling in centre, coming home to the body, a sense of safety, where we rest into the pause.
4. On the inhale, feel the natural softening and expansion down into the belly, which subsequently lifts the lumbar arch, without tension.
5. On the exhale, allow the waist and lumbar spine to soften and release to the floor. The tailbone may naturally lift.
6. Allow the movement of the spine and belly to be fluid, undulating, lengthways. The breath leads, the body follows and the mind observes.
7. The head and neck may move to 'counter'; on the inhale, as the lumbar lifts, the cervical spine can arch, head dropping back, opening

the throat. As the lumbar softens on the exhale, the chin draws in towards the chest, lengthening the cervical spine. This has a pumping effect in the lymphatics around the diaphragm and draining out from the neck and throat through the collarbone.

8. Allow each part of the breath to conclude naturally, noticing the pause (page 50) before 'tipping over' into the next stage. On the inhalation, the mobilising tone of the nervous system tends to be opening, more active, to receive and expand the ventral body. The exhale is where we come to the protective curling response and it's more dorsal, releasing into a more nurturing and 'not doing' tone. Relating spinal movements with the breath can be incredibly supportive to the immune system, through autonomic nervous system regulation (see Part 2).

9. Reduce the movement little by little, coming to stillness naturally, and tuning into the natural motions left simply from the presence of the breath and these mammalian forward-back spinal movements.

Body rocking diaphragm release

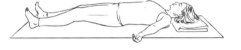

- Exploring extension of the legs out from the belly and through the psoas up to the diaphragm – feeling out that space to notice differences between left and right.
- Helpful after movements softening into the psoas, to lengthen out through it (the diaphragm down to the legs) and bringing awareness to the relationship with the lower back, feeling movement of the legs up into the body.

1. Lengthen out the legs to pause in *savasana* (corpse pose) for as long as you need to, to feel the body expanding over the ground.
2. Flex the feet loosely up to the ceiling.
3. Rock side to side on the heels, quite bouncily, so that the pelvis elastically rolls. The head may spontaneously move too.
4. Notice any holding in the diaphragm, separating the upper and lower body, common in held stress patterns, and regulate the movement (even lessening it or slowing down) to find where the diaphragm is happy to join in and doesn't need to partition off the lower body in self-protection.

5. Settle back to centre, noticing murmurs of autonomic release in the body and breath. Allow *prana* (energy, *chi*) to assimilate as you orient back to the central axis.

6. Rock the toes in and out gently from the midline, so that each leg is moving towards and away from each other. Keep it fluid, moving lymphatics around the groin and lower colon, which can be very stagnant from sedentary living.

7. Drop back down into the space of *savasana*.

Supine sliding leg tree

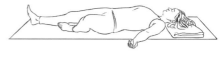

1. Take one knee out to the side, drawing up towards the pelvis, allowing the pelvis to roll to that side and keeping space between the foot and the extended leg.

2. Take this movement side to side, allowing the head to move too, the whole body included as it naturally joins in, but not forcing anything.

3. Stay attentive to the quality of the breath and the tones and textures of the sensations, so you find the stride of your movement – not too little, not too much.

Rolling *supta baddha konasana* (supine bound angle pose)

- Opening out the belly space between the hip bones, to feel a containment in the lower back. Freeing the mid-body, squeezing the organs and opening the rotational, diagonal lines.

- Engaging the root of the feet coming together, awakening the channels of the inner legs. Rolling that place for a massaging effect up the lymphatics of the outer thighs.

1. Slide both heels up towards the pelvis, knees and hips externally releasing, soles of the feet coming towards each other but not too

close into the groin so you retain space in the lower back, and ease in the belly.

2. Roll the legs side to side, pelvis rolling with the movement so one outer leg at a time meets the ground, opening the psoas, creating movement around the organs.

3. Rest back in CRP with the hands on the belly to tune into this area you've been awakening, offering kindness there.

Apanasana (wind-relieving pose) with hug

- A place to orient back to the 'home' of the midline; like other places organised there to come to the pause – for example, CRP, *adho mukha svanasana* (down-face dog), *balasana* (child's pose), *tadasana* (mountain pose).

- Taking the scenic, meandering route to draw the knees in, to feel out the needs of the lower back with self-massage and bodily enquiry.

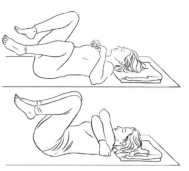

- Gathering back into the heart and the belly via a journey through the lower back and belly. The proprioceptive compassion of the hug, releasing the soothing 'love molecule' oxytocin.

1. Draw each leg into and away from the chest, exploring and feeling what is in the lower body before drawing in towards *apanasana*; take your sweet time in this self-massage.

2. Reach the arms right around the opposite shoulder and settle into a protective, nurturing position around the heart. This calms, activating the soothing vagus nerve alongside oxytocin release. Our proprioceptive senses are stimulated around the torso by the arm bind, and we find room to breathe into the heart space.

3. Repeat with the arms in the opposite cross of the hug. Notice the response of the breath and the nervous system with your shifting perception and adaptation to even a simple change.

Wringing out dishcloth to twist

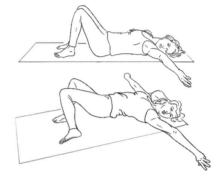

- Waking and mobilising deep into the shoulder girdle and scapulae, to support freeing into the neck, throat and jaw.
- Reaching through this proprioceptive waking of the shoulder, cheek and neck space to tune into 'interesting' feelings there, without reactivity or judgement – breathing space around them.
- Brings in orientation via *drishti*, with a soft, focused gaze tracking the point of focus as the hand initiates the feelings into the shoulder girdle.
- In the twist, gathering into the back body illuminates connection from the whole spine out to the arms and hands.

1. From CRP, on the inhalation, turn the head to the right as the arm rotates the 'awkward' way, that is, the thumb moves down towards the ground, the little finger side of the arm lifting.
2. Exhale back to centre, letting the head rotate back to neutral, both palms facing upwards. Take the head to the left and then move side to side, inhaling into the movement, exhaling out.
3. Add in the turning of the opposite arm in the 'easy' way, that is, the thumb rotates to the ceiling to bring the palm downwards. Moving that either side, feel a 'wringing out' sensation through the shoulders and upper chest, as the arms rotate in opposite directions. Spend time with that movement, feeling the arms spiralling one way and then the other as one long line, through the chest, out to all of the fingers.
4. If or when comfortable, let the legs drop away in the opposite direction to the head, arching up into the back, creating a squeeze, and release through the fascia and the lymphatics as you gather the shoulder blades in towards the chest. You may even feel drawn in to hold and stay in the inhale position on each side, to explore different feeling tones of the lungs moving over the shoulder blade area, freeing the fascia there.
5. Return to centre, allowing simply 'being', non-reactivity, coming to whichever neutral position (CRP, *apanasana* (wind-relieving pose), *savasana* (corpse pose)) around the midline that allows you to breathe into the shoulder and chest area in the aftermath of innervating there.

Feldenkrais half-bridge roll

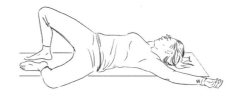

- Offers the support to notice and release each side of the psoas (soft tissues to the inside of the hip bones), feeling as one matrix with the diaphragm.
- Helps coax out a back bend and explore towards *setu bandha sarvangasana* (bridge pose), one side at a time, to feel differences in soft tissues around the psoas and groin.
- Feels out the lines through the belly, across the diagonals (hip to opposite shoulder) – follow in towards the natural motion of a reach.

1. From CRP with arms open to where the shoulders can drop, on an inhalation, let one knee drop out to the side, rolling onto the side of that foot, then easily exhale it back, decompressing back to the centre. Then move to the other leg, so the motion alternates side to side, just behind the breath.
2. Feeling rooted through the foot on the ground, the other outer leg drops fully to the ground as you allow the opposite side of the pelvis to lift, letting the belly roll in the direction of whichever knee is dropping to the side. In this way, as you inhale and open the chest, a back arch evolves, and you can lift up into the heart, squeezing between the shoulder blades as invited with each in-breath. Resist back with the inside of the knee staying pointed up to the ceiling to lengthen the fascial line from there to the chest as you create space in between the hip bones.
3. The head can move in the opposite direction to the dropped leg, opening across the diagonal.
4. On the inhale, open and lift the chest, squeezing between the shoulder blades to awaken, rolling open the ribs.
5. Press the foot on the ground to lift the hip bone on that side without gripping into the buttock and pulse through that side, listening in to the soft tissue – the dense lymphatic area in the groin. This also allows lymphatic flow against gravity as there is a little inversion, bringing malleability and hydration to the psoas, which allows full diaphragmatic movement.

By exploring fluid micromovements with an open awareness, a small pulsation sparks a living inquiry into a timeless presence that has the power to converse with the primordial. Pioneering somatic educator Emilie Conrad recognises that by "entering our own terrain, we have large capabilities of nourishment that enrich our options in how we engage with life." Undulating fluids become meaningful through deep levels of satisfaction, which awakens our consciousness to the diversity of intelligent life inviting us to participate in a larger conversation.

Liz Koch[30]

Moving *setu bandha sarvangasana* (bridge pose)

- Rising up through the heart, soft eyes and jaw allow the rising *prana* with *sukha* (ease). Feeling the falling *apana* quality of the exhale as the spine rolls down (page 93).
- On the rise, *pada bandha* (foot lock) (lifting the arches of the feet) to gather up tissues into the inner thighs; *jalandhara bandha* (chin to chest), purifying around the throat (page 336).
- A counter foetal shape to the side allows release into the back body in a fully curled out, primal shape.

1. Remove any support from under the head.
2. Feel out where there is good traction for all four corners of the feet on the ground: not too close to the buttocks, spine long.
3. Inhale to slide the arms up in 'angel wings' around the side of the body to articulate into the ribs; exhale to draw the arms down the same way.
4. On the next inhale raise the arms at the same time as raising the pelvis and spine in a fluid movement, feeling buoyancy in the filling lungs, supported by grounding the base of the big toe.

---

30   Koch (2019).

5. With the release of the exhale come back down to earth, vertebra by vertebra.
6. Holding the next raise, lift the chest and the heart, moving one knee further away from the pelvis at a time by pressing that footprint into the ground. Gather more muscular strength and form into the midline after more fluid, fascial practices, but without gripping the buttocks or pushing out the lower ribs. Find where the inhale supports the pose without over-efforting.
7. Coming to rest, don't rush to counter; rather, spend time in CRP, allowing the back muscles to release before coming to curl onto your side, breathing into the back body that has just contracted, curling the knees in slowly.

Bhujangasana (cobra pose) with reptilian opening

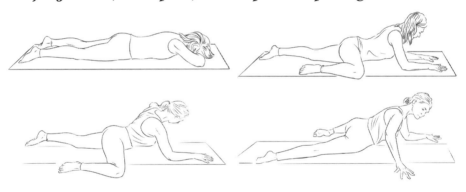

- Reptilian movement is lower to the ground and limbs away to the side, creeping and low crawling; this stage within the evolution of our species (and personal, from the womb) is linked to the primal, instinctual lower brain, and developing the back and neck strength to lift the head.
- Many somatic and primal movements come back to this stage to revisit any patterns laid down here, especially for trauma in the early years of life.
- Allows us to tune into the breath at the belly as the inhalation creates compression into the organs, exhalation, then the following release, flooding fluids through the tissues and releasing tension.

1. Lie on the belly, the ventral aspect of the body held by the ground. Here we can feel the inhalation into the back of the lungs and sacrum, whilst compression of the belly into the ground is relieved with the exhale. Feeling these edges clearly, we can cultivate awareness of our boundaries (see Part 4).

2. Come into *bhujangasana* (cobra pose), arms far enough forwards or holding the opposite elbow to lengthen the erector spinae muscles and not feel you are levering into the lower back.

3. Slide one bent leg up, then the other, rolling the pelvis side to side naturally, allowing the body to organise itself, to find where there is the possibility of release in the psoas. Allow the head and neck to move concurrently to look towards the moving knee, playing with the pace responsively. This awakens the core sheath, kidney meridian and *ida/pingala nadis*.

4. Next, bring the same arm as the bent leg out to shoulder height, elbow bent, lifting from the fingertips up into the palm, so that the arm is energised. Explore fluid, undulating movements through the spine and across the shoulders, allowing the head and neck to move freely.

5. Repeat with the opposite arm to the leg, then with the other leg and each arm position, noticing how it is with each combination of limbs through the pelvis and up into the back.

6. Drop back to the belly, rolling the pelvis side to side.

Bridging to *balasana* (child's pose)

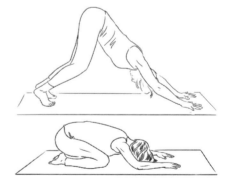

- After somatic practices where we focus on fluidity over form, gathering up from the ground to feel how we organise intelligent containment.
- In an explorative *adho mukha svanasana* (down-face dog), rooting through the palms and base of the index fingers to find the most effort-less lines of support, through space explored in the spine, shoulders and rib cage.
- Deciding via your body rather than your mind when to earth down into the primal shape of *balasana* (child's pose).

1. Listening to your body, expand through a playful *adho mukha svanasana* without focus on 'getting the heels down' but allowing bend and play through the legs to find length between the pubic and breast bones, movement from the ribs – with any sighs or noises that invite release.
2. Listening in to 'enough', ease yourself into *balasana*, cradled between the thighs, as you were in the womb. Arms forward supports the neck to draw the chin lightly into the throat with the full primary curve of this foetal shape.
3. Rest and breathe into the back body, diaphragm and sacrum. Breathing into the more parasympathetic fibres in the back and bottom of the lungs.
4. Roll the forehead side to side, activating the trigeminal nerve there (which soothes the body via connection with the vagus nerve, and also innervates the skin, mucous membranes and sinuses).

Cross-legged twist

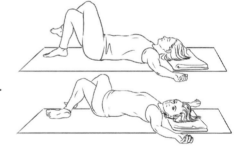

- Coming into revolution into the organ body, the squeeze and release of deep lymphatic material and the gut wall – sites of immune potential.
- Bringing keen awareness to the diaphragm and ribs as places inviting breath to occupy and move.
- A useful twist after opening the hips in a preceding practice, as we roll them back in, gather towards the centre after opening out, and feel connection with the legs at the midline.

1. From supine, take the left leg over the right (right foot on the floor).
2. Breathe, rooting into the left arm and shoulder as the legs drop to the right, using support (cushion, etc.) if needed to be able to hold and stay through guidance of the breath.
3. Inhale to draw the knees back to centre and take the time to swap the cross of the legs, coming to the other side.

Savasana (corpse pose) – with smooth transition out

Lying fully supine is always available and recommended at the end of any practice. Alternative positions are offered throughout the rest of the book, but however you complete your practice, it is courageous (heartful) to stay in this place of reflection, where we can feel profound integration and meeting of our vulnerability. The considerations for mindfulness that follow are an inherent part of *savasana* and, indeed, any part of our physical practice, kind attention, refined awareness and attunement.

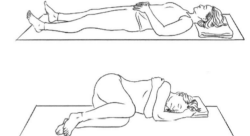

- Throughout the practice that comes before, we differentiate and focus on specific body parts; *savasana* is where we integrate and bring ourselves 'back' to the whole that we always were.
- This can be practised at the end of a physical or enquiring meditative time, or as a standalone practice to allow the day's thoughts and activities to be processed.

Take your time moving out from the side; smooth transition in practice supports how we adapt in all areas of life.

1. Coming into *savasana*, attend to any pinching in the back with support under the knees. Hands can be on the belly if that supports steadying your attention.
2. Allow the top of the back and chest to feel equanimity rather than adjusting shoulders down the back.
3. Breathe space between the ribs, kind attention to the diaphragm.
4. Bring any subtle practice or focus on the breath to guide you into the interior (*pratyahara*) – an anchor to come back to as you then move to simply be, to be breathed.
5. After 10–15 minutes, awaken from the periphery (fingers, toes, jaw) to enliven, and then intuitively roll to whichever side feels right into a foetal position, drawing in around the belly and the heart, resourced by the inner tide of the breath.

SUBTLE PRACTICES: MINDFULNESS OF BREATHING

Within Tibetan Buddhism, *rigpa* is the knowledge that ensues from recognising one's nature, awareness or knowledge of the innermost nature of the mind – similar to the yogic or Hindu term *vidya*. The opposite of *rigpa* is *marigpa* (like *avidya*, ignorance) – a hindrance, affliction or obstacle (*klesha*).

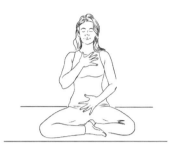

Bringing one hand on to the heart (compassion) and the other on to the belly (awareness) can support our journey inward.

Anapanasati (mindfulness of breathing)

In Tibetan, *dzogchen* means 'great perfection'. This is the meditative state in which we sit, recognising the true nature of the mind. This is pure awareness, *rigpa*, unaffected by the experiences or feelings that arise, simply reflecting with openness and compassion: 'The practice of mindfulness...is living your life as if it really mattered from moment to moment. The real practice is life itself.'[31]

The yogic path emphasises the development of concentration on a highly refined object, such as the breath, to drop into profound states of absorption. The Buddhist path, on the other hand, focuses on a mindfulness of all events as they unfold in the stream of consciousness, where you can experience what is arising or revealing without clinging to it or aversion. So what is the difference between breathing with awareness – consciously, deliberately, attentively, intently – and the breathing that occurs automatically at all times?

Mindful breathing means knowing that you are breathing, not in an abstract or conceptual way, but immediately, viscerally and uninterruptedly – moment by micro-moment. Bringing the breath into conscious awareness also regulates the autonomic nervous system. We will look at bringing particular attention to the exhale as the antidote to the dominance of the inhalation with the constant 'doing' in our very active society, and how this relates to the stress response, in Part 2.

---

31   Kabat-Zinn (2004).

Foundations of anapanasati practice

Anapanasati consists of 16 formal stages or contemplations, divided into four steps. As teachers we can practically apply the focus of each stage and consider through both still and moving practices:

- Mindfulness of the body, breath and sensation – *annamaya* and *pranamaya koshas* (page 150). The first stage focuses on conditioning the body through the breath. Truly being 'where we are' (grounding, orientation) drops us beneath illusion and plants us into a place from where we can grow into the true, present experience. When teaching we can come back to body and breath – placing hands on our own body, making audible breaths and joining in with practice to model and co-regulate.
- Mindfulness of mind – the second stage brings attention to our mind habits, categorisations and judgements, so we can begin to recognise that 'our thoughts are not us'. We can also then see that feelings and thoughts are continually interwoven and feed into each other when left to roam without discernment. Thoughts about feelings, and feelings about thoughts, can create an endless loop unless we intercept and choose to get off that particular merry-go-round. When teaching this means not imposing our self and story on a student or client.
- Mindfulness of feelings or *vedana* – sensations from internal sense organs and how they meet the external world (page 262). In a world of external sensory overload, this third stage can help us step away from the reactivity born of high expectation and imposition of ideals and 'shoulds'. It guides us into the reality of 'what is' here in this moment and supports interoceptive processing (how we sense inwardly; page 258), helping to address many modern chronic conditions. We become able to attune more quickly and directly to the needs of another, beneath what they may be presenting as a coping strategy.
- Mindfulness of mental formations (the characteristics of reality; events and outer circumstances) that are impersonal, impermanent and unsatisfactory. This fourth stage is where practice 'on the mat' translates into our lives beyond – observing how we relate to others, react to difficulty and disagreement and navigate life. As a teacher,

studio atmosphere, outside noise and relations with others can take us out of mindful, kind attention – we come back to our own body and breath.

According to The Middle Length Discourses of the *Buddha, A Translation of the Majjhima Nikaya*:

> He abides contemplating in feelings their nature of arising, or he abides contemplating in feelings their nature of vanishing, or he abides contemplating in feelings their nature of both arising and vanishing. Or else mindfulness that "there is feeling" is simply established in him to the extent necessary for bare knowledge and mindfulness. And he abides independent, not clinging to anything in the world. That is how a bhikkhu abides contemplating feelings as feelings.[32]

Mindfulness of breathing within our physical practice

The first two stages on the previous page can be felt within the experience of a moving practice, particularly when that is less concerned with how much we can do or how far we can get, but rather dropping beneath such goal-oriented behaviour and towards listening in to the nuances and shifts as shown by the breath. Further exploration into spine undulations in Part 2 brings clarity to the tones and differing sensations of the inhale–exhale continuum.

Awareness and compassion

Mindfulness draws together two key aspects: awareness and compassion. Awareness is the quality of attention we bring, breath by breath, moment to moment. Compassion is the act of bringing kindness into that awareness; without it, we can simply be vigilant and come from a fear-based rather than expansive viewpoint. Compassion without awareness can mean that we don't necessarily meet the more difficult aspects of the practice; experiencing the present often means looking at thoughts or feelings that can feel downright icky or scary. Bringing these two together helps allow vulnerability, a brave step that takes steadiness and kindness for us to hold.

---

32 The Teachings of the Buddha (1995).

Seven pillars of mindfulness

Using these pillars to guide us, we can begin to draw back to our body's present experience *breath by breath, moment to moment*, at any given time. This can provide a guide for these qualities that were suggested by Jon Kabat-Zinn as part of the more recent, secular Mindfulness movement (although, of course, they draw on more historic routes):

- *Non-judging*, being an impartial witness to our own experience. This requires awareness of, and stepping back from, the stream of judging and reacting to inner and outer experiences. This habit of categorising into 'good and bad' or 'positive and negative' locks us into mechanical reactions that we are not aware of and that often have no objective basis at all. An interesting enquiry is to observe over 10 minutes how much you are preoccupied with liking and disliking what you are experiencing.
- *Patience* demonstrates that we understand and accept that all things unfold in their own time. Practising mindfulness provides the opportunity to offer time and space to our own unfolding experience. Why rush to the next 'better' moment when each one is our very life in this moment? Patience (for instance, in the pause in our practice) isn't waiting for something to happen, but rather, allowing the moment to unfold, without expectation or imposition.
- *Beginner's mind*, seeing everything as if it was for the first time, and not allowing our illusion of 'knowing' to prevent us from being present to our experiences. This can show up clearly within a yoga or other physical practice that you have gained experience or 'knowing' within, rushing to 'side two' or into a familiar position. Taking time to arrive in this moment, we can tune into the clear view that nothing is a repetition and comes with different nuances to any other time. To come back to beginner's mind in daily life, next time you meet someone you know well, try and see something new in this person, or look for the wonder and change in places you visit often. Looking with fresh eyes is a reminder that everything is always in flux, change – impermanence (*anicca* in Buddhism, *anitya* in Sanskrit). This frees us up from gripping onto things 'as they are', rather allowing things to spontaneously arise, as they invariably will, even if we are putting in fruitless energy trying to stop them!

- *Trust* – developing basic trust in oneself and feelings is an integral part of any meditation practice, including fostering autonomy and agency, rather than getting caught up in the reputation or authority of teachers. It is impossible to become like somebody else – your only hope is to become more fully yourself. As teachers, we can let students know that we cannot make any assumptions on how they feel or respond; we can only hold a compassionate space for them to explore their own journey.

- *Non-striving* – where almost everything we do is for a purpose, meditation, yoga and play are 'purposeless', which can be a challenge to the conditioned mind. Although meditation takes dedication and energy, it is about non-doing. It has no goal other than for you to be your true nature. The irony is that you already are...we cannot practise towards a goal of becoming relaxed, enlightened or sleep better, but rather we have to learn to carefully see what is happening and accept it. These may come as side effects along the way, but the measuring of practice against them will change its very nature.

- *Acceptance*, which often follows periods of intense emotional turmoil and anger. These states use up energy in the struggle instead of facilitating healing and change. We are much more likely to know what to do and have the inner conviction to act when our vision is not clouded by the mind's self-serving judgements and desires or fears and prejudices. Acceptance is not putting up with that which we should not. It is observing healthy boundaries (page 227) while noticing where we can offer compassion, ease and a loosening of holding on to outworn ego stories or goals that do not serve us.

- *Letting go* – when we pay attention to our inner experience, we discover that there are certain thoughts, feelings and situations that the mind seems to want to hold on to. If pleasant, we try and prolong our experience; if unpleasant, we try and avoid them. In meditative practice, we try to intentionally put aside the tendency to elevate some aspects of our experience and reject others. Letting go isn't getting rid of stuff, but rather loosening our grip on that which we might have tightened around; we may view it differently when it has more space.

Four-stage breathing

The particular form – in four stages – is found in the *Visuddhimagga* (*Path of Purity*) of the great Theravadin scholar Buddhaghosa, who lived in 5th-century India and Sri Lanka.[33] Practise each stage for 5–10 minutes:

1. Bring attention to the physical sensations of the breath, and internally count each exhale just after it has ended. Count ten out-breaths, and then another ten, and so on. If distracted, begin the process of counting, starting over from one.
2. Change the count to the beginning of the inhale.
3. Pay attention to the breath, but drop the counting, noticing that the breath is a continuous process, a never-ending flow of sensation.
4. Narrow the sphere of attention, focusing in on the more subtle and refined sensations found around the rims of the nostrils.

Anapanasati (mindfulness of breathing) is a practice that may allow the state of *vipassana* (deep seeing, truly seeing the nature of reality) to arise. This includes insight of our attachment to pleasurable states: 'Some of the commonest manifestations of rapture, or *piti*, are rushes of energy, or tingling, or pleasant sensations in various parts of the body. While these sensations arise, the meditator should simply observe them, without becoming elated by them.'[34]

Self-enquiry questions

Take your time to explore these questions in your practice, journaling your responses over time. You may come back to them time and time again and notice any shifts.

1. How do you see where the barriers and boundaries of the immune and respiratory systems meet? Both theoretically, and where you feel it bodily and through your breath?
2. How does *anapanasati* (mindfulness of breathing) draw you into the present moment experience of not only your breath, but also other aspects of your bodily feelings and mind states?
3. How do you feel that awareness of the pauses (*kumbhaka*; page 50)

---

33 Wildmind Meditation (no date).
34 Luders *et al.* (2011).

between each tone of the breath helps you notice the physical experience and embodied awareness?

4. What do you observe within the larger pauses for integration and assimilation after somatic practices?

5. How can you experience and describe self-protection within calm states? How does this differ to feeling more defensive in stressed, survival mode?

Further resources

Joanne Avison (2021) *Yoga: Fascia, Anatomy and Movement*, 2nd edn. Pencaitland: Handspring Publishing Ltd.

Donna Farhi (1996) *The Breathing Book: Vitality and Good Health Through Essential Breath Work*. New York: Henry Holt & Co.

Stanley Keleman (1989) *Your Body Speaks Its Mind*. Berkeley, CA: Center Press.

Dr Jenna Macciochi (2022) *Your Blueprint for Strong Immunity: Personalise Your Diet and Lifestyle for Better Health*. London: Yellow Kite.

James Nestor (2021) *Breath: The New Science of a Lost Art*. London: Penguin Life.

Whole Health classes and webinars with Charlotte Watts: www.charlottewattshealth.com

References

ASTRO (no date) 'Innate and adaptive immunity.' Available at: www.astro.org/Patient-Care-and-Research/Research/Professional-Development/Research-Primers/Innate-and-Adaptive-Immunity. Accessed March 2022.

Avison, J. (2021) *Yoga: Fascia, Anatomy and Movement*, 2nd edn. Pencaitland: Handspring Publishing Ltd.

Bradley, H. and Esformes, J. (2014) 'Breathing pattern disorders and functional movement.' *International Journal of Sports Physical Therapy 9*(1), 28–39. Available at: www.ncbi.nlm.nih.gov/pmc/articles/PMC3924606

Bush, Z. (2021) 'Innate immune system.' YouTube, 8 January. Available at: www.youtube.com/watch?v=oWT3dcz4QlU

Bush, Z. and Cummings, P. (2021) 'The innate immune system.' Available at: https://zachbushmd.com/innate-immune-system

Candore, G., Colonna-Romano, G., Balistreri, C.R., Di Carlo, D., *et al.* (2006) 'Biology of longevity: Role of the innate immune system.' *Rejuvenation Research 9*(1), 143–148. Available at: https://pubmed.ncbi.nlm.nih.gov/16608411

Centers for Respiratory Health (2021) 'Lung capacity: What does it mean?' 7 September. Available at: https://centersforrespiratoryhealth.com/blog/lung-capacity-what-does-it-mean

De Ronne, N. (2010) 'Management of fever in children younger than 3 years.' *Journal de pharmacie de Belgique 3*, 53–57. Available at: https://pubmed.ncbi.nlm.nih.gov/21090380

Dranoff, G. (2004) 'Cytokines in cancer pathogenesis and cancer therapy.' *Nature Reviews. Cancer 4*(1), 11–22.

Flutter, J. (2006) 'The negative effect of mouth breathing on the body and development of the child.' *International Journal of Orthodontics – Milwaukee 17*, 31–37.

Gardiner, M. (2013) 'The window in: Following the breath – by Donna Farhi.' Manaia Yoga & Wellbeing, 22 September. Available at: https://manaiawellbeing.co.nz/the-window-in-following-the-breath-by-donna-farhi

Gardner, J. (2012) 'Is fever after infection part of the illness or the cure?' *Emergency Nurse 19*(10), 20–25, quiz 27. Available at: https://pubmed.ncbi.nlm.nih.gov/22519079

Hadley, H. (2019) 'The power of pandiculation.' Total Somatics Blog, 17 April. Available at: https://totalsomatics.com/the-power-of-pandiculation

Hanna, T. (2004) *Somatics: Reawakening the Mind's Control of Movement, Flexibility, and Health*. Cambridge, MA: Da Capo Press.

Kabat-Zinn, J. (2004) *Wherever You Go, There You Are: Mindfulness Meditation for Everyday Life*. London: Piatkus Books.

Koch, L. (2019) *Stalking Wild Psoas: Embodying Your Core Intelligence*. Berkeley, CA: North Atlantic Books.

Koizumi, S., Minamisawa, S., Sasaguri, K., Onozuka, M., Sato, S. and Ono, Y. (2011) 'Chewing reduces sympathetic nervous response to stress and prevents poststress arrhythmias in rats.' *American Journal of Physiology – Heart and Circulatory Physiology 301*, 4, H1551–H1558. Available at: https://journals.physiology.org/doi/full/10.1152/ajpheart.01224.2010

Leutenegger, S. (no date) *Moshé Feldenkrais Concise Biography*. The Feldenkrais Method®. Accessed 31/05/2022 at https://feldenkraiscork.com/biography-of-moshe-feldenkrais-and-his-life

Liang, G. and Bushman, F.D. (2021) 'The human virome: Assembly, composition and host interactions.' *Nature Reviews. Microbiology 19*(8), 514–527. Available at: https://pubmed.ncbi.nlm.nih.gov/33785903

Luders, E., Clark, K., Narr, K.L. and Toga, A.W. (2011) 'Enhanced brain connectivity in long-term meditation practitioners.' *Neuroimage 57*(4), 1308–1316.

Mischke-Reeds, M. (2018) *Somatic Psychotherapy Toolbox*. Eau Claire, WI: PESI Publishing.

Moskalev, A., Stambler, I. and Caruso, C. (2020) 'Innate and adaptive immunity in aging and longevity: The foundation of resilience.' *Aging and Disease 11*(6), 1363–1373. Available at: www.ncbi.nlm.nih.gov/pmc/articles/PMC7673842

Nestor, J. (2020) *Breath: The New Science of a Lost Art*. London: Penguin Life.

Owen, J., Punt, J., Stranford, S. and Jones, P. (2018) *Kuby Immunology*, 8th edn. New York: W.H. Freeman.

Paolantonio, E.G., Ludovici, N., Saccomanno, S., La Torre, G. and Grippaudo, C. (2019) 'Association between oral habits, mouth breathing and malocclusion in Italian pre-schoolers.' *European Journal of Paediatric Dentistry 20*, 204–208.

Purssell, E. (2007) 'Treatment of fever and over-the-counter medicines.' *Archives of Disease in Childhood 92*(10), 900–901. Available at: https://pubmed.ncbi.nlm.nih.gov/17522164

Schünemann, H.J., Dorn, J., Grant, B.J., Winkelstein Jr, W. and Trevisan, M. (2000) 'Pulmonary function is a long-term predictor of mortality in the general population: 29-year follow-up of the Buffalo Health Study.' *Chest 118*(3), 656–664. Available at: https://pubmed.ncbi.nlm.nih.gov/10988186

Sharma, J.N., Al-Omran, A. and Parvathy, S.S. (2007) 'Role of nitric oxide in inflammatory diseases.' *Inflammopharmacology 15*(6), 252–259. Available at: https://pubmed.ncbi.nlm.nih.gov/18236016

Stirk, J. (2021) *Deeper Still: Authentic Embodiment for Yoga Teachers*. Pencaitland: Handspring Publishing Ltd.

The Teachings of the Buddha (1995) *The Middle Length Discourses of the Buddha, A Translation of the Majjhima Nikaya*. Translated by Bhikkhu Ñāṇamoli and Bhikkhu Bodi. Somerville, MA: Wisdom Publications.

Wildmind Meditation (no date). *Learn the Mindfulness of Breathing Meditation Practice*. Wildmind: learn meditation online. Accessed 31/05/2022 at www.wildmind.org/mindfulness

PART 2

STRESS AND INFLAMMATION

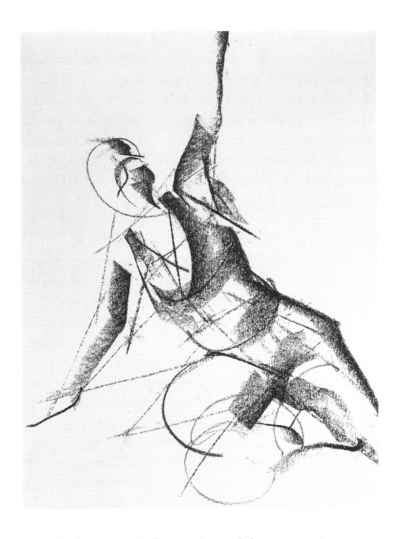

In this part we look at stress, inflammation and the autonomic nervous system in relation to breath and immunity – looking through the lens of the psycho-social stress that can dominate much of the modern, human experience.

When considering practices for the modern human, we need to place our bio-chemistry within the context of how we are living. As we have wandered away from direct and constant interrelating with the wild (what we now call 'nature', as if it were something other than us) and towards more psycho-social stress, we are seeing the health concerns that accompany this 'domestication' – often referred to as 'diseases of Western civilisation'. These ripple through all body systems, with the immune and respiratory systems large players and orches-trators in our struggle to adapt to what we were not designed for – sedentary lives, over-stimulus, technology and living outside the cohesion of the tribe.

The result is so often chronic stress that shows up as a protective response – inflammation. A paper on 'Life stress and health' noted the following: 'There is emerging evidence showing that stressors involving interpersonal loss and social rejection are among the strongest psychosocial activators of molecular processes that underlie inflammation...individuals who are more neurally sensitive to social stressors may mount greater inflammatory responses to social stress.'[1]

To understand these responses and the part that compassionate embodied awareness can play in relieving them, we come to the autonomic nervous system, where immunity and respiration receive many of their signals for response.

The autonomic nervous system (ANS)

The ANS is part of the peripheral nervous system, which is outside the central nervous system (CNS); the brain and spinal cord. It supplies smooth muscle and glands and influences the function of our internal organs.

Most of the action that goes on in the body is unconscious. The ANS is regulated by integrated reflexes through the brainstem to the spinal cord, and out to organs that are constantly communicating with the CNS. It comprises sympathetic and parasympathetic branches but also the enteric nervous system (ENS), often referred to as the second brain, housed in the gut wall (page 196).

Figure 2a shows the ANS, which responds to our limbic system, the 'emo-tional centre' of the brain, and behaviour and motivation that comes from our emotional landscape. Much of that is from unconscious drivers, the buried long-term memory stuff and associations laid down for future survival. It is also prompted by olfaction (smell), which is why we have such profound asso-ciations with aromas. However, we are visually dominant creatures, so what comes in through our eyes has a massive (and often overriding) effect on the

---

1   Slavich (2016).

ANS and is emotionally subjective – we view and remember things differently, according to our mood and how safe we felt.

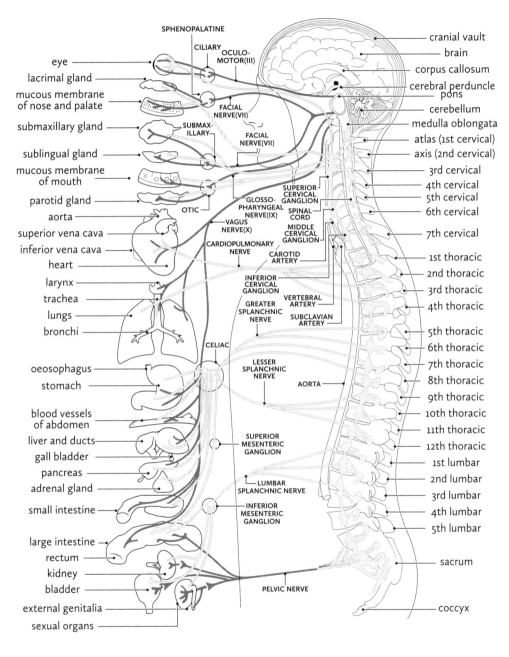

eye
lacrimal gland
mucous membrane of nose and palate
submaxillary gland
sublingual gland
mucous membrane of mouth
parotid gland
aorta
superior vena cava
inferior vena cava
heart
larynx
trachea
lungs
bronchi
oeosophagus
stomach
blood vessels of abdomen
liver and ducts
gall bladder
pancreas
adrenal gland
small intestine
large intestine
rectum
kidney
bladder
external genitalia
sexual organs

SPHENOPALATINE
CILIARY
OCULO-MOTOR(III)
FACIAL NERVE(VII)
SUBMAX-ILLARY
FACIAL NERVE(VII)
OTIC
SUPERIOR CERVICAL GANGLION
GLOSSO-PHARYNGEAL NERVE(IX)
VAGUS NERVE(X)
SPINAL CORD
MIDDLE CERVICAL GANGLION
CARDIOPULMONARY NERVE
CAROTID ARTERY
INFERIOR CERVICAL GANGLION
VERTEBRAL ARTERY
GREATER SPLANCHNIC NERVE
SUBCLAVIAN ARTERY
CELIAC
LESSER SPLANCHNIC NERVE
AORTA
SUPERIOR MESENTERIC GANGLION
LUMBAR SPLANCHNIC NERVE
INFERIOR MESENTERIC GANGLION
PELVIC NERVE

cranial vault
brain
corpus callosum
cerebral perduncle
pons
cerebellum
medulla oblongata
atlas (1st cervical)
axis (2nd cervical)
3rd cervical
4th cervical
5th cervical
6th cervical
7th cervical
1st thoracic
2nd thoracic
3rd thoracic
4th thoracic
5th thoracic
6th thoracic
7th thoracic
8th thoracic
9th thoracic
10th thoracic
11th thoracic
12th thoracic
1st lumbar
2nd lumbar
3rd lumbar
4th lumbar
5th lumbar
sacrum
coccyx

PARASYMPATHETIC  SYMPATHETIC

FIGURE 2A. AUTONOMIC NERVOUS SYSTEM (ANS)

The nerves marked in light grey in Figure 2a are the sympathetic fibres; they are more active, mobilising fight-or-flight. They connect to the spinal cord, so are more related to the hypothalamus–pituitary–adrenal (HPA) axis down the HPA line. The parasympathetic fibres (in darker grey) are associated with cranial nerves, including the vagus nerve – this is our more ancient, visceral response, including the freeze response – and from the spinal cord down into the intestines, kidneys, bladder and the sexual organs. This can be quickly influenced by sympathetic behaviour.

The ANS runs in the background, self-regulating us in relation to our external and internal landscapes. Any idea that mind and body are separated is completely overridden by the fact that the ANS is highly responsive to our emotional state. In the words of Bessel van der Kolk: 'You begin to experiment with changing the way you feel. Simply noticing what you feel fosters emotional regulation, and it helps you to stop trying to ignore what is going on inside you. Once you start approaching your body with curiosity rather than fear, everything shifts. Body awareness also changes your sense of time.'[2]

Functions of the ANS
The ANS regulates:

- Digestion
- Blood pressure
- Heart rate
- Urination and defecation
- Pupillary response
- Breathing (respiratory) rate
- Sexual response
- Body temperature
- Metabolism
- Electrolyte balance
- Production of body fluids including sweat and saliva
- Emotional responses

What is not always mentioned in terms of ANS function is the immune component: 'Neurotransmitters released by sympathetic and parasympathetic nerve

---

2   van der Kolk (2015).

endings bind to their respective receptors located on the surface of immune cells and initiate immune-modulatory responses.'[3]

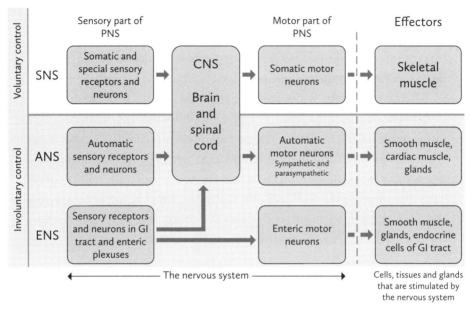

FIGURE 2B. BRANCHES OF THE NERVOUS SYSTEM
Source: This illustration first appeared in Yoga Therapy for Digestive Health *by Charlotte Watts*

The ANS has a continual effect on the appropriate/inappropriate regulatory immune landscape, that is, the balance between not too much and not too little, where we find the equilibrium we call health.

Figure 2b shows a scheme of the nervous system: the bottom two-thirds in the light grey background is the stuff of involuntary control and the unconscious, separate to the brain and spinal cord and from the ENS. The top third is voluntarily controlled. The 'SNS' here is the somatic nervous system rather than the sympathetic nervous system, that of soma, body, of movement – more voluntary. This is influenced by our unconscious drivers, our gestures and our body language, out of our remit of awareness or control.

THE SOMATIC NERVOUS SYSTEM

How we move, express and reach out into the world is in the hands of our somatic nervous system. It is part of the peripheral nervous system,

3   Kenney and Ganta (2014).

which is basically everything outside of the brain and spinal cord, our central nervous system (CNS). Specifically, the somatic nervous system is responsible for how we can affect the muscles in a voluntary way, that is, we can be conscious this is happening, move as we need and choose in a process known as a reflex arc. There is constant communication through nerve impulses between the CNS and out via the peripheral nervous system to skeletal muscles, fascia, skin and sensory organs.

The primary role of the somatic nervous system is to connect the CNS to the organs, muscles and skin. This allows us to perform complex movements and behaviours. The somatic neurons carry messages from the outer areas of the body having to do with the senses. It is like a passageway from the environment to the CNS. Sensory/afferent neurons carry the impulses to the CNS and the brain. After being processed by the CNS, the somatic motor or efferent neurons take the signal back to the muscles and sensory organs.

The sympathetic nervous system (SNS)

The SNS is governed by hormones – adrenaline (aka epinephrine) and cortisol – which tend to be referred to as 'stress hormones' and are more inflammatory in nature. When something stressful is sensed, hormones immediately send a cascade down from the brain to the adrenal glands through a route called the HPA (hypothalamic–pituitary–adrenal) axis, to release stress hormones, increasing our heart rate and sending blood coursing around our muscles ready for effective physical reaction.

Adrenaline is a protein-based hormone produced for instant effect, which we only need and produce at moments of excitement, motivation, activity, threat or perceived danger. Adrenaline is such rocket fuel (with the potential to damage tissues and DNA) that if the stimulus for stress goes on past around an hour, cortisol takes over to keep up the response as a less intense solution.

Cortisol is a long-term, steroid-based (fat) hormone. We need steroid hormones in the blood at all times, as they regulate metabolism, immunity and wake/sleep cycles. Cortisol is what gets us up in the morning, what motivates us – ideally within the active parts of our circadian rhythm.

The adrenal glands also produce noradrenaline (aka norepinephrine), which is also a mood and motivation neurotransmitter or brain chemical. It works with other neurotransmitters, for example with serotonin, to influence mental behaviour patterns, while dopamine is involved in movement – going through with an action.

The SNS used to be called 'excitory' but it has the opposite effect in the guts and sexual regions, where it enervates and dampens down action. We need to be in parasympathetic states for digestion or for sexual arousal to occur. The SNS is our quick-response, mobilising system; it gets us going and creates motivation, excitement and vigilance. It is known as the fight-or-flight response – standing our ground or running away. We'll talk about that more in terms of polyvagal theory[4] and the vagus nerve in Part 3.

This response (in balance with the parasympathetic) is important and healthy: fast, effective, motivated and directed, with a purpose and clarity that can come with reactivity, impulsiveness and judgemental behaviours, which are vital when we need to make quick decisions within a survival situation. However, when much of our modern stressors are emotional and psychological, this full-body response can be more than the situation requires, and leave us struggling to come down again, or left in agitation, irritability and anxiety.

It is when nervous system states are not balanced, when the SNS dominates and we are running on constant alert, fear or worry, that there is a negative impact on other body systems. In terms of yoga theory, sympathetic dominance has the *rajasic guna* (page 274) quality of irritability, aggression, intolerance, even addiction, and more compulsive behaviours. We have less impulse control and become hypervigilant, where the nervous system is upregulated into constant fear-based mind states and survival mode.

Neither the parasympathetic nor sympathetic nervous systems are good or bad; we need them in balance and to be acting appropriately, to be able to move and to rest. The same applies to inflammation (part of the SNS response) – it is neither good nor bad; it is when it gets stuck 'on' that problems arise, which we will discuss later.

The phrenic nerve

The phrenic nerve (*phren* is Greek for 'diaphragm') is the main nerve of the respiratory system and can be associated to some extent with the SNS, with the vagus the main nerve of the parasympathetic nervous system (PNS). The phrenic nerve runs between the neck and the diaphragm, with two branches that pass through the heart and lungs. It passes motor information to the diaphragm and receives sensory information from it, regulating breathing.

---

4   Porges (2009).

Without a functioning phrenic nerve, there is no breath, no life. Medical students might learn this rhyme: 'C3, C4, C5, keeps the diaphragm alive', as the phrenic nerve connects to the cervical spine, the neck. In the words of researchers Sohaib Mandoorah and Therese Mead: 'The phrenic nerve is among the most important nerves in the body due to its role in respiration. The phrenic nerve provides the primary motor supply to the diaphragm, the major respiratory muscle.'[5]

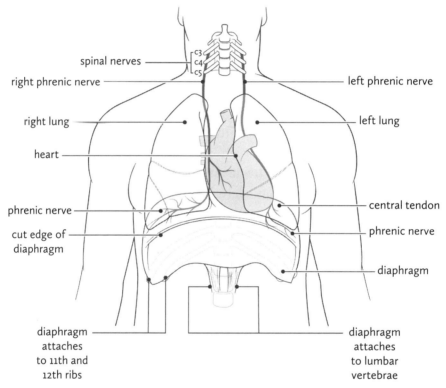

FIGURE 2C. PULMONARY CENTRES

The stress response

Stress in and of itself is not a judgement; it is simply a provocation to challenge, a call to act or react. It is 'doing' as opposed to 'not doing'. It is how we come down after that suggests whether it is unhealthy or helpful. Do we experience constant stress responses, and if so do we have the requisite recovery afterwards? Can we balance the motivational, doing drive with a sense of ease? A good example is in *virabhadrasana II* (warrior II pose) where we have

---

5   Mandoorah and Mead (2021).

strength in the legs but are easeful in the upper body: steadiness with ease, *shtira-sukha-asanam*.[6] This posture offers a potentially good stress (eustress), challenging with weight bearing on the front knee. We need some stress as a challenge, but not too much, otherwise it becomes wearing and can keep us in inflammatory states.

Secondary (thoracic) breathing

When we're stressed or the diaphragm can't move fully, our breath moves to the upper chest and shoulders, which can mimic and set off the fight-or-flight response. Poor movement in the diaphragm gives us the signal that we need to stay in a stress response, creating a vicious cycle when the diaphragm becomes less mobile and the breath moves into the upper chest and the shoulders, where they can get stuck in sensory motor amnesia (page 53). People who are in heightened stress response states can tend to have tight shoulders held up to the ears and carry tension up into the jaw and the base of the skull insertions, related to headaches and neck, upper back and lower back pain. This is why 'soft eyes and jaw' is a key instruction in practice to bring awareness to these areas and begin the processing of unravelling habitual tension.

In this vital survival response, we need quicker, shallow breaths for quick oxygenation to the brain, our main organ of survival. We need to have that mental currency, to have our senses online and acute, which is why, when we stay up in sympathetic mode, we can get overwhelmed by sensory overload, as noise, light and even touch sensitivity. Getting stuck in that pattern uses up a huge amount of energy – through inefficient breathing and holding physical tension. This can be related to jaw clenching – bruxism (teeth grinding) – another common place for sensory motor amnesia, related to secondary breathing holding patterns, sometimes with accompanying cramps.[7,8]

This can create forced rather than easeful exhalation (Figure 2d), where the internal intercostals and abdominal muscles get co-opted in to compensate for lack of diaphragmatic movement, which is more energetically tiring. This can also evolve from overdoing *uddhiyana bandha* (upward flying lock), when the abdominal muscles are held in tension, because the belly can't move easily enough with the breath, so the exhalation becomes forced, and that that feeds into the pattern of the whole being held in secondary breathing.

---

6   Bryant (2009, *Yoga Sutra* 2.46).
7   Hanna (2004).
8   Peterson (2015).

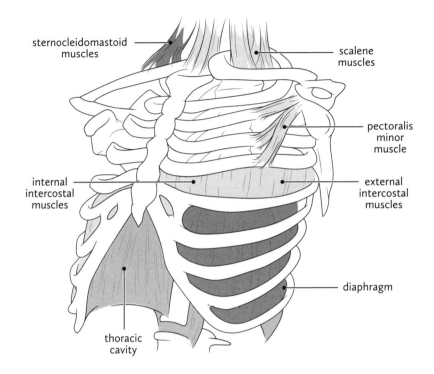

Principal inspiration
diaphragm
external intercostal muscles

Forced inhalation
sternocleidomastoid muscles
pectoralis minor muscles
scalene muscles

Forced exhalation
abdominal muscles
internal intercostal muscles

FIGURE 2D. MUSCLES OF FORCED BREATHING

The parasympathetic nervous system (PNS)

The PNS is the opposing opposite branch of the ANS, which brings us down from the sympathetic. It is anti-inflammatory and drops us down from a heightened survival response, so the immune system doesn't need to be on high alert. It is governed by the neurotransmitter acetylcholine, one of our main memory neurotransmitters – one of many reasons why memory issues are often part of stress-related conditions. The PNS takes marginally longer to work than the adrenal hormones and used to be referred to as inhibitory because it puts the brakes on, dampening down heightened responses, but again, that's not absolute as it innervates gut action and sexual arousal. It is often referred to as a more slowly activating dampening system, but the 'slowly' is relative to the SNS. Prolonged survival modes can also create slower stress responses.

Also known as 'rest and digest' or the less poetic 'feed and breed', the PNS is where we detoxify, heal, build things up. This is when our ancestors would have been able to stop, have a meal and procreate. It is where we can be open-minded; see more sides of a story or an argument. It is more spacious internally, more relaxing, and the quality is that of deeper consciousness and awareness.

Again, we need balance. Where it is really good to drop into relaxed states, we don't get much done, it doesn't get us up in the morning or motivate us. Too much can leave us *tamasic*, dull and lacklustre (page 274). If we are continually caught in sympathetic states, we can drop over into 'adrenal fatigue' and even experience 'leisure sickness' – where we go on holiday and stress hormones suddenly drop and there is a flood of cytokines (signalling molecules that regulate immunity and inflammation; page 88), resulting in low-grade flu symptoms. This is when the body shuts down as a reaction to doing, doing, doing, so that the immune system can get on with healing. Habitual patterns of doing loads by day before crashing in the evening (without the parasympathetic balance of something like yoga, breath practices or the conscious relaxation of going for a walk or a bath, etc.) is not a sustainable plan and the body will eventually force the issue and tip over into crash or burnout.

The relaxation response

This is the opposite tone to the stress response, a generalised reduction in both cognitive and somatic arousal. Coming down from arousal – that is, calming the mind and body – is to modify and regulate activity of the HPA axis (the hypothalamus in the limbic system, pituitary and the adrenal axis) and the ANS. In early yoga research on its effects on the ANS, Basu Bagchi says: 'Physiologically, yogic meditation represents deep relaxation of the autonomic nervous system without drowsiness or sleep.'[9] Ideally the relaxation response is not a crash; rather, it has an awareness and clarity. Meditation is a different experience to flopping on the sofa.

---

9   Wenger, Bagchi and Anand (1961).

Primary (diaphragmatic) breathing

Within the ANS, primary breathing is most efficient, using the diaphragm with an easy exchange of filling and emptying the lungs, chest and belly expanding, diaphragm moving downwards to inhale, rising back up without co-opting any muscles to do it as the chest drops to exhale. Lying down, as in constructive rest position (CRP; page 55), is really useful to be able to notice that rhythm. It is the most energy-efficient oxygenating breath and the least stressful for the muscular system, using up the least energy.

Sympathetic dominance

Sympathetic dominance is a term used in naturopathy or functional medicine. It keeps our inflammatory responses up as part of survival: injury or infection are the most dangerous threats for a wild animal (our primal setting), and inflammation seals a wound to stop us bleeding out or brings immune components to the site.

Sympathetic dominance is often kept up even in a low-grade way, with this 'constant alert' a most usual state. We may have spent a lifetime this way if we grew up without feelings of safety – this is then the experience of 'normal' and can take time and embodiment for rest states to feel familiar and safe.

We might experience this upregulation of the SNS in the skin or joints, the fascia, as pain, in the digestive tract or the reproductive tissues as endometriosis...anywhere in the body. When stress influences our inflammatory survival tones, it also lowers our existing resistance to other infection, particular stresses which are chronic or long-term, and we tend to go into either inflammatory or fighting off disease mode. The mind-body expects to come down from the stress response and rest overnight in a parasympathetic state (where we can heal and recover), but that can often be pushed aside and we get stuck in an inflammatory loop when we tend towards sympathetic dominance.

Cytokines are immune messengers that set off the inflammatory cascade and keep that alert going when we're in sympathetic dominance. We've seen cytokine storms within the COVID-19 pandemic (page 103): those who have the worst symptoms or even die tend to be those who have the most inflammatory responses, where the body is not able to drop down into anti-inflammatory tone, but moves into 'hyperinflammation.'[10]

---

10   Gustine and Jones (2021).

Mitochondria

Survival functions are mediated by mitochondria – organelles within cells that convert energy from food and oxygen into cellular energy (ATP (adenosine triphosphate)), in order to regulate cellular respiration, inflammation, immunity, hormone production and cellular life and death. These mitochondrial responses require energy, so where an illness or infection persists without replenishment, the original problems may persist, cascading to increased inflammation and immune reactivity.[11]

Mitochondria enact the survival mechanism 'cell danger response' (CDR), which has three stages:

1. Active inflammatory/immune response: detecting and removing intruders and toxins, damage control and containment with inflammation. This diversion of energy is why we often experience fatigue at the beginning of an illness.
2. Repair: replacing dead or damaged cells, containing damaged tissue, recruiting stem cells to heal.
3. Reform: cell differentiation and tissue remodelling, detoxification, cueing adaptive immune responses and metabolic memory, sensory and pain modulation and sleep tuning.

When this cycle of healing is complete, cell-to-cell communication reinstates. The process is linear, sequential and ATP-intensive (requiring a continuous supply of energy), so if a secondary infection occurs during the process, it can be derailed. Mitochondrial metabolism is at the root cause of persistent disease, where the availability of energy hinders the body's ability to progress through healing cycles. Certain vitamins (C and B), minerals (such as magnesium and iron) and the antioxidant nutrient co-enzyme Q10, and exercise – along with low stress – are crucial for healthy mitochondria.[12,13,14]

This is crucial for immune rejuvenation (page 91); Dr Mark Hyman states:

The best example (of rejuvenation) involves mitochondria. These are cell components where energy is processed and stored. But energy isn't easy to handle – think of electricity – and mitochondria can age rapidly from this wear

---

11   Bratic and Aleksandra (2010).
12   Sweet and Zastre (2013).
13   Hood (2009).
14   Monda *et al.* (2017).

and tear. This brings us to mitophagy, a rejuvenation process for renewing damaged mitochondria...[15],[16] Optimal immunity takes expert coordination of energy production, so this is a big deal.[17]

Inflammation response

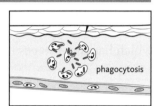

ONE OF THE FIRST RESPONSES	STIMULATED BY CHEMICAL FACTORS RELEASED BY INJURED CELLS	
Macrophages and mast cells release chemical signals such as histamine.	Local inflammatory response: capillaries widen. Fluid containing antimicrobial proteins enter the tissue. More phagocytes invade the site.	Phagocytic cells digest pathogens, and the tissue heals.

SYMPTOMS

redness, heat, swelling, pain and possible
dysfunction of the organs or tissues involved

FIGURE 2E. INFLAMMATION

Inflammation is one of our first, most ancient responses, part of our innate immunity (page 27). It is stimulated by chemical factors released by injured cells. Most well known of these is maybe the hormone histamine, which increases the permeability of capillaries to white blood cells and some proteins, allowing them to engage pathogens in infected tissues. Histamine is also an excitory neurotransmitter that keeps us alert and active, which is why increased inflammation, and especially chronic low-grade inflammation, is associated with anxious and depression states. Those with inflammatory (atopic) conditions – such as asthma, eczema, hay fever, migraines, arthritis and psoriasis – can experience the racing mind, worry and hypervigilance that reflect the histaminic, fear-based nature of the fight-or-flight response.

When we are injured, inflammation involves bringing large molecules like macrophages and mast cells (page 32) to wound sites. This response helps to

---

15 Xu, Shen and Ran (2020).
16 Gkikas, Palikaras and Tavernarakis (2018).
17 Hyman (2021).

stop bacteria entering through the skin into the bloodstream as well as sealing up the wound, with redness, heat and swelling. In Ayurveda, this is the *dosha pitta* – 'that which cooks' (page 276) – heated, irritable, with an element of fire.

Growth or protection – thrive or survive

Key to understanding our system organisation is that we can be either in growth or protection state. In parasympathetic mode, we are building back up again, in an anabolic state of healing, repairing tissues that have been torn down in exercising muscle, for instance, or replenishing immune components. In sympathetic dominance, we are primed for survival, in a catabolic state of breaking things down. We cannot be in both simultaneously. We need to consciously come down from doing to be able to restore and thrive. When we consciously notice the states and habits where we are caught in excitory states, we access our body and mind's inherent default towards recovery, the energy conservation that is so important in the wild.

Immuno-rejuvenation in relation to COVID-19

Dr Jeff Bland (founder of the Functional Medicine model) calls the damage that accumulates in our immune system as we age 'immuno-senescence' – old, tired 'zombie' cells drag us down into dysfunction and disease. Its opposite is 'immuno-rejuvenation' – where instead of blindly boosting a damaged immune system (exaggerating defects), rejuvenation uses our built-in programming to rebalance and reboot the system's optimal function – a more foundational and longer lasting solution. As we've explored, 'boosting immunity' is a problematic phrase anyway, as immune issues are so often around poor modulation (page 26), with some parts stuck on over-reaction, especially inflammation.

Dr Bland's colleague, Dr Mark Hyman, states:

> Modern immune systems face unprecedented challenges, like accumulated toxins in the environment, calorie-rich diets that provide little nutrition, and global sharing of microbes, to name just a few.[18] Repeated exposure to stressors like these can skew immune function, creating an imbalance between our immune systems' core capabilities to play offense and defense. Over time, this can set the stage for inflammation, susceptibility to infection, hypersensitivities, and other signs of immune imbalance.[19]

---

18 Haahtela (2019).
19 Hyman (2021).

These epigenetic factors – those factors within our lifetimes that affect our gene expression (also including psycho-social stress and trauma) – are those we can affect and that are constantly influencing our immune cells. These turn over fast, so as Hyman says, 'we can essentially build an entirely new immune system every few months', the question he puts being: 'would you rather recreate the old one, or build a better one?'[20]

This is in line with the work of the Human Cell Atlas initiative, whose mission is to create comprehensive reference maps of all human cells – the fundamental units of life – as a basis for both understanding human health and diagnosing, monitoring and treating disease. Their work on a scientific understanding of SARS-CoV-2 and COVID-19[21] (as reported in the *Integrated Healthcare & Applied Nutrition* magazine[22]) has included comparing people showing COVID-19 with no symptoms and those with more serious reactions, who had raised levels of immune cells, monocytes and killer T cells (page 32) – in those hospitalised, these were at the uncontrolled levels that lead to lung inflammation. In those with no symptoms, they found increased levels of B cells (that produce antibodies), found in mucus passages such as the nose, missing in those with serious symptoms. Those with mild to moderate symptoms had high levels of B cells and helper T cells (that fight infection), the part of the immune system that failed in those with severe disease. Boosting imbalanced or poorly trained immune cells will only amplify immune dysfunction.[23]

Immuno-rejuvenation is our bodies' natural system of refreshing immune cells for optimal immune function. Rejuvenation only happens when you let it, when dropping stress hormones allows this growth potential – eating well, staying active (that is, not sedentary), supporting resilience with 'good stress' (eustress; pages 101 and 155) and getting the rest we need to optimise rejuvenation capacity – quality sleep and conscious relaxation (such as restorative practice; see Part 5).

Adding in an epidemic of mouth-breathing tendencies (page 168) as a key epigenetic factor, as cited in an article titled 'Lessons learned with long-COVID', focus on the breath regulation is now seen within many therapies as the key place to regulate the nervous system, activate that vagus nerve and

---

20 Hyman (2021).
21 www.humancellatlas.org/covid-19
22 Wellcome Trust Sanger Institute (2021). Original study: Stephenson *et al.* (2021).
23 Gruver, Hudson and Sempowski (2007).

alter 'stress chemistry'. As the author put it: 'On a very basic survival level, if you can't breathe, how is your body meant to know it is safe to heal?'[24]

So appropriate to this balance is *Yogas citta-vrtti-nirodhah*, translated as 'yoga is the stilling of the changing states of the mind'.[25] This is referring to hypervigilance, to the rumination, to the main states of tensity prevalent when we are in sympathetic, fear-based responses. Even if that doesn't feel like heightened anxiety, it can manifest when we are at the whim of the mind running the show and not able to drop into more reflective states – 'racing mind'. Another translation is: 'Yoga is the control of the modifications of the mind field. Then the seer rests in its very true nature.'[26] So, for instance, when we clamp the jaw or hold the diaphragm, these are feeding into *granthi*, or knots (page 153), which can be translated as doubts in the mind, where we tend to hold energy from habitual mind states we loop around.

In Ayurveda, this is related to *vata* dominance (page 276), where the whirlwind energy of the mind cannot drop down to allow energy into the heart or the belly and feel a sense of compassion, cut off from interoception as thoughts dominate. Many people hold themselves in this state because they don't want to feel what's going on below; meeting our essence nature or the unconscious down into the belly is the more difficult stuff of vulnerability.

The vayus in balance

This also relates to the *vayus*, or vital winds in yoga: *prana* and *apana* (see more on page 285). These are examples of polarities – things we may view as opposite but that are actually both necessary parts of the cycle that cannot exist with each other – neither is better or worse, right or wrong. We cannot have up without down, stress without relaxation (yin without yang) – we need both, and we need them in balance, which is the yogic path.

Prana (with a small 'p' rather than *Prana* as life force) and *apana* are in this constant polarity cycle within our body (and all *koshas*; page 150). *Prana* lifts up the front of the body, force rising up from the ground, where *apana* drops us back down to gravity, earths us, releasing. *Apana* is related to the moon and the feet, where *prana* correlates to the sun, stimulated by standing. Our society is over-stimulating; we so often need the regulatory cooling of the moon, which is why *chandra bhedana pranayama* (moon-piercing breath practice) is included on page 131.

---

24 Sehinson (2021).
25 Bryant (2009).
26 Swami Rama, quoted in Bharati (no date).

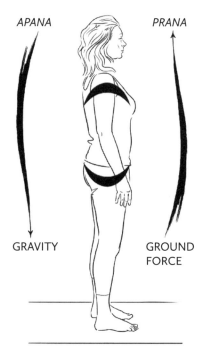

FIGURE 2F. THE POLARITY OF *PRANA* AND *APANA VAYUS*
Source: This illustration appeared in Yoga Therapy for Digestive Health *by Charlotte Watts*

The breath as immune regulator

Our respiratory centre, which regulates breathing, is in the old, primal parts of the brainstem (medulla and pons). It receives input from chemoreceptors, chemical signalling throughout the body, as well as mechanoreceptors, responsive to whether we are in active stress states or passive, where we need to metabolise at a different rate, or where we are holding ourselves in patterns. Contracting our shoulders, for example, keeps us at a higher breath rate.

The input of the respiratory centre is stimulated from different actions:

- *Involuntary/unconscious*, from altered levels of oxygen (O_2), carbon dioxide (CO_2) and blood pH, which is constantly buffering for our acid/alkaline levels in the body. These need to be slightly alkaline (apart from very acidic stomach acid), so that enzymes work most efficiently. So O_2 and CO_2 balance kidney function and mineral exchanges are all working to regulate homeostasis, stable blood pH. This is also related to hormonal changes that are in constant communication with stress levels – what's excitory, where we can come down from that, and in response to strong emotions like anxiety or pain. This all registers through the ANS, and the part of the brain that tracks what is happening in the respiratory centre ends up at the ANS; they are constantly feeding into each other.

- *Voluntary/conscious*, where we get involved in our breath within our ANS expression. It didn't used to be believed this self-control was possible until studies on yogis from the 1920s to 1960s (measuring the brainwaves of meditators) revealed that conscious breath practices could change the qualities, expressions, the rates of breathing and the ANS signalling through the cerebral cortex.

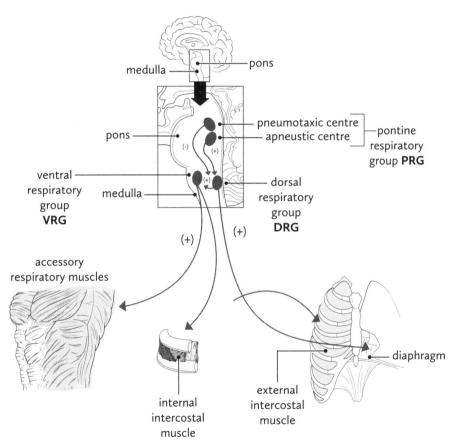

FIGURE 2G. RESPIRATORY CENTRES OF THE BRAIN

Oxygen as life force

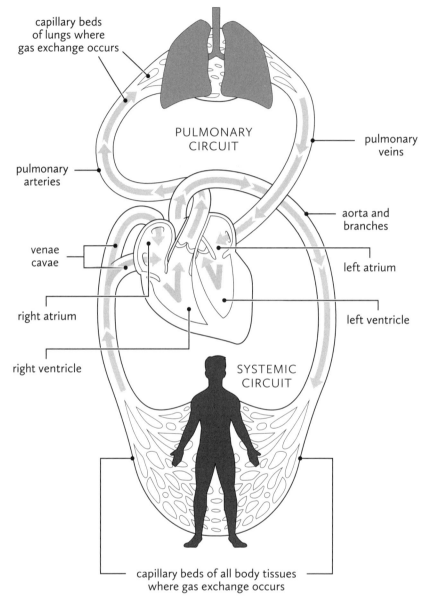

capillary beds
of lungs where
gas exchange occurs

PULMONARY
CIRCUIT

pulmonary
veins

pulmonary
arteries

aorta and
branches

venae
cavae

left atrium

right atrium

left ventricle

right ventricle

SYSTEMIC
CIRCUIT

capillary beds of all body tissues
where gas exchange occurs

FIGURE 2H. PULMONARY SYSTEMIC CIRCUITS

Oxygen is our vital energy, one aspect of *Prana*, life force. The human body comprises about two-thirds O_2, incorporated into things such as carbohydrates, our organic chemistry. The end-product of O_2 being brought in from the lungs to the heart and sent to all cells where it is incorporated into haem, haemoglobin (making the red colour of blood), is cell respiration. This is O_2 coming to all cells and burning off the energy in our power stations, mitochondria (page 89), the by-products of which are CO_2 and water.

Yoga practices affect the efficiency of oxygen coming in, slowing down our metabolic rate, which is beneficial when we relate to the body's ability to rest and heal. *Pranayama* (yogic breath consciousness; page 307) is associated with longevity, giving us more time to resolve our *samskaras* (habits; pages 153 and 279). Where we are running at a high level, caught in sympathetic responses, the heartbeat is raised and we metabolise faster, creating more CO_2 and by-products in respiration as well as using up more nutrients. This is why sighing out is such a regulatory natural process for ANS regulation – it blows off excess CO_2 that can build up from stress, as well as a vibratory release.

Carbon dioxide controls breathing

Even though we don't want too much, this doesn't mean that CO_2 is not simply bad or a 'waste product' as it used to be referred to. This would be like saying *apana* is releasing stagnant energy, which it does, but it's also an important part of elimination, moving things through. Our holding of CO_2 in the body, our tolerance of it – where we pause at the top of the inhalation – is an important part of our relationship with O_2. When CO_2 reaches a certain level in the body at the end of the exhale, a signal is sent to the brainstem, to the breathing muscles, triggering an inhalation. Exhaling CO_2 signals a new breathing cycle, the space for the new to enter. CO_2 is produced in every cell, every nanosecond, and we exhale the build-up. The more active we are, or the more stress we experience, the more CO_2 is produced, working the nervous system more, making the heart pump faster. We breathe more and faster in sympathetic tone and the O_2/CO_2 balance can be disrupted.

Holding CO_2 consciously into the body actually allows it to have beneficial effects:

- Anti-bacterial: a Swedish study[27] showed that growth of the Staphylococcus bacteria was 1000 times higher when exposed to normal air for 24 hours compared with exposure to air saturated with CO_2.
- Increased oxygenation: we need CO_2 to use air – the Bohr effect, where CO_2 forces oxygen to leave the blood to enter muscles and cells for utilisation and prompts our ability to oxygenate.
- Widens smooth muscles: vasodilation, a widening and relaxing effect

---

27 Persson *et al.* (2005).

on smooth muscle – the muscles in the intestines, bladder, womb, etc. – can't be controlled consciously.

James Nestor cites various conscious breath-holding practices and therapies where CO_2 is purposefully inhaled as beneficial for symptoms as broad ranging as anxiety, pneumonia, asthma and epilepsy, rebalancing chemoreceptors.[28]

Normal breathing, within healthy parameters, which would be measured after about 7 to 15 minutes of not doing or being active, is about 8 to 12 breaths a minute. Over-breathing is like a low-grade form of hyperventilation, which is more like 18 to 25 breaths a minute. This upsets the O_2 and CO_2 balance, and we end up with too much O_2 in the body but also exhaling too much CO_2 because the system is swamped.

Balanced immune system

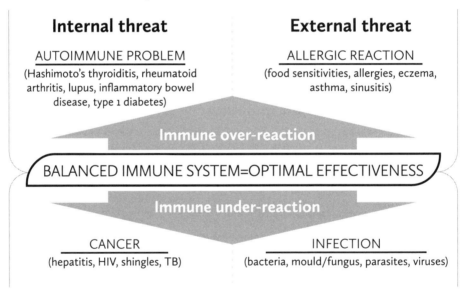

FIGURE 21. BALANCED IMMUNE SYSTEM

The immune system relies on a balance between parasympathetic and sympathetic for an appropriate response in immune modulation. Put very simply, too much and we are caught in the over-reaction of sympathetic dominance; too little and we struggle to deal with bacterial or viral loads – for example, HIV, shingles, coronaviruses – and they can hang around unchallenged.

28 Nestor (2020).

We are constantly exposed to bacteria, mould, fungus, parasites and viruses – these are part of our internal landscape. Constant adaptation to their presence and mutations is a key part of our immune behaviour and depends on the health of our innate immunity. Severity of symptoms to pathogenic variants of these can depend if we're meeting something for the first time, where the response is going to be higher than where we have memory of it (acquired immunity) and the reaction will be less. It is part of a healthy response to have some kind of symptomology showing an immune response, but that is resolved rather than persists. Under-reaction can mean that we can't hold back the invasion and a call to attend to our innate immunity (and microbiome; page 208) and stress levels.

Over-reactivity can show up as allergic reaction, food sensitivity or intolerance, or atopic conditions such as eczema, asthma, sinusitis, dermatitis and rhinitis – '-itis' at the end of a word describes inflammation there. This is often a body region in English or Latin – for example, 'derma' means skin, 'rhino' is nose and pleuritis is another term for pleurisy, inflammation of the tissue between the lungs and rib cage (pleura).

Constant (inappropriate) reaction to things that aren't life threatening keeps us in unresolved loops. In autoimmune conditions, our immune system attacks our own body, as we are not able to recognise self from not-self – for example, type 1 diabetes attacking cells in the pancreas, or inflammatory bowel disease attacking parts of the colon. In Part 4, we explore the role the microbiome has in determining appropriate immune response and signalling from the gut wall, a key factor in autoimmunity.

Incidence of suffering from some kind of atopic (inflammatory) disease such as atopic dermatitis, allergic asthma, hay fever or food allergy is shown to 'have reached epidemic proportions during the past decades in industrialized and, more recently, in developing countries'.[29] Poor-quality nutrition, physical inactivity, psychological stress, trauma and circadian disruption (from jet lag, shift work or artificial light) are known to influence the development of and progression of atopic disease. Some (like allergic conditions, including rhinitis) involve response to bacteria and viruses, but it is healthy innate immunity that determines how we respond to these. Exploring these factors as well as any measures to reduce infection or exposure are key to reducing such conditions. Improving circadian rhythms by altering light/dark exposure (timing and type

---

29   Thomsen (2015).

of light), meal and exercise timing, and work schedules could emerge as important in atopic disease remedy.[30,31]

The sedentary nature of modern life is a major environment–gene interaction that also increases risk of chronic disease.[32] Exercise offers potent
anti-inflammatory effects and modulation of gut microbiome–host immune
interactions.[33] Intervention studies in asthmatic children and adults have
been shown to benefit atopic conditions (with both total and allergen-specific
immune antibody levels) to improve respiratory function and enhance disease
control and quality of life.[34,35]

Chronic inflammation

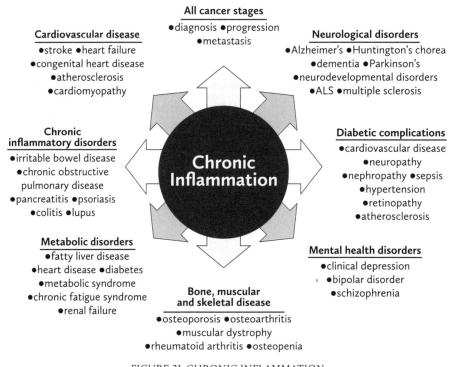

FIGURE 2J. CHRONIC INFLAMMATION

Chronic inflammation can be a massive part of inappropriate responses, at the

---

30   Roenneberg and Merrow (2016).
31   Nakao (2020).
32   Ruegsegger and Booth (2018).
33   Mendes *et al.* (2011).
34   Wanrooij *et al.* (2014).
35   Eichenberger *et al.* (2013).

heart of what we now call 'diseases of Western civilisation', including hypertension, diabetes, cancer, stroke, kidney disease and cognitive impairment. Conditions such as osteoporosis have a low-grade inflammatory component – here, impairing the regeneration of bone. We cannot be in rest and survival mode at the same time, so if in sympathetic dominance, healing is compromised. Bone is a matrix that is alive; it needs constant regeneration, which is signalled by the 'good' stress (eustress) of weight-bearing exercise. Being in the eustress of contact with nature (physical demands, the elements, cold, some discomfort, natural fasting) has a regulatory effect on all of our body systems, including our immune and respiratory systems; it is how we evolved.[36]

Anxiety and stress can be the result of separation with nature and they impact significantly on inflammatory responses: 'Psychological stress is reported to modulate cytokine production, suggesting potential relevance of this mediator to mental health. In fact, cytokine signalling in the brain is known to regulate important brain functions including neurotransmitter metabolism, neuroendocrine function, synaptic plasticity, as well as the neural circuitry of mood.'[37]

> Yoga (as mind-body therapy) has shown through many studies to be effective at reducing inflammatory cytokines, through (as one review of the literature states) "the resulting alterations in neuroendocrine, neural and psychological and behavioural processes".[38]

Yoga to cool inflammation

Inflammation is an urgent overheating, so cooling (*langhana*) yoga practices have the capacity to soothe and reduce it via the nervous system. Modern life includes much psycho-social stress, leading to intolerance, irritability and fear-based reactivity. Practices that stoke fires (*brahmana*, heating), that encourage *agni* (digestive fire), can be useful as we need that motivation of metabolic processes, but awareness of having just enough and not too much is vital.

Part of encouraging self-regulation is the ability to recognise and interocept when we feel heated, when we feel busy around the head, tight in the temples, the heartbeat rises or the breath quickens. Then, when we need cooling, we can respond by consciously fostering the soothing parasympathetic response,

---

36 Pruimboom and Muskiet (2018).
37 Salim, Chugh and Asghar (2012).
38 Bower and Irwin (2016).

focusing on self-compassion and embodied awareness, where we register being in our body, an important part of being able to register safety. The brain can panic when it is not aware of where the body is in relation to the world around us, when we are not grounded.

A growing body of research clearly shows that yoga is effective at reducing inflammatory response, often determined by inflammatory cytokines as markers. Cytokines include a broad range of small proteins, produced by many cells that act as immunomodulating agents. They act through cell surface receptors, including on the epithelium (page 206), are producing body-wide and by immune cells.

RESEARCH ON YOGA AND CHRONIC OBSTRUCTIVE PULMONARY DISEASE (COPD)

An estimated 24 million Americans may have COPD, which includes chronic bronchitis, emphysema or both. Patients with COPD have trouble pushing used air out of their lungs, making it difficult to take in healthy new air. Although there is no cure for COPD, a patient's quality of life can be improved by controlling symptoms, such as shortness of breath. COPD, most commonly caused by cigarette smoking, affects both men and women, and often, symptoms are seen in people in their 40s.

'COPD is a systemic inflammatory disease that causes difficulty breathing,' said study presenter Randeep Guleria, MD, professor and head, Department of Pulmonary Medicine and Sleep Disorders. 'We investigated to see whether simple, structured yoga training affects the level of inflammation, shortness of breath, and quality of life in patients with stable COPD.'[39]

The study included 29 stable patients with COPD who received yoga training in a format that included the use of physical postures (*asanas*), breathing techniques (*pranayama*), cleansing techniques (*kriyas*), meditation and a relaxation technique (*savasana*, corpse pose) for one hour, twice a week, for four weeks. Following the four-week period, patients were trained for one hour every two weeks, with the remaining sessions completed at home. Patients were evaluated on

---

39   Quoted in American College of Chest Physicians (2013).

assessment of lung function, breathing, quality of life and inflammation status. All parameters showed significant improvement at the end of the 12-week period.

'We found that yoga can be a simple, cost-effective method that can help improve quality of life in patients with COPD,' stated Dr Guleria.

Inflammation cascade

Where pro-inflammatory cytokines are essential during the process of fighting off infection, severe inflammation can cause a cytokine cascade or storm, leading to multisystem organ failure and death, as we have seen in COVID-19 'hyperinflammation' (page 88). Because cytokines affect the microenvironment of nearby tissues and cells, they also create 'an optimal environment for tumorigenesis (tumor formation) and chronic inflammatory diseases'.[40] As a foreground to the COVID-19 pandemic, chronic inflammation has become a prevalent factor in Western civilisation.

Inflammation and ageing = inflammaging?

'Inflammaging', a contraction of inflammation and ageing, coined by Italian researcher Claudio Franceschi in 2000, refers to the low-grade chronic inflammation that characterises ageing. This process may partially explain why some older people become more ill with COVID-19. Beyond this pandemic, many refer to the creeping symptoms related to inflammation as a sign of ageing, as if they are inevitable, an example being acceptance of joint pain and loss of mobility: 'Ageing is often described as the progressive accumulation of deleterious changes over time leading to a loss of physiological aptitude and fertility, an increased susceptibility to disease, and ultimately to death.'[41]

While ageing is a process of degeneration, having an awareness of where we can engage in our regeneration capacity (and immuno-rejuvenation, page 91) also stems from where our body systems meet the stresses placed on them.

Geroscience, the science of ageing, considers the intertwining processes of disease. Four of the seven recognised factors of ageing also tie into processes of disease that push the balance of regeneration to degeneration (the natural cycle of life and death):

---

40 Cavaillon and Adib-Conquy (2002).
41 Tosato *et al.* (2007).

- *Decreased adaptation to stress* causing anxiety, overwhelm, sensory overload or other 'stress-related symptoms' such as fatigue, insomnia, irritability, depression, inflammatory conditions and weight gain (through increased appetite and the stress hormone cortisol that raises insulin and switches on fat storage).[42]

- *Epigenetic dysregulation*, where behaviours and environment change the way our genes express themselves.[43] For example, pathogens – from smoking to germs – can weaken our immune system. Epigenetics is a broader way of viewing how our gene expression is influenced by factors over our lifespan (and from that down the generations): stress, trauma, disease, lifestyle, exercise, diet, etc. 'Increasing evidence shows that epigenetic deregulation is a common mechanism in cancer.'[44]

- *Macromolecular damage.*[45] Macromolecules are large molecules, most commonly proteins, nucleic acids and carbohydrates. Neurodegenerative diseases, which have been linked to the oxidisation and aggregation of proteins, increase with age. Data also shows that macromolecular damage may be causative in ageing as damaged proteins can change the 'signalling in cells/tissues, which can alter cellular functions and appear to play a role in a variety of age-related diseases – e.g., cardiovascular disease, cancer, Parkinson's disease, and diabetes'.[46,47] This damage is from oxidative stress, which is an imbalance between free radicals (unstable, damaging molecules, for example in sunlight, fried foods, certain pesticides and cleaners, radiation, pollution, cigarette smoke) and antioxidants (immune-supporting compounds in food (page 106), vitamins A, C and E, minerals zinc and selenium) in your body.[48]

- *Derangement of metabolism.*[49] Before the onset of farming, humans ate predominantly complex carbohydrate (plant) foods that release sugars into the bloodstream slowly. The refined sugars of modern diets upset our natural blood sugar balance, causing glucose highs and lows, rather than the sustained, constant energy feed that all of our

---

42 Tan *et al.* (2020).
43 Campisi *et al.* (2011).
44 Muntean and Hess (2009).
45 Franceschi and Campisi (2014).
46 Maggio *et al.* (2006).
47 Richardson and Schadt (2014).
48 Schöttker *et al.* (2015).
49 Maggio *et al.* (2006).

body cells require. This can set off inflammatory responses, and sugar directly causes inflammation via AGEs (advanced glycation end-products or glycotoxins), especially when eaten with fats, for example in pastries and cakes.

With stress and inflammation clearly involved, we can see a route to engaging with our own health and quality of life, essentially having some agency with our own epigenetics – how we move, breathe and relate to our own inner narratives and relationships with others. Adding in awareness of our responses to stressors – and how mindful attention, practices and compassion can transform these – and ripple effects through the other factors can be observed.

Dr Helen Lavretsky studies geriatric psychiatry at UCLA, investigating the microbiotic role in mood and cognitive functions in elders. Her studies have shown that mind-body disciplines such as yoga and tai chi have helped to reduce cognitive decline and mood disorders in an ageing population, helping to modulate nervous system function, metabolism and immunity.[50] See more on the microbiome in Part 4.

Cellular senescence
Cellular senescence is the biological mechanism where the DNA of a cell is damaged and it stops dividing due to stressors – for example, drugs (especially cancer medications), radiation, oxidative stress, mitochondrial dysfunction or elevated glucose levels – so it cannot grow, but remains metabolically active.[51] It is how wounds initially repair themselves, and is vital to the body's process of halting cancer development. A healthy immune system would usually eliminate senescent cells. Where there is excessive inflammation, however, signalling is disrupted and a continuous inflammation loop evolves. Internal stem cells are less able to replace damaged cells to maintain normal oxygen function. Senescent cells rapidly release inflammatory mediators that negatively affect surrounding tissues, which can lead to organ dysfunction, and is at the root of many age-related chronic diseases. Tissue can become fibrotic, where excess collagen is produced in an exaggeration of the wound healing process: '45% of all mortality is associated with significant fibrosis'.[52]

Preventative measures include a diet rich in omega-3 fatty acids and polyphenols (such as quercetin) – antioxidant-rich micronutrients that occur

---

50 Lavretsky (2019).
51 Campisi (2013).
52 Wynn (2008).

naturally in some plant-based foods such as cocoa powder, dark chocolate, green tea, ginger, garlic, berries, turmeric, chilli and cruciferous vegetables (broccoli, cabbage, etc.).[53,54,55,56]

The thymus gland

Immunosenescence is the changes to the immune system that evolve with ageing, the consequence of the progressive atrophy of the thymus gland. This lymphoid organ of the immune system is located behind the sternum, in front of the heart. It facilitates the maturation of protective T cells (the 'T' stands for thymus-derived; Figures 1a and 1b). The ageing thymus declines in its capacity to eliminate self-reactive T cells and to produce immature T cells, reducing the diversity of the T cells that assist in defence against various invaders and disrupt the cells' homeostasis.[57]

Nearly two decades post inflammaging theory, Franceschi added 'garb-ageing', which links chronic stress, the microbiota–gut–brain axis and an increased inflammatory state into a unified body–brain–mind framework that can be used to understand ageing and age-related diseases.[58] In short, our ageing cells stop replicating, have impaired ability to clean up debris and damage (garbage), stop going through apoptosis (cell death) and start secreting proinflammatory markers. At the same time, our immune system becomes weaker at warding off harmful bacteria, viruses and cancer.

Inflammation and resolution

Initial inflammation has to be reduced, resolved and the damage repaired to remain well and delay the development of chronic disease. Inflammation and resolution are separate active pathways of an overall balanced inflammatory response.[59,60,61,62,63,64] Remember, we cannot resolve or repair in stress mode.

53 Gutiérrez, Svahn and Johansson (2019).
54 Tauseef Sultan et al. (2014).
55 Gorzynik-Debicka et al. (2018).
56 Mlcek et al. (2016).
57 Fülöp et al. (2016).
58 Franceschi et al. (2017).
59 Serhan (2014).
60 Spite, Claria and Serhan (2014).
61 Chiang et al. (2012).
62 Morita et al. (2013).
63 Ramon et al. (2014).
64 Hotamisligil (2017).

According to inflammation researcher Dr Barry Sears[65], inflammation, when not resolved, sparks a dangerous reaction of further inflammation, which can become chronic. The creation of scar tissue in organs or senescent cells which increase the ageing of organs can disrupt metabolism and lead to chronic disease. This in turn can drastically reduce quality of life as well as life expectancy.

CASE STUDY: YOGA AND RHEUMATOID ARTHRITIS

Rheumatoid arthritis (RA) is an example of an inflammatory autoimmune condition where research has shown yoga to be beneficial in promoting physical and emotional shift:

> Our findings show measurable improvements for the patients in the test group, suggesting an immune-regulatory role of yoga practice in the treatment of RA. An intensive yoga regimen concurrent with routine drug therapy induced molecular remission and re-established immunological tolerance. In addition, it reduced the severity of depression by promoting neuroplasticity.[66]

A systematic inflammatory disease: COVID-19

COVID-19 is a virus that acts like an inflammatory disease, causing an uncontrolled release of cytokines and an imbalanced immune response.[67] ACE2 (angiotensin-converting enzyme 2) is a receptor in many cells – including oral and nasal mucosa, lungs,[68] stomach, skin, colon, kidneys, liver, spleen and brain – and acts as the receptor-binding domain for the distinguishing protein spikes of the virus SARS-CoV-2, which causes COVID-19.

ACE2 is infected by SARS-CoV-2, which then replicates itself and releases copies around the cells. Affected cells die and leak into the intercellular space, triggering an anti-inflammatory response, a cytokine cascade and an inflammatory feedback loop. The myriad symptoms of the virus are testament to the widespread presence of ACE2 receptors throughout the body, and many come from the damage caused by inflammation, including difficulty breathing, muscle and joint pain, headache or dizziness and blood clots. Usually, the body

---

65   DrSears.com (no date).
66   Gautam *et al.* (2019).
67   Ye, Wang and Mao (2020).
68   Mo *et al.* (2020).

limits infection with a quick-fire inflammatory response, developing long-term acquired immunity 7–10 days after exposure to a virus.[69] The exacerbated inflammatory response of COVID-19, however, when not downregulated, can lead to tissue damage and organ failure.

Severe COVID-19 also disproportionally affects those with inflammaging (page 103), older people with multiple comorbidities – including hypertension, diabetes and obesity – and children with severe multisystem inflammatory syndrome.[70] All can be linked back to stress, for example hypertension is continually raised blood pressure – part of the sympathetic response – raising circulation ready for survival action, and the heart beats faster to send blood to muscles and brain. Hypertension has been shown to 'delay viral clearance and exacerbates airway hyperinflammation in patients with COVID-19'.[71]

Another factor of the SARS-CoV-2 virus is the inflammasome, an intercellular structure that is turned on and produces inflammatory cytokines. Inflammasome activation causes excessive blood clotting, which can damage the veins, leading to less oxygen in the blood. People who already suffer from chronic issues, where the inflammasome is already upregulated, will be more susceptible to the damaging effects.[72]

Growing scientific evidence shows that fat tissue aggravates COVID-19, pooling SARS-CoV-2, thus increasing viral load. It is suspected that substances are released into the bloodstream by fat cells that further increase the inflammatory response: 'A cytokine storm resulting in systemic inflammation similar to sepsis occurs in some severe COVID-19 patients. We believe these inflammatory factors come from adipose tissue. It's been shown that when adipocytes expand too much, they can cause inflammation throughout the body, even the brain.'[73]

Post-viral fatigue and long COVID

Long COVID may be used in diagnoses where chronic fatigue syndrome/myalgic encephalomyelitis (CFS/ME) could have been previously recorded,[74] recognising that previous exposure and infection from a virus can leave a

---

69 García (2020).
70 Bektas *et al.* (2020).
71 Trump *et al.* (2021).
72 Yanuck *et al.* (2020).
73 Silverio *et al.* (2021).
74 NICE (2020).

lingering post-viral illness.[75] From a systemic (psycho-neuro-immunological; page 153) perspective, these illnesses are the 'straw that broke the camel's back', coming into a system already experiencing trauma or chronic stress, making it more likely for a viral overload to be poorly challenged by the immune system.

The inflammatory environment created by stress leaves us compromised in our ability to fight off invaders and can contribute to autoimmune conditions, in essence, attacking ourselves. Upregulation, where cytokine production stays stuck on, causes low-grade constant inflammation (sometimes high in conditions such as arthritis, skin issues or inflammatory bowel disease (IBD)), is exhausting and interferes with the ability to reach deep states of rest where recovery can occur.

Long COVID includes both ongoing symptomatic COVID-19 (from 4 to 12 weeks) and post COVID-19 syndrome (12+ weeks).[76] The most common long-term manifestation is a higher resting heart rate and a greater than usual increase in exercise heart rate, with lower cardiac utilisation of oxygen, leading to fatigue and lightheadedness. About 50 per cent of patients who survive an intensive care unit (ICU) also suffer post-intensive care syndrome, which can include debilitating cognitive, mental and physical impacts, and can severely delay recovery.[77]

UK studies have shown that almost 70 per cent of young, low-risk individuals (average age 44) experiencing long COVID or ongoing symptoms have some organ dysfunction.[78] A study by University College London and Great Ormond Street Children's Hospital suggests that even patients who had been asymptomatic or experienced mild symptoms were experiencing an inflammatory 'long tail' of COVID-19. The virus also causes mitochondrial stress, amplifying fatigue and reducing immunity.[79]

Holistic care for COVID-19 and long COVID

In the prevention phase, it's useful to think about ways to reduce sources of non-purposeful inflammation. This would include adequate sleep and lowering stress levels. A low glycemic diet and minimising alcohol will also help.[80] There has been much research into how yoga can reduce the stress hormone cortisol, which can help to reduce both weight and inflammation.[81]

---

75   Wostyn (2021).
76   Wostyn (2021).
77   Brown (2021).
78   Dennis *et al.* (2021).
79   Doykov *et al.* (2020).
80   Yanuck *et al.* (2020).
81   Watts (2018).

Yoga, lifestyle and nutrition can be advantageous when working with the symptoms of the COVID-19 aftermath. Breath work increases oxygen in the arteries, reducing respiratory effort and the burden on the heart. *Pranayama* strengthens the diaphragm and increases lung capacity.[82] Exercising and diaphragmatic support benefits any postural syndrome or inflamed physiology, as well as activating the soothing PNS.

Because there may be variabilities in blood pressure after COVID-19, yoga sequences should move between planes slowly, for example staging movements from the ground upwards mindfully – to avoid dizziness when blood flow to the head can't catch up immediately with the raised height off the ground.

When we practise yoga *asana* we contract muscles, which leads to the release of interleukin 6 (IL-6), considered to be one of the most important protective cytokines during infections.[83] It acts as an anti-inflammatory, triggering the repair of muscle fibres and the production of anti-inflammatory cytokines, inhibiting proinflammatory cytokines.[84,85] This shows how muscles communicate with cells and organs to downregulate inflammation on a molecular level. Post-COVID-19, there are likely to be musculoskeletal weaknesses, stiffness and immobilisation that can be gently expanded with conscious movements.

Whatever your situation has been, it is a sense of uncertainty that creates a baseline of anxiety and distress. We know that meditation practices help us notice that fear doesn't have to dictate our actions and take over our heart space.[86] Self-care as nourishment and lifestyle factors are also key for recovery and the sense that we can play a role in our health:

- *Food.* It is not only the vitamin and mineral content of organic, heirloom foods (those from ancient crop varieties rather than modern, genetically modified forms) that are superior to modern, processed foods. These food types also contain higher levels of compounds shown to reduce inflammation and modulate immune response. A low-sugar diet is also key to healthy immunity (meta-analyses have shown that metabolic issues are significantly associated with the development of severe COVID-19).[87] Working alongside a nutritional therapist is advised.

---

82 Szcygiel *et al.* (2018).
83 Velazquez-Salinas *et al.* (2019).
84 Pederson (2011).
85 Pederson (2012).
86 Black and Salvich (2016).
87 Yanai (2020).

- *Lifestyle.* The immune system works best when the starting point is regulated. Reducing 'non-purposeful inflammation' could include reducing everyday stress and sleeping well. Stress reduction and ANS regulation is key to bringing these metabolic and immune imbalances towards homeostasis. Where stress or poor sleep are unavoidable, adaptogens can aid stress tolerance and positively support body chemistry. Adaptogenic herbal supplements such as rhodiola, ashwagandha, ginseng and schisandra can support regulation in the HPA axis, the stress response.[88]

NUTRITIONAL IMMUNOLOGY RESEARCH FOR LONG COVID

A growing body of evidence points towards how nutritional immunology could have a role to play in modulating immune function, attenuating inflammation, inhibiting viral replication and supporting the gut, liver and a healthy bloodstream. Interventions using an extended array of nutrient and plant bioactive combinations would be worthwhile in the context of long COVID-19 to determine whether these could help to restore health, wellbeing and quality of life to what was once 'pre-COVID'. Of note, vitamin D, zinc and zinc ionophores, selenium, glutathione, curcumin, EGCG, quercetin and bioactive combinations appear to show particular promise – balancing immune response, attenuating inflammation and inhibiting SARS-CoV-2 activity.[89,90,91,92,93]

Dr Emma Derbyshire[94]

---

88 Please refer to a healthcare professional before taking supplements, particularly if you are taking medication. For more information, see Charlotte's Whole Health webinars at www.charlottewattshealth.com

89 Ibid.

90 Alexander *et al.* (2020).

91 Antwi *et al.* (2021).

92 Guloyan *et al.* (2020).

93 Mrityunjaya *et al.* (2020).

94 Dr Emma Derbyshire, taken from a continuing review of over 2000 relevant papers, published by researchers, at https://long-covid-recovery.org/pages/vitamin-nutrient-toolkit-for-long-covid (accessed February 2022).

PHYSICAL PRACTICE: UNDULATING AND TWISTING

We tune into the autonomic nervous system (ANS) via the breath, offering us an insight into how we can regulate and play a part in noticing and shifting our states (we can also equate this with the qualities of the *gunas*, page 274). In this way, when experiencing any health issue, we can engage not with a disease that is simply happening to us (as if the mind is viewing the body as something separate), but as a call for awareness and self-care.

In this practice we explore spine undulations, as a route into this awareness and self-regulation, as well as natural movements that ease out areas where the protection of the stress response tends to hide out. This rhythmic pumping moves fluids from the centre out, squeezing organs, supporting fascial hydration and pliability, lymphatic movement and a loosening of tensions held within sympathetic dominance (page 88). Recognising where the pressure valve of the exhalation can be found is a vital starting point, and many who have been held in chronic stress or trauma need movement to be able to feel this.

Ventral and dorsal – the rhythm of spine undulations

- Inhaling, we expand the front spine, chest, ribs, lungs and belly: the energising, sympathetic tone of the breath can be related to opening the ventral, front body. The ventral aspect is where, when opened, we are saying 'approach', that we feel safe enough to reveal the soft, vulnerable parts of the throat, heart and belly. It is part of our psychological makeup as bipedals (two-legged animals) to not hide those parts; other animals protect them on all-fours.
- Exhaling, we close around the belly and the heart, open the back body, back of the diaphragm, lungs and base of the skull: coming into the dorsal aspect, opening the back, more protective tones of curling into dorsiflexion, into the foetal position, is more parasympathetic in tone. This is a gesture of self-protection, calming the sympathetic. When we tend towards the curling response, this may signal a holding pattern of shame, trauma or even heart depletion, cut off from the fullness to be able to open up and meet the world.

We need both the opening courage of the sympathetic inhalation, and the calming release of the parasympathetic exhalation; moving with them can help us find this balance. Knowing we have the 'coming home' of the exhalation, we can feel able to open to the world in the inhalation. We can, of course, move in other relations to the front and back body, and need to shift and adapt within our practice, but coming here to establish the root of a moving *anapanasati* (mindfulness of breathing; page 69) can attune us to our nervous system states.

There are changing effects depending on the plane of the spine and the positions of the arms and legs in relation to gravity. We can bring them into practice to arrive and loosen, and sequence them into any practice, particularly as we move between planes, for example coming from the ground to all-fours. There are also examples in a lunge (page 180) and many standing variations in Part 4.

It is easy to lead with the chin as we inhale in spine undulations, especially when postural habits shape many of our movement patterns. Leading instead with the belly, heart and collarbone retains space in the back of the neck and base of the skull and creates self-soothing possibilities via the vagus bundle, including a sense of softness in the front brain. The lying spine undulations in Part 1 differ with a counter motion between lumbar and cervical spines.

Marjaryasana-bitilasana (cat-cow pose, spine undulation on all-fours) is maybe the best known and so useful before moving into *adho mukha svanasana* (down-face dog) as movement is suspended between the shoulder and hip joints, allowing free movement and breath up the whole spine.

Autonomic self-regulation through the guide of the breath

As we have seen, stress can tend to have us breathing in over the end of an exhalation; awareness of allowing a complete out-breath is the signal for an easeful inhalation to enter simply to fill space, with just enough effort needed, and no more. Resting into the still point of the *bahya kumbhaka* (pause at the end of the exhalation; page 50), we can allow completion of the recovery before the action of the inhalation. Through this continuum we find the spinal tide of breath and movement synchronicity, soothing mind-body. We can see the unfolding of the beginning, middle and end of each, and the natural pause of potential as one hands over to the other, supporting embodied practice where we feel rather than think our way through movement.

Where we move into spine undulations, it allows us to marry up the tones of the ANS with the breath, and that synchronicity helps us self-regulate. It can also help those with sensory motor amnesia, holding up in secondary breathing (page 85). Noticing the breath is enlightening where there is lack of access, an unavailable feeling inwardly – where there's no sense of the inhale or exhale – so mindful breathing with motion helps identify those different tones. These movements allow us to physically feel where our boundaries lie, not crash into them, adopting appropriate adaptive responses. As Tias Little says: 'If the yogi does not regulate the adrenal charge through both physical and psychological means and direct it toward altruistic and spiritual activities, then he or she is at the whim of instinctual and impulsive drives.'[95]

Twisting through the viscera

Twists, focusing mindfully on how (with length in the spine, space between discs) rather than how far, are key to how our central body connects to the periphery, torso to limbs. Experience within them will be dependent on the entire story of the breath and the body, as much as the movement around the spine. Too little rotational capacity and our organs become fused and lack differentiation, even becoming collagenous like tendons, stuck in place with the diaphragm.

The spiral lines

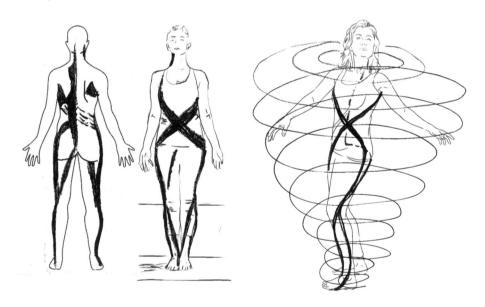

---

95   Little (2016).

Within Thomas Myers' Anatomy Trains®[96] system, the myofascial (muscle and fascia) meridian lines of force transmission through the body offer us a useful map of the body in motion.

Myers describes the spiral lines in the torso crossing over at the front, just above the navel. The fascial researcher Robert Schleip describes these as diagonal torso lines.[97]

These allow us to twist and express rather than shut down and harden around the waist, with movement in the limbs an integral reach out from the belly. They cross over at the midpoint, our line of function between the top and bottom body, where forces move across and then reach down the side of the hips, down the sides of the legs to the ankles. At the back, they cross over at the bottom of the sacrum, the tailbone, and then reach up either side of the spine to cross over and reach into the base of the skull.

Bigger rotational twists move through the fascial spiral lines reaching diagonally across the abdomen to the opposite hip. In any twisting motion, space between the vertebrae is more important than how far we turn. Simply turning without length in the spine can create compression in the discs, with pain and nerve impingements. Twists focused on quality over quantity can help to relieve such issues and create the awareness of turning in from the belly.

Following our spiralic forms

Spirals are the movement of life – within the helix of DNA, of growing and self-organising shapes and throughout force transmission in body fascia. There are no straight lines (or levers) in biologic forms, and following our innate curves and spirals releases tissue tension, fatigue held into fascia, and helps open up the central core of the body and space around the organs.

The Sanskrit word *kundalin* translates as 'circular' or 'coiled'. *Kundalini* or 'coiled snake', originating from the *Shaiva Tantra*, is believed to be the divine feminine energy, or *shakti*, located at *muladhara* (the root *chakra*), at the base of the spine. Hatha yoga has included *Kundalini* practices since the 9th century, in which twisting, spiralling and rotational movements around the spine – alongside meditation, mantra and *pranayama* – can awaken this upward movement of prana (vital energy) through *sushumna* (the central *nadi* or channel), transforming consciousness. Physically this is likened to the feeling of surging current rising up which correlates to the physiological stimulation

---

96   Myers (2013).
97   Schleip with Bayer (2021).

of the blood, lymphatic and nervous systems brought about by the fluidity of spiralling movements.

BENEFITS OF UNDULATIONS AND TWISTING FOR THE IMMUNE SYSTEM

- Opening into the front, back and sides of the ribs, lungs and diaphragm.
- Bringing us into presence (ventral vagus tone; page 162), for neural conditioning to be able to come back to a safe, engaged space, where the process of healing can begin.
- Unwinding and unravelling patterns laid down in the body from stress, trauma, movement habits, sitting, etc.
- Encouraging the lymphatic flow that supports immunity and vitality – through the groin, abdomen, diaphragm, collarbone and throat.
- Opening up neurovascular channels (nerves alongside blood vessels) that nourish and communicate through the body.
- Supporting healthy digestion through diaphragmatic movement, moving fluids through fascia, making space for organs and relieving compression and stagnation into the lower abdomen and organs there.
- Creating slide-and-glide through fascia, which encourages fluidity, adaptation and responsiveness, as well as loosening lesions and adhesions created by lack of movement, inflammation, surgery, injury, trauma and the chronic tension of long-term stress (page 145).

Spinal fluidity for gut–brain flow

We can experience the polarity between the base of the skull and the sacrum directly; these two areas are in constant dialogue and mirror each other's responses. Considering the positioning of the main soothing vagal input to digestive organs from the skull (Figure 2a), spine undulations (where we follow the natural motion of the breath through the spine) can help to balance the cranio-sacral rhythm, assisting parasympathetic action and reducing tension via gut–brain feedback.

These physical movements are also associated with improving digestion in many cultural practices (for example qi gong and Kundalini yoga). They create awakening and fluidity in the abdominal region, massaging the organs and softening the deep hip flexors. They allow us to feel the relationship with the rib cage and the pelvis for postural awareness and easing of digestive issues through pelvic stability and reducing psoas tension. They also support gut motility and balance of the immune and respiratory regulating microbiome in the gut, as well as the throat, respiratory tract and the lungs (Part 4), through the health of tissues there.

Constructive rest position with jaw release

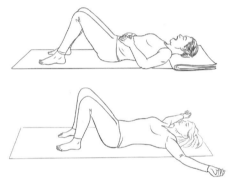

- Arriving to the ground, we can notice the continuing relationship with regions at the top and bottom of the spine:
- Skull and sacrum – lower back responding to opening space into the base of the skull (vagus and brainstem area).
- Belly and jaw – the route of the gut–brain axis and vagus.
- Diaphragm, heart and throat between – breath here allows movement and communication bottom-up to the brain.

We can also have a little rebound here in constructive rest position (CRP) (and other planes), a bouncing through tissues (shimmying on the back up and down) to liberate fluids through tissues, lymphatic flow and in CRP, awakening in the dorsal body to connect all the places mapped above.

1. In CRP (page 55), bring the hands to the belly, arriving in to breathe there, inviting movement of the diaphragm. Take time to notice how the upper and lower jaws can release from each other. Open the mouth as wide as is comfortable, and then slowly allow it to close softly. Repeat two more times, allowing the mouth to close in very slow increments so that the brain and the central nervous system (CNS) register that there is no need to hurry.

2. Allow the arms to expand to shoulder level, for a sense of openness around the lymphatics of the throat, collarbone and armpits.

Adrenal response exercise

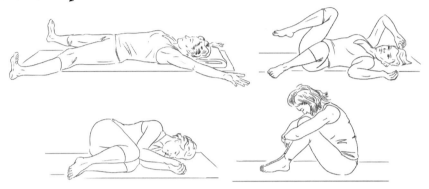

- This exercise can be done as part of a sequence or on its own, when reactivity is showing as inflammation, sensory overwhelm, anxiety, irritable bowel syndrome (IBS) or insomnia.
- Inhaling to open, exhaling to close, we relearn appropriate and adaptive nervous system states.
- To reset heightened responses, do this around the same time every day (about 20 minutes for a full cycle on both sides), for instance on waking or returning from work. These are transitional times where we may struggle to adapt.

Babies are hyper-sensitive to stress – the Moro reflex is where the arms shoot outwards to alert a caregiver – but beyond about a year, we mostly curl inwards for self-protection and stronger reactions to changes in light, movement, touch, sound, temperature, hunger, thirst are inhibited. Those with early trauma, lack of attachment or attunement when young (or, it is theorised, maybe illness) may not fully develop these filters and continue to respond to even subtle change as if it were danger.

Meditation has been shown to lessen this retained primitive startle response in adults,[98] and rolling movement such as the adrenal response exercise helps to reset the head, neck and shoulder responses to nervous system input. It also creates a conscious imprint of the different tones of the breath. Those with

98 Levenson, Ekman and Ricard (2012).

chronic stress can often be disconnected from when they are breathing in and out, registering that connection around the belly imprints this on a visceral level. Spine undulations also have this effect, but here we open the entire front body to meet the world while held by the safety of the ground.

1. Open up into a star shape on the ground, reaching out through fingers and toes as is comfortable, wider than the sides of a mat.
2. Marry up the tone of the breath with the ANS, opening up through the front body on the inhale, on the exhale curling onto one side to come into a foetal position. Reopen all the way back out to centre, meeting the world with the inhale. Exhale back over onto the other side. Follow this pattern side to side, noticing the shift between the protective foetal curling and the reaching out to occupy your whole self in this large body print. Find fluid transitions in motion.
3. The next time you come into a foetal position on one side, hold that there, to protect the belly and heart, breathing into the back of the lungs, back of the ribs and lower back.
4. Roll up easefully from the side and resume the foetal position seated in an upright plane, soothing the parasympathetic nervous system (PNS), curling inwards in a gesture of restoration and healing.

Z-legs loosening sequence

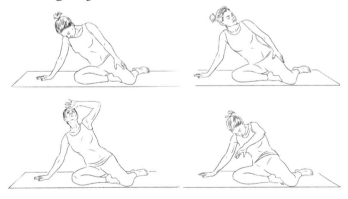

*   Z-legs is a primal position, as one we might naturally come to as part of our design.
*   These are examples of movements we may explore from here, but the possibilities are endless; it is a wonderful place from which to

explore movement into the arm, through the shoulders and ribs, from the belly.

- We are rooted on the leg turned in here – the other hip and buttock are allowed to lift off the ground, leaving us free to move from the tailbone up.

1. Come to this z-legs position where, if the left leg is bent in, the right leg is turned out. Do not try to sit equally on the sitting bones; rather, let the weight drop onto the left sitting bone, bringing the left arm out to the side, dropping the head without rushing to feel any need to lift up through the front of the spine. An easy uplift on the chest doesn't need to be braced or rigid. The head can be heavy as you arrive.

2. Take some rotations with the top shoulder, inhaling it forward and up towards the ears, exhaling it down and round. Allow the right arm to move and the hand to just slide around the right thigh, the full weight of the arm taken from the shoulder, moving around as it needs to make space. Let any movement curve through the shoulders and ribs from the pelvis without holding the torso in position, letting whatever is to be moved, simply move – down into the belly and hips.

3. This is starting to create a spine undulation; follow that in by taking the bent right arm in front of the collarbone as you reach it up and over the face (palm out), with softness around the heart area and throat. Let the eyes softly track the hand so there is a sense of self-organisation through the whole upper body.

4. Exhale to draw the arm back round and in front of the belly as you open the lower back. This may have a bit of a pandiculation response (pages 56 and 290), prompting a yawn.

Z-legs settling in

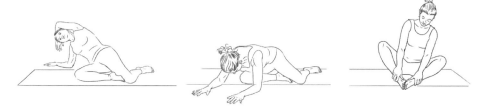

From a place of safety, fluidity and connection, we can then move out from the centre to larger gestures out to the periphery. In older-style yoga practices, a *pranayama* practice like *bastrika* may have been recommended to open the core first, but more recent body workers (such as Ida Rolf) recommend opening the periphery first to move safely in towards any trauma held in the centre. Outer movement can create more malleability and ultimately less tension at the axial core – movement on the outside to soften the inside.

1. Slide the bottom hand a little bit further away and out on the diagonal. Take the right arm up and over, and hang it over the head. Find where both sides of the neck are evenly lengthened up away from the shoulders, drawing the channel a little into the throat, so it is still possible to breathe space in the base of the skull, space between the back teeth, around the eyes.
2. Drop down into a version of *balasana* (child's pose) supported over the left thigh. Come to where feels comfortable, not just necessarily how far it is possible to go. On all levels, what is appropriate to maintain space? Particularly if compressing into the belly, the diaphragm or the chest, we can feel different levels of proprioception, for example into the digestive system or the diaphragm.
3. Roll back up through the body, drawing the belly into the spine, head coming up last. Come into this loose *baddha konasana* (bound angle pose), not needing to come up 'straight' or grasping to bring the legs in closer, simply a relaxed, fluid version, rocking a little side to side to feel into it.
4. Repeat on the other side, allowing the curiosity of beginner's mind (page 72), not simply repeating a learned story from the first side.

Lymphatic pump spinal undulation with twist

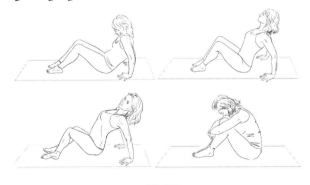

- The back and front body never truly meet except through the sacral point at the belly, where digestion is most happy in the balance between non-doing and doing. Punctuating forward–back spine undulations with twists in practice helps open this channel.
- Here we bring them together to explore occupying the ventral and dorsal aspects of the body, with the changing involvement with the arms – supporting on the exhalation, press-lifting up from the ground to open the chest on the inhalation.

1. Sit on the floor with a similar relationship between the feet and the buttocks as we would have had in CRP – feet about hip-width apart, so feet, knees and hips are in line. Hands on the ground, at least as wide as the shoulders, fingers pointing forward, although the position can be changed according to what feels right if that is too compressive into the wrists. The wrists can be supported with palms on a block for soft fingers that allow space in the carpal tunnel.
2. On the exhale, round the back, letting the chin drop in and bending the elbows, opening between the shoulders.
3. Inhale to press-lift into the hands and open the front body. Lengthen the back of the neck, to avoid hingeing the head or leading with the chin or the eyes, which can dominate experience. Lift the heart and feel a squeeze between the shoulder blades – awakening this thoracic area which can tend to get quite 'concretised'.
4. Follow just behind the breath, curling in on the exhale, allowing the weight of the lumbar to drop to the floor, lifting up to expand the ventral body on the inhale – creating suppleness through the spine, back and chest. Feel moving to the front aspect of the sitting bones on the inhale, back aspect on the exhale.
5. On the next inhale to the upwards arch, let the knees drop to the right to twist (moving hand position if you need to). There may be more of a squeeze under and around the left shoulder blade, where taut tissues can contribute to neck and shoulder pain. Exhale to centre, as before, and inhale knees to the left as the chest lifts, alternating sides with each in-breath. Notice the sensations around the thoracic spine, taking space from any compression in the lumbar. The exhale brings release, dropping down as much as necessary with elbows bent. This pumps lymphatics drainage at the ends of the collarbone, around the diaphragm and the groin, whilst mobilising the ribs.

6. Rest sitting, to hug the knees and come back to releasing the jaw.

Reaching from the belly

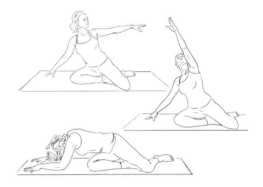

- With more connections between the brain and hands than any other body part, hands are our most important tool, shaping how we work, express and play. Tension in the fingers and wrists from constant contact with technology feeds directly into rigidity in the jaw, diaphragm and belly.
- Reaching out through the right hand reaches up through the liver, left through the stomach and heart. This is not to feel anything particular, but rather to remind us of the asymmetrical nature of the viscera and fascia in our torso, where tightness may be felt through the structure to the periphery. Also, that each side is a fresh experience.

1. Starting from z-legs, left leg inwards and right outwards, lean towards the left, using the left arm for support. Lift the spine up through the shoulders, retaining space in the left shoulder. Take the right arm out to the side and focus the gaze on it, spending a few moments here to fully place the mind into the hand, as you soften that shoulder.
2. With full breath/body attention into that hand, sweep the arm down and past the body to create full circles, reaching up and over, back through the starting point. Following that sweep with the eyes (*drishti*) on the hand for movement out from the navel, allow the motion to reach from the belly, through to the chest, shoulders, neck and head with most fluidity, feeling it through the hips, the whole of the fascial web.
3. Drop down into the belly, connecting to the ground physically to move up from it.
4. Change to the other side, taking time to feel difference and therefore presence.

5. Lift and lean to the side, coming to the elbows, finding a place that feels even through the shoulders to release the head. Breathe into the side body, the ribs, finding a position where an easeful dropping down is allowed. Roll up through the belly, head coming up last.

6. Repeat on the other side.

REACH AS A SOMATIC GUIDE

Reaching motions mimic those we naturally make towards something we want to touch, take or request. Movement follows the direction of gaze and desire, a motivation to find organisation through the path of least resistance, with most ease and grace. It is part of aliveness in our psyche to sense that once a reaching action is completed, if we have acquired something, we feel the contentment of pulling it towards us – satisfaction we feel in the belly.

This is the point where the circle is complete and we can then yield and feel safe to let go. The hand represents the present moment, the focus in time and space: a steady eye connection there can feel as though we are placing our mind into our hand. When the mind is not running the show in terms of pace (that conditioned urge to speed up), we can find the 'flow' where the speed is determined by the quality of presence.

Seated undulation to twist

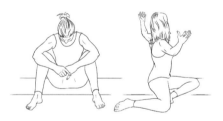

-   Moving side to side, in and out of z-legs, rolls the thigh bones in and out of the hip sockets, freeing that space and encouraging lymphatic motion there.

-   Forwards motion can result from the undulating side to side on the sitting bones, which has similarities in terms of walking, perambulating forwards, legs driven by the spine. If you find your toes and feet reaching forward, move with it and travel.

1. Sitting with feet about mat-width apart, in an open, foetal position, loosely bind elbows around the front of the knees and let the head go. With a broader, wider triangle base, there is the invitation to feel

into the qualities of having a different relationship with the ground in terms of space, the footprint of the body.

2. Rising up from the belly, start to move with the breath again into another spinal undulation, this time as we inhale moving the knees to one side to come back into z-legs. Open the arms out to the side, soft elbows to drop the shoulders and breathe into the chest, long back and sides of the neck rather than leading with the chin. Exhale back to centre. Move side to side from the belly.

Seated spinal undulation 1

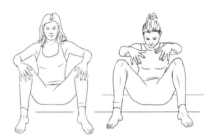

- Shoulder blades can rise up the back with the exhalation, to inform us where to move down the back with the inhalation, offering space to open the chest as the lungs fill.
- This highlights that what happens in one place always has a differing or opposite effect somewhere else.
- Hands to knees on the inhalation provides the purchase to rise up through the front of the spine.

1. From the same position as the previous twist, as you curl back with the exhalation, hold the knees or open the arms in a soft, wide bowl. Feel the expansion between the dorsal aspect of the vertebrae from the tailbone all the way up into the base of the skull.
2. On the inhalation, feel the movement initiated from the tailbone, lifting back up through the arc of the ventral body.

SHIFTING BREATHING PATTERNS FOR NEUROPLASTICITY

We might get used to doing one pattern – inhaling in, exhaling out, with directional movement – but it's really good to play with the opposite breath patterns so that we build neuroplasticity, our ability to adapt with ease. We can either feel the different qualities of switching breath assigned to movement or simply move without assigning a specific breath tone, just breathing feeling to different sensations through the nervous system with a sense of play and curiosity.

Upavistha konasana (wide-seated angle pose) to z-legs twist

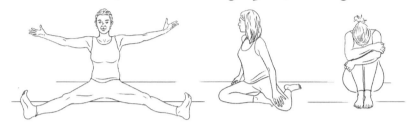

- Opening the limbs out further from the centre to twist into z-legs, when coming to rest, a tighter bundle of a foetal position can feel like the containment – more proprioceptive gathering back into the central axis.
- This is just one possible arm positioning; you might find yourself coming to others, for example switching arm motions (and even breath) around. Some days it might feel more attuned to your emotional states or energy needs to keep the arms lower. Some days you may feel more able to meet the world around and open out from the centre more. You can also switch, shift and adapt within a single practice.

1. Taking the legs wider, bend your knees if you don't easily sit up here through the front of the spine (or onto the front of the sitting bones), feet still flexed for support. Here, the lengthening, lifting up through the spine, and broadening, opening the chest, is on the inhale.
2. On the exhale twist into z-legs, arms low. On the inhale come back to centre, open the ventral body before exhaling to the other side.
3. Come back to centre in a more compact, foetal position, and allow the head to release, breathing quiet into the base of the skull after strong action.

Seated spinal undulation 2

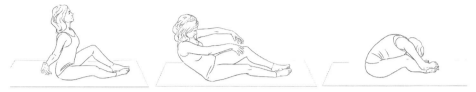

- This is another seated spine undulation because these are so useful for bringing us up through the planes; here, asking for more uplift and activity as we strongly shift the pelvic angle over the front and back aspects of the sitting bones.
- Feel the neck positioned as a continuation of the spine up from the tailbone, avoiding shunting the chin forward and compressing the soothing space at the base of the skull.
- Another foetal shape allows us to rest into the midline, but lengthening the legs a little more is evolving towards the more extended leg position that allows babies to eventually come to stand. This illustrates that forward bends with extended legs (such as *uttanasana* (standing forward bend) and *paschimottanasana* (seated forward bend)) represent the 'grown-up' form of this embryological shape.

1. Sitting upright, feet hip-width apart, let the legs bend and easefully drop out to the side, keeping that outward rotation. Inhale to open the arms and chest, lifting in and up between the shoulder blades.
2. On the exhalation, drop the belly backwards and scoop the arms forward, as if holding a large ball, keeping the arms rounded, hands apart and head dropping. Come back to where it feels possible to easily lift up through the belly and the heart without feeling that that snaps or pulls into the lower back. The thighs are not engaged to root us down; we are engaging the belly for support.
3. On the inhale, return to the first position, lifting from the belly and heart. Move between the two, arm and hand movements fluid and expressive, shoulders soft for less stress in the belly.
4. Keep the feet where they are and allow the lower arms to drop down to the shins; let the head go into another centrally organised foetal shape. Breathe into the lower back.

Anapanasati (mindfulness of breathing) to *chakravakasana* (sunbird)

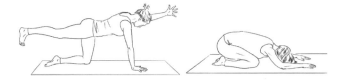

- The breath wants to slow down, wants to conserve energy, a large part of survival. Allowing this guide when we begin to move our weight more off the ground can meet (notice and soothe) the mind's want to go faster with the mobilisation that is related to the 'getting going' of the sympathetic nervous system.
- This moving meditation allows us to feel the tones of the breath, to guide the motion up from the belly so that there is the rise of the breath with the upwards movement, the rise of the *prana* up through the front of the spine, and then down the spine the releasing quality of *apana* drops us back down towards the ground.

I. From *balasana* (child's pose), rise up to all-fours on an inhalation, reaching out the right arm and left leg. Follow behind the breath to exhale back down into *balasana*, then inhale up to the other side, lifting the left arm, right leg. Find where the neck is comfortable for softness in the temples, so looking down rather than forward, where our human head and neck are most naturally organised above the shoulders. On the inhale, gather the lower ribs towards the sky from the waist, then settling back down into *balasana* between sides, becoming relatively heavy in relation to gravity.

THE WISDOM OF TAILBONE CIRCLING

From all-fours, circling the tailbone, limiting the motion in the shoulders so it is directed into the pelvis and the abdomen, is a key movement for fascial slide and glide (page 146) and loosens the spinal and lower back tissues in preparation for *adho mukha svanasana* (down-face dog pose). After some time, let the shoulders and head get involved, so the tailbone is still the origin of the movement and the rest of the body is being moved in any way that spirals upwards towards the head. Allow a fluid quality, playful, explorative, without agenda or interpretation. Soften around the jaw and the eyes, and stick out the tongue, moving the face and the jaw. If this feels chaotic, minimise the motion at the top of the body and come back to the origin of the tailbone rotating. Feel the rotational movement through the viscera, the movement of the pelvic floor. Allow the breath (or sounding; see Part 6) to express what has been released up from the root to the upper body and move any tension out; this is autonomic release. Lion's breath (page 362) can feel helpful here.

Take the movement in the opposite direction, noticing which way feels more automatic, natural. The second side may be 'going against the grain' and meeting the more interesting stuff of *granthi* (knots or doubts; page 153), or psychic knots, in the body. It may also be going against the tide of movement in the colon, so create resistance there that supports its muscular function (and the microbiome; page 208).

You can explore circling the tailbone in many positions for similar and differing effects – in constructive rest position (CRP), a soft lunge, standing, *adho mukha svanasana*, z-legs, seated and more...

Bridging in *adho mukha svanasana* (down-face dog pose) towards prone *savasana* (corpse pose)

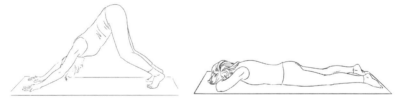

- In prone positions (face down), the inhale doesn't have space to move forwards of the body, so we can feel its presence as compression into the organs. The following exhale releases and creates a nourishing flood of fluids through the tissues and softening into the fascial sacs around the organs.
- This lack of space to move forward also sends the breath into the back body, which sometimes gets left out of the breathing process. We can focus breathing into the backs of the lungs (especially the lower part, where there are more parasympathetic fibres) and allow motions of the breath into the sacrum.

- It is quite common for people with trauma to have tense holding patterns or for those with sedentary habits to lose movement of the sacrum with the breath – cranio-sacral therapy can help reintroduce lost connections and release sensory motor amnesia there.

1. If it feels appropriate, come to *adho mukha svanasana* (down-face dog pose) with an attitude of moving towards rest. Rather than pedalling backwards and forwards, slide the tailbone side to side, heels can follow, so the body opens the sides of the spine, opening the core fascial sheath, through the mid-line of the body – like an apple core.
2. Come onto the belly for prone *savasana* (corpse pose), with hands underneath the forehead, palms down. Feel what is needed to be comfortable and happy here. Perhaps have a little roll through the pelvis, lifting the feet above the knees and rolling side to side for a little deeper movement, twisting through the lower back to settle.
3. Tuck the toes under when returning to prone to engage the legs, drawing the strong muscles at the front of the body up so that when we finally come to drop down there is an acquiescence, a yielding to the ground.
4. Feet can be as wide as the lower back needs, so if there is any compression in the lower back in back arches, take the feet wider (this probably suggests a wider sacrum – our bones are as individual as we appear from the outside) to allow the heels to naturally drop out, opening space across the lower back.
5. Find ease in the belly where the body meets the ground, a guide to tune into the breath there, at our physical centre, radiating out into all parts of our body and aspects of our being (*koshas*; page 150).

SUBTLE PRACTICES: BREATHING FOR REGULATION

Chandra bhedana pranayama (moon-piercing breath)

This is a cooling practice to reduce sympathetic dominance (page 88), the opposite of *surya* (sun) breath.

1. Inhale through the left nostril (*ida*, moon).
2. Exhale through the right nostril (*pingala*, sun).

We can add an optional internal *mantra*: '*Ahum*' ('I am') while inhaling through the left; '*Shanti*' ('Peace') exhaling through the right. This can be practised with or without the *mudra* used in *nadi shodhana* (alternate nostril breathing) on page 318. See more in-depth guidance around *pranayama* in Part 5.

Coherent breathing

In *The Healing Power of the Breath*, Richard Brown and Patricia Gerbarg state: 'Belly breathing and Coherent Breathing...shift the nervous system response into a healthier balance by activating the healing, recharging part of the nervous system while quieting the defensive, energy-burning parts.'[99]

On average, humans breathe erratically, using only around 10 per cent of the available diaphragm range, allowing sufficient gaseous exchange for survival but not to thrive. Coherent breathing aims to increase this to 40–60 per cent of our diaphragmatic range in a rhythmic manner, optimising gaseous exchange, allowing the nervous system to rest, restore and rebalance. During coherent breathing, blood circulates somewhere between once per minute (resting) and six times per minute (exercise), although the body remains at rest. The rhythm of the breath is regulated to a count of six on the inhale and six on the exhale (counting in time with seconds in a minute), so one complete breath is 12 seconds long, reducing the breathing rate to five breaths per minute. This helps to coordinate the thoracic and heart pumps, reducing the load on the vascular system. This count can, of course, be reduced if any force is felt, practising *ahimsa*.

The heart rate is a good indicator of nervous tone. The heart rate fluctuates

---

99 Brown and Gerbarg (2012).

continually depending on many factors including environmental stressors, thought processes, etc. The optimal differentiation between heart rate variability (HRV) on inhalation and exhalation is 20–30 beats. When a person is caught in a stress loop affecting breath rate, rhythm and quality, this will have a negative impact on HRV. Normally, when someone is stuck in this pattern, the breath is short and inhale-dominant, which increases the heart rate and sympathetic tone, causing the whole body to go into flexion, which might be equated with *sthira*, with a need for the balancing ease of *sukha*. This puts a strain on the pulmonary pump (as the thoracic pump is not being used optimally), which reduces optimal gaseous exchange and puts a strain on all body systems. Slowly introducing this practice can begin to undo this patterning and allow for a more balanced reality to unfold physiologically, which reverberates throughout the being on a cellular level.

It is of great scientific importance how deeply beneficial slow breathing can be as a long-term practice. In *The Physiological Effects of Slow Breathing in the Healthy Human*, Russo, Santorelli and O'Rourke expand that slow breathing 'appears capable of achieving optimal sympathovagal balance, and enhancing autonomic reactivity to physical and mental stress', rather than simply reducing sympathetic nervous tone'.[100]

People who have been breathing rapidly for many years will find a relaxed state of being more difficult to access, as it will be contrary to their established breathing pattern. It is important to go slowly and patiently when introducing this (or any breathing) practice. Noticing the subtle signs of tension building (in the jaw, eyes, throat, temples, base of skull, diaphragm, chest, hands, etc.) is a vital part of the mindful practising of such specific breath counts. This avoids them simply becoming something that 'we do', and that doing them well or correctly supersedes the feeling tones and nuances.

It is easy to get caught up in the clear boundaries of such a practice that can make us feel safe, but we need to be cultivating whole body (global) relationships with the effects and how to modulate to build up with body intelligence; these cannot be rushed. We also need to recognise that 'progression' isn't simply linear, but we will feel different responses on different days – this is not being better or worse at a practice, but rather offers us insight into our nervous system states at that time in space, which is very useful information in and of itself.

---

100 Russo, Santarelli and O'Rourke (2017).

Coherent breathing practice

1. Sit upright and supported (able to easily rise up through the front spine), resting the whole body for a few breaths, releasing the jaw and around the eyes.
2. Follow a couple of full inhales and exhales to stretch out the diaphragm and the primary breathing muscles, noticing the natural breathing pattern.
3. Become aware of the exhalation, noticing how long, how smooth, how steady it is.
4. Now begin to count your exhalation, gradually lengthening it to a count of six (if this isn't easeful for any reason, reduce the count). Counting for yourself can be a good place to start as you will self-regulate to need, but it won't likely be exactly five breaths per minute – see the timers below (or use a soft metronome to avoid technology in your practice space) for exact counts.
5. Do a few rounds and then relax and allow the breath to be totally natural.
6. Resume the count on the exhale, noticing any physical sensations.
7. Add the count on the inhale: in for six, out for six (or less), for a breath or two, attentive to how it feels. If there is any strain, go back to counting the exhalation only, freeing the inhalation.
8. Go carefully and easefully with an attitude of curiosity about the breath and how you feel.

LINKS WITH SET CHIMES FOR FIVE BREATHS PER MINUTE

Search for videos online with the following titles:

*   Coherence Breathing Clock – Visual Focus.
*   Coherent Breathings Iconic 2 Bells – with Sinusoidal Pacing.

Self-enquiry questions

Explore these questions from an experiential point of view, bringing the poetic, descriptive felt sense into any analysing or describing from an anatomical or biomechanical standpoint. Find how this enquiry can help you translate the theory of body systems into the real, individual experience of yourself and your students.

1. Describe the feelings, bodily and in the present – tones, textures and flavours, rather than the story – of your breath, pulses, tone of skin, muscle, fascia, etc.
2. Can you tune into the capacity for self-regulation of the autonomic nervous system via your breath?
3. What differences to your inner experience can you notice with regular attention to freeing movements in the jaw within any form of practice?
4. Which emotional resonances do you notice differing between opening the front and back (ventral and dorsal) aspects of the body?
5. What do you notice about the positioning of your head and your nervous system responses?

Further resources

Fiona Agombar (with contributions from Leah Barnett) (2020) *Yoga Therapy for Stress, Burnout and Chronic Fatigue Syndrome*. London and Philadelphia, PA: Singing Dragon.

Dr Jeffrey S. Bland (2015) *The Disease Delusion: Conquering the Causes of Chronic Illness for a Healthier, Longer, and Happier Life*. New York: HarperWave.

Richard Brown and Patricia Gerbarg (2012) *The Healing Power of the Breath: Simple Techniques to Reduce Stress and Anxiety, Enhance Concentration, and Balance Your Emotions*. Boulder, CO: Shambhala Publications.

Daniel Lieberman (2014) *The Story of the Human Body: Evolution, Health and Disease*. London: Penguin.

Charlotte Watts (2015) *The De-Stress Effect*. London: Hay House.

References

Alexander, J., Tinkov, A., Strand, T.A., Alehagen, U., Skalny, A. and Aaseth, J. (2020) 'Early nutritional interventions with zinc, selenium and vitamin D for raising anti-viral resistance against progressive COVID-19.' *Nutrients 12*(8), 2358. Available at: https://pubmed.ncbi.nlm.nih.gov/32784601

American College of Chest Physicians (2013) 'Yoga practice beneficial to patients with COPD.' Science Daily, 28 October. Available at: www.sciencedaily.com/releases/2013/10/131028114836.html

Antwi, J., Appiah, B., Oluwakuse, B. and Abu, B.A.Z. (2021) 'The nutrition–COVID-19 interplay: A review.' *Current Nutrition Reports 10*(4), 364–374. Available at: https://pubmed.ncbi.nlm.nih.gov/34837637

Bektas, A., Schurman, S.H., Franceschi, C. and Ferrucci, L. (2020) 'A public health perspective of aging: Do hyper-inflammatory syndromes such as COVID-19, SARS, ARDS, cytokine storm syndrome, and post-ICU syndrome accelerate short- and long-term inflammaging?' *Immunity & Ageing 17*, 23. Available at: http://dx.doi.org/10.1186/s12979-020-00196-8

Bharati, S.J. (no date). *Yoga Sutras of Patanjali Interpretive Translation*. Available at: https://swamij.com/pdf/yogasutrasinterpretive.pdf

Black, D.S. and Salvich, G.M. (2016) 'Mindfulness meditation and the immune system: A systematic review of randomised controlled trials.' *Annals of the New York Academy of Sciences 1373*(1), 13–24. Available at: https://doi.org/10.1111/nyas.12998

Bower, J.E. and Irwin, M.R. (2016) 'Mind-body therapies and control of inflammatory biology: A descriptive review.' *Brain, Behavior, and Immunity 51*, 1–11. Available at: www.ncbi.nlm.nih.gov/pmc/articles/PMC4679419

Bratic, I. and Aleksandra, A. (2010) 'Mitochondrial energy metabolism and ageing.' *Biochimica et Biophysica Acta (BBA) – Bioenergetics 1797*(6–7), 961–967. Available at: www.sciencedirect.com/science/article/pii/S0005272810000058

Brown, B. (2021) 'Enhanced ACE2 expression, pre-existing endothelial dysfunction and procoagulant state.' *Integrative Healthcare & Applied Nutrition* magazine, March.

Brown, R.P. and Gerbarg, P.L. (2012) *The Healing Power of the Breath: Simple Techniques to Reduce Stress and Anxiety, Enhance Concentration, and Balance Your Emotions.* Boulder, CO: Shambhala Publications.

Bryant, E.F. (2009) *Yoga Sutras of Patanjali.* New York: North Point Press.

Campisi, J. (2013) 'Aging, cellular senescence, and cancer.' *Annual Review of Physiology 75*, 685–705. Available at: https://pubmed.ncbi.nlm.nih.gov/23140366

Campisi, J., Andersen, J.K., Kapahi, P. and Melov, S. (2011) 'Cellular senescence: A link between cancer and age-related degenerative disease?' *Seminars in Cancer Biology 21*(6), 354–359. Available at: http://dx.doi.org/10.1016/j.semcancer.2011.09.001

Cavaillon, J.M. and Adib-Conquy, M. (2002) 'The pro-inflammatory cytokine cascade.' *Immune Response in the Critically Ill, Update in Intensive Care Medicine*, 37–66. Available at: https://link.springer.com/chapter/10.1007%2F978-3-642-57210-4_4

Chiang, N., Fredman, G., Bäckhed, F., Oh, S.F., *et al.* (2012) 'Infection regulates pro-resolving mediators that lower antibiotic requirements.' *Nature 484*(7395), 524–528. Available at: https://pubmed.ncbi.nlm.nih.gov/22538616

Dennis, A., Wamil, M., Alberts, J., Oben, J., *et al.* (2021) 'Multiorgan impairment in low-risk individuals with post-COVID-19 syndrome: A prospective, community-based study.' *BMJ Open 11*(3), e048391. Available at: https://pubmed.ncbi.nlm.nih.gov/33785495

Doykov, I., Hällqvist, J., Gilmour, K.C., Grandjean, L., Mills, K. and Heywood, W.E. (2020) '"The long tail of Covid-19" – The detection of a prolonged inflammatory response after a SARS-CoV-2 infection in asymptomatic and mildly affected patients.' *F1000Research 9*, 1349. Available at: https://pubmed.ncbi.nlm.nih.gov/33391730

DrSears.com (no date). *Resolution Response™.* DrSears.com. Accessed 31/05/2022 at: https://drsears.com/the-resolution-response-managing-inflammation-dr-sears

Eichenberger, P.A., Diener, S.N., Kofmehl, R. and Spengler, C.M. (2013) 'Effects of exercise training on airway hyperreactivity in asthma: A systematic review and meta-analysis.' *Sports Medicine 43*(11), 1157–1170. Available at: https://pubmed.ncbi.nlm.nih.gov/23846823

Franceschi, C. and Campisi, J. (2014) 'Chronic inflammation (inflammaging) and its potential contribution to age-associated diseases.' *Journals of Gerontology, Series A: Biological Sciences and Medical Sciences 69*(S1), S4–S9. Available at: https://pubmed.ncbi.nlm.nih.gov/24833586

Franceschi, C., Garagnani, P., Vitale, G., Capri, M. and Salvioli, S. (2017) 'Inflammaging and "garb-aging".' *Trends in Endocrinology and Metabolism 28*(3), 199–212. Available at: http://dx.doi.org/10.1016/j.tem.2016.09.005

Fülöp, T., Dupuis, G., Witkowski, J.M. and Larbi, A. (2016) 'The role of immunosenescence in the development of age-related diseases.' *Revista de Investigacion Clinica 68*(2), 84–91. Available at: https://pubmed.ncbi.nlm.nih.gov/27103044

García, L.F. (2020) 'Immune response, inflammation, and the clinical spectrum of COVID-19.' *Frontiers of Immunology 11*, 1441. Available at: https://doi.org/10.3389/fimmu.2020.01441

Gkikas, I., Palikaras, K. and Tavernarakis, N. (2018) 'The role of mitophagy in innate immunity.' *Frontiers in Immunology 9*, 1283. Available at: www.ncbi.nlm.nih.gov/pmc/articles/PMC6008576

Gorzynik-Debicka, M., Przychodzen, P., Cappello, F., Kuban-Jankowska, A., *et al.* (2018) 'Potential health benefits of olive oil and plant polyphenols.' *International Journal of Molecular Sciences 19*(3), 686. Available at: https://pubmed.ncbi.nlm.nih.gov/29495598

Gruver, A.L., Hudson, L.L. and Sempowski, G.D. (2007) 'Immunosenescence of ageing.' *J Pathol 211*, 144–156. Available at: https://pubmed.ncbi.nlm.nih.gov/17200946

Guloyan, V., Oganesian, B., Baghdasaryan, N., Yeh, C., *et al.* (2020) 'Glutathione supplementation as an adjunctive therapy in COVID-19.' *Antioxidants (Basel) 9*(10), 914. Available at: https://pubmed.ncbi.nlm.nih.gov/32992775

Gustine, J.N. and Jones, D. (2021) 'Immunopathology of Hyperinflammation in COVID-19.' *The American journal of pathology 191*(1), 4–17. Available at: https://pubmed.ncbi.nlm.nih.gov/32919977

Gutiérrez, S., Svahn, S.L. and Johansson, M.E. (2019) 'Effects of omega-3 fatty acids on immune cells.' *International Journal of Molecular Science 20*(20), 5028. Available at: https://pubmed.ncbi.nlm.nih.gov/31614433

Haahtela, T. (2019) 'A biodiversity hypothesis.' *Allergy 74*(8), 1445–1456. Available at: https://pubmed.ncbi.nlm.nih.gov/30835837

Hanna, T. (2004) *Somatics: Reawakening the Mind's Control of Movement, Flexibility, and Health.* Cambridge, MA: Da Capo Press.

Hood, D.A. (2009) 'Mechanisms of exercise-induced mitochondrial biogenesis in skeletal muscle.' *Applied Physiology, Nutrition, and Metabolism 34*(3), 465–472. Available at: https://pubmed.ncbi.nlm.nih.gov/19448716

Hotamisligil, G.S. (2017) 'Inflammation, metaflammation, and immunometabolic disorders.' *Nature 542*(7640), 177–185. Available at: https://pubmed.ncbi.nlm.nih.gov/28179656

Human Cell Atlas (no date). *HCA Research on Covid-19.* Human Cell Atlas. Accessed 31/05/2022 at: www.humancellatlas.org/covid-19

Hyman, M. (2021) 'The difference between rejuvenating and boosting your immune system.' Blog, 1 November. Available at: https://drhyman.com/blog/2021/11/01/the-difference-between-rejuvenating-and-boosting-your-immune-system

Kenney, M.J. and Ganta, C.K. (2014) 'Autonomic nervous system and immune system interactions.' *Comprehensive Physiology 4*(3), 1177–1200. Available at: https://pubmed.ncbi.nlm.nih.gov/24944034

Lavretsky, H. (2019) 'Yoga and meditation can help improve cognitive functioning in older adults with mild cognitive impairment and dementia.' *The American Journal of Geriatric Psychiatry 27*(2), 198–199. Available at: https://pubmed.ncbi.nlm.nih.gov/30538073

Levenson, R.W., Ekman, P. and Ricard, M. (2012) 'Meditation and the startle response: A case study.' *Emotion 12*(3), 650–658. Available at: www.ncbi.nlm.nih.gov/pmc/articles/PMC3742737

Little, T. (2016) *Yoga of the Subtle Body: A Guide to the Physical and Energetic Anatomy of Yoga.* Boulder, CO: Shambhala Publications.

Little, T. and Little, S. (no date) SATYA (Sensory Awareness Training for Yoga Attunement) [course training manual]. Accessed 2019.

Maggio, M., Guralnik, J.M., Longo, D.L. and Ferrucci, L. (2006) 'Interleukin-6 in aging and chronic disease: A magnificent pathway.' *Journals of Gerontology, Series A: Biological Sciences and Medical Sciences 61*(6), 575–584. Available at: https://pubmed.ncbi.nlm.nih.gov/16799139

Mandoorah, S. and Mead, T. (2021) 'Phrenic nerve injury.' StatPearls. Available at: www.ncbi.nlm.nih.gov/books/NBK482227

Mendes, F.A.R., Almeida, F.M., Cukier, A., Stelmach, R., *et al.* (2011) 'Effects of aerobic training on airway inflammation in asthmatic patients.' *Medicine and Science in Sports and Exercise 43*(2), 197–203. Available at: https://pubmed.ncbi.nlm.nih.gov/20581719

Mlcek, J., Jurikova, T., Skrovankova, S. and Sochor, J. (2016) 'Quercetin and its anti-allergic immune response.' *Molecules 21*(5), 623. Available at: https://pubmed.ncbi.nlm.nih.gov/27187333

Mo, X., Jian, W., Si, Z., Chen, M., *et al.* (2020) 'Abnormal pulmonary function in COVID-19 patients at time of hospital discharge.' *The European Respiratory Journal 55*(6), 2001217. Available at: www.ncbi.nlm.nih.gov/pmc/articles/PMC7236826

Monda, V., Villano, I., Messina, A., Valenzano, A., *et al.* (2017) 'Exercise modifies the gut microbiota with positive health effects.' *Oxidative Medicine and Cellular Longevity 2017*, 3831972. Available at: https://pubmed.ncbi.nlm.nih.gov/28357027

Morita, M., Kuba, K., Ichikawa, A., Nakayama, M., *et al.* (2013) 'The lipid mediator protectin D1 inhibits influenza virus replication and improves severe influenza.' *Cell 153*(1), 112–125. Available at: https://pubmed.ncbi.nlm.nih.gov/23477864

Mrityunjaya, M., Pavithra, V., Neelam, R., Janhavi, P., Halami, P.M. and Ravindra, P.V. (2020) 'Immune-boosting, antioxidant and anti-inflammatory food supplements targeting pathogenesis of COVID-19.' *Frontiers in Immunology 11*, 570122. Available at: https://pubmed.ncbi.nlm.nih.gov/33117359

Muntean, A.G. and Hess, J.L. (2009) 'Epigenetic dysregulation in cancer.' *The American Journal of Pathology 175*(4), 1353–1361. Available at: www.ncbi.nlm.nih.gov/pmc/articles/PMC2751531

Myers, T. (2013) *Anatomy Trains: Myofascial Meridians for Manual and Movement Therapists*, 3rd edn. Edinburgh: Churchill Livingstone.

Nakao, A. (2020) 'Circadian regulation of the biology of allergic disease: Clock disruption can promote allergy.' *Frontiers in Immunology 11*, 1237. Available at: https://pubmed.ncbi.nlm.nih.gov/32595651

Nestor, J. (2020) *Breath: The New Science of a Lost Art.* London: Penguin Life.

NICE (National Institute for Health and Care Excellence) (2020) *COVID-19 Rapid Guideline: Managing the Long-term Effects of COVID-19.* London: NICE. Available at: https://pubmed.ncbi.nlm.nih.gov/33555768

Pederson, B.K. (2011) 'Muscles and their myokines.' *Journal of Experimental Biology 214*(2), 337–346. Available at: http://dx.doi.org/10.1242/jeb.048074

Pederson, B.K. (2012) 'Muscular interleukin-6 and its role as an energy sensor.' *Medicine and Science in Sports and Exercise 44*(3), 392–396. Available at: https://pubmed.ncbi.nlm.nih.gov/21799452

Persson, M., Svenarud, P., Flock, J.I. and van der Linden, J. (2005) 'Carbon dioxide inhibits the growth rate of Staphylococcus aureus at body temperature.' *Surgical Endoscopy 19*(1), 91–94. Available at: https://pubmed.ncbi.nlm.nih.gov/15529188

Peterson, M. (2015) 'The mystery of "muscle knots" solved: Sensory motor amnesia.' Pain Relief Through Movement, 18 July. Available at: https://essentialsomatics.wordpress.com/2015/07/18/muscle-knots-are-another-word-for-sensory-motor-amnesia

Porges, S.W. (2009) 'The polyvagal theory: New insights into adaptive reactions of the autonomic nervous system.' *Cleveland Clinic Journal of Medicine 76*(Suppl 2), S86–S90. Available at: https://pubmed.ncbi.nlm.nih.gov/19376991

Pruimboom, L. and Muskiet, F.A.J. (2018) 'Intermittent living; the use of ancient challenges as a vaccine against the deleterious effects of modern life – A hypothesis.' *Medical Hypotheses 120*, 28–42. Available at: https://pubmed.ncbi.nlm.nih.gov/30220336

Ramon, S., Baker, S.F., Sahler, J.M., Kim, N., *et al.* (2014) 'The specialized proresolving mediator 17-HDHA enhances the antibody-mediated immune response against influenza virus: A new class of adjuvant?' *Journal of Immunology 193*, 6031–6040. Available at: www.ncbi.nlm.nih.gov/pmc/articles/PMC4258475

Richardson, A.G. and Schadt, E.E. (2014) 'The role of macromolecular damage in aging and age-related disease.' *The Journals of Gerontology. Series A, Biological Sciences and Medical Sciences 69*(1), S28–S32. Available at: https://pubmed.ncbi.nlm.nih.gov/24833583

Roenneberg, T. and Merrow, M. (2016) 'The circadian clock and human health.' *Current Biology 26*(10), R432–R443. Available at: https://pubmed.ncbi.nlm.nih.gov/27218855

Ruegsegger, G.N. and Booth, F.W. (2018) 'Health benefits of exercise.' *Cold Spring Harbor Perspectives in Medicine 8*(7), a029694. Available at: https://pubmed.ncbi.nlm.nih.gov/28507196

Russo, M.A., Santarelli, D.M. and O'Rourke, D. (2017) 'The physiological effects of slow breathing in the healthy human.' *Breathe (Sheff) 13*(4), 298–309. Available at: www.ncbi.nlm.nih.gov/pmc/articles/PMC5709795

Salim, S., Chugh, G. and Asghar, M. (2012) 'Inflammation in anxiety.' *Advances in Protein Chemistry and Structural Biology 88*, 1–25. Available at: https://pubmed.ncbi.nlm.nih.gov/22814704

Schleip, R. with Bayer, J. (2021) *Fascial Fitness: Practical Exercises to Stay Flexible, Active and Pain Free in Just 20 Minutes a Week*, 2nd edn. Chichester: Lotus Publishing.

Schöttker, B., Brenner, H., Jansen, E.H.J.M., Gardiner, J., *et al.* (2015) 'Evidence for the free radical/oxidative stress theory of ageing from the CHANCES consortium: A meta-analysis of individual participant data.' *BMC Medicine 13*, 300. Available at: www.ncbi.nlm.nih.gov/pmc/articles/PMC4678534

Sehinson, C. (2021) 'Lessons learned with long-COVID – An integrative medicine approach.' *Integrative Healthcare & Applied Nutrition* magazine, May, 30–34.

Serhan, C.N. (2014) 'Pro-resolving lipid mediators are leads for resolution physiology.' *Nature 510*(7503), 92–101. Available at: https://pubmed.ncbi.nlm.nih.gov/24899309

Silverio, S., Gonçalves, D.C., Andrade, M.F. and Seelaender, M. (2021) 'Coronavirus disease 2019 (COVID-19) and nutritional status: The missing link?' *Advances in Nutrition 12*(3), 682–692. Available at: https://academic.oup.com/advances/article/12/3/682/5911598

Slavich, G.M. (2016) 'Life stress and health: A review of conceptual issues and recent findings.' *Teaching of Psychology 43*(4), 346–355. Available at: https://pubmed.ncbi.nlm.nih.gov/27761055

Spite, M., Claria, J. and Serhan, C.N. (2014) 'Resolvins, specialized pro-resolving lipid mediators, and their potential roles in metabolic disease.' *Cell Metabolism 19*, 21–36. Available at: www.ncbi.nlm.nih.gov/pmc/articles/PMC3947989

Stephenson, E., Reynolds, G., Botting, R.A., Calero-Nieto, F.J., et al. (2021) 'Single-cell multi-omics analysis of the immune response in COVID-19.' *Nature Medicine 27*(5), 904–916. Available at: https://pubmed.ncbi.nlm.nih.gov/33879890

Sweet, R.L. and Zastre, J.A. (2013) 'HIF-1α-mediated gene expression induced by vitamin B1 deficiency.' *International Journal for Vitamin and Nutrition Research 83*(3), 188–197. Available at: https://pubmed.ncbi.nlm.nih.gov/24846908

Szcygiel, E., Blaut, J., Zielonka-Pycla, K., Tomaszewski, K., *et al.* (2018) 'The impact of deep muscle training on the quality of posture and breathing.' *Journal of Motor Behavior 50*(2), 219–222. Available at: https://pubmed.ncbi.nlm.nih.gov/28820662

Tan, L., Wang, Q., Zhang, D., Ding, J., *et al.* (2020) 'Lymphopenia predicts disease severity of COVID-19: A descriptive and predictive study.' *Signal Transduction and Targeted Therapy 5*, 33. Available at: www.nature.com/articles/s41392-020-0148-4

Tauseef Sultan, M., Butt, M.S., Qayyum, M.M. and Suleria, H.A.R. (2014) 'Immunity: Plants as effective mediators.' *Critical Reviews in Food Science and Nutrition 54*(10), 1298–1308. Available at: https://pubmed.ncbi.nlm.nih.gov/24564587

Thomsen, S.F. (2015) 'Epidemiology and natural history of atopic diseases.' *European Clinical Respiratory Journal 2.* Available at: www.ncbi.nlm.nih.gov/pmc/articles/PMC4629767

Tosato, M., Zamboni, V., Ferrini, A. and Cesari, M. (2007) 'The aging process and potential interventions to extend life expectancy.' *Clinical Interventions in Aging 2*(3), 401–412. Available at: www.ncbi.nlm.nih.gov/pmc/articles/PMC2685272

Trump, S., Lukassen, S., Anker, M.S., Chua, R.L., *et al.* (2021) 'Hypertension delays viral clearance and exacerbates airway hyperinflammation in patients with COVID-19.' *Nature Biotechnology 39*, 705–716. Available at: https://pubmed.ncbi.nlm.nih.gov/33361824

van der Kolk, B.A. (2015) *The Body Keeps the Score: Brain, Mind, and Body in the Healing of Trauma.* London: Penguin.

Velazquez-Salinas, L., Verdugo-Rodriguez, A., Rodriguez, L.L. and Borca, M.V. (2019) 'The role of interleukin 6 during viral infections.' *Frontiers in Microbiology*, Opinion article. Available at: www.frontiersin.org/articles/10.3389/fmicb.2019.01057/full

Wanrooij, V.H.M., Willeboordse, M., Dompeling, E. and van de Kant, K.D.G. (2014) 'Exercise training in children with asthma: A systematic review.' *British Journal of Sports Medicine 48*(13), 1024–1031. Available at: https://pubmed.ncbi.nlm.nih.gov/23525551

Watts, C. (2018) *Yoga Therapy for Digestive Health.* London and Philadelphia, PA: Singing Dragon.

Wellcome Trust Sanger Institute (2021) 'Differing immune responses discovered in asymptomatic cases vs those with severe COVID-19.' ScienceDaily, 20 April. Available at: www.sciencedaily.com/releases/2021/04/210420121500.htm

Wenger, M.A., Bagchi, B.K. and Anand, B.K. (1961) 'Experiments in India on "voluntary" control of the heart and pulse.' *Circulation 24*, 1319–1325. Available at: https://pubmed.ncbi.nlm.nih.gov/14006121

Wostyn, P. (2021) 'COVID-19 and chronic fatigue syndrome: Is the worst yet to come?' *Medical Hypotheses 146*, 110469. Available at: https://pubmed.ncbi.nlm.nih.gov/33401106

Wynn, T.A. (2008) 'Cellular and molecular mechanisms of fibrosis.' *The Journal of Pathology 214*(2), 199–210. Available at: https://pubmed.ncbi.nlm.nih.gov/18161745

Xu, Y., Shen, J. and Ran, Z. (2020) 'Emerging views of mitophagy in immunity and autoimmune diseases.' *Autophagy 16*(1), 3–17. Available at: https://pubmed.ncbi.nlm.nih.gov/30951392

Yanai, H. (2020) 'Metabolic syndrome and COVID-19.' *Cardiology Research 11*(6), 360–365. Available at: www.ncbi.nlm.nih.gov/pmc/articles/PMC7666594

Yanuck, S.F., Pizzorno, J., Messier, H. and Fitzgerald, K.N. (2020) 'Evidence supporting a phased immuno-physiological approach to COVID-19 from prevention through recovery.' *Integrative Medicine (Encinitas) 19*(1), 8–35. Available at: www.ncbi.nlm.nih.gov/pmc/articles/PMC7190003

Ye, Q., Wang, B. and Mao, J. (2020) 'The pathogenesis and treatment of the "cytokine storm" in COVID-19.' *The Journal of Infection 80*(6), 607–613. Available at: https://pubmed.ncbi.nlm.nih.gov/32283152

PART 3

FLUID ADAPTATION

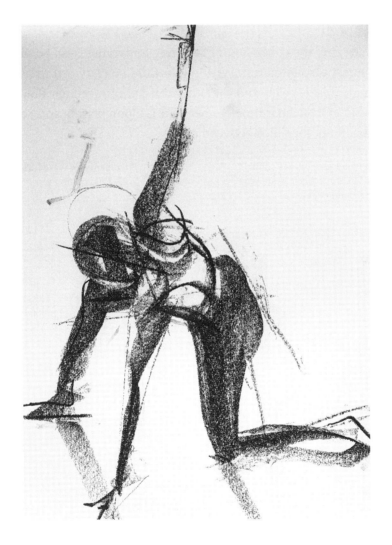

A journey through the ways in which our bodily fluids and fascia are part of the whole orchestration of breath and immunity. Exploring how these relate to the vagus nerve and nasal breathing for adaptive regulation and our full-on systemic response – how we cope with stress, how we move through life.

Settling into fluid qualities within our embodied practice is tapping into ancient rhythms and tides, back to the sea and the amniotic fluid that we evolved in suspension within; on species and personal levels. As Tias Little states: 'Water, like an awakened mind, has the capacity to encompass all things. This is Big Mind, also called the ocean of the heart. Like a mind that stays fluid and avoids fixation, the water way is boundless'.[1]

The fluid body

We are fluid – in fact, 55 per cent of the body for women, and 60 per cent in males. The rest is solid matter. Within that fluid body, two-thirds are intra-cellular fluids (inside cells), and the other third is extracellular fluid (outside cells). Of that extracellular fluid, 20 per cent is blood plasma and 80 per cent is interstitial fluid, the fluids between cells.

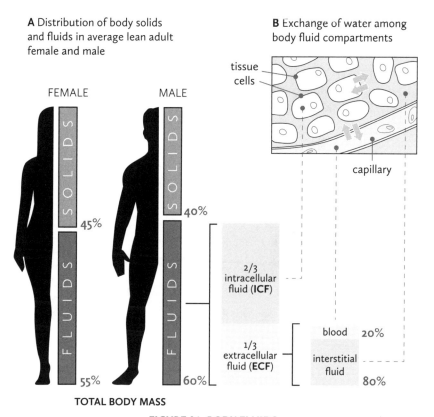

FIGURE 3A. BODY FLUIDS

---

1   Little (2010).

All these fluids must be kept in balance while providing nutrients to body cells. Homeostasis means keeping things the same within a functioning parameter, the process of keeping an organism alive and functioning by recalibrating balance according to the circumstances, environment, the moment. A more accurate term may be 'allostasis'; rather than this balance being one fixed point, recognising that equilibrium shifts and changes. Balance is subjective and relative, according to our changing energies and needs.

Extracellular fluid – minor components

Extracellular fluids move water and electrolytes throughout the body; the latter are the minerals sodium, potassium, calcium and magnesium, those that we need for electrical impulses through the nervous system. Of that extracellular fluid, minor components are lymph within lymphatic vessels (lymphatic fluid, including its immune components, lymphocytes; see Part 1) and transcellular fluid 'moving across', for example cerebrospinal fluid (CSF) in the spine, intraocular fluid in the eye, synovial fluid in the joints. Then we have protective fluids such as pericardial fluid around the heart, intrapleural fluid between the lungs, peritoneal fluid, which lines the abdomen and pelvic cavity, and digestive fluids. Hydration and fluid movement means smooth motion between the organs, 'slide and glide', for optimal function and ease of motion.

Interstitial fluid

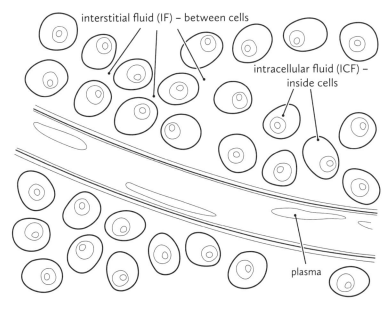

FIGURE 3B. PLASMA AND INTERSTITIAL FLUID

Around 11 litres of our body fluid is interstitial fluid – 26 per cent of our total body water – surrounding and between cells (extracellular). Considering we only have five to six litres of blood, it is a prominent aspect of the fluid body.

Interstitial fluid has the properties of a gel: striated with collagen fibres, it has protein as part of its structure, filled with tumbleweed-like proteoglycan filaments, all of which bind the water in (99 per cent of the water in interstitial fluid is 'trapped'), giving it structure and cohesion. The interstitial fluid structure also contains white blood cells for immune protection; something that is so prominent in the body needs to have this protective factor.

The interstitial organ

The interstitial organ, like the fascial organ (page 144), used to be overlooked, because when you cut into a body in dissection, these shrink away in the presence of oxygen. The interstitial organ is body-wide, but not boundaried (except by the 'edges' of skin) or easily drawn or quantified.

It connects to the lymphatic system, and current research points to it as a way that cancer cells spread throughout the body.[2] Evidence is growing in samples from people with cancer that various tumour types travel along the interstitium to different tissue layers (including lymph nodes). This may help to explain why cancers that start in one spot end up somewhere far away, despite having no clear path to do so.[3]

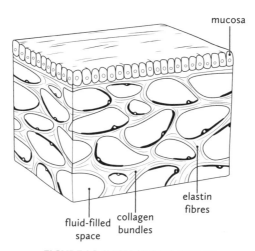

FIGURE 3C. INTERSTITIAL ORGAN

The interstitial organ is an effective 'highway' of fluid-filled spaces, and acts as a 'shock absorber' in places where the body expands and contracts, for example the lungs, aorta, digestive tract and bladder.

2   Yi *et al.* (2021).
3   Cenaj *et al.* (2021).

Lymph to interstitial fluid

Fluids are constantly moving through the body, changing their functions (and therefore what we call them) according to where they are contained. For example, 20 litres of plasma flow through the body's arteries, smaller arteriole blood vessels and capillaries every day. As blood circulates through the body, blood plasma leaks into tissues through the thin walls of the capillaries. Here it becomes interstitial fluid, delivering oxygen, glucose and nutrients needed to tissue cells.

After this nutrient delivery and removal of waste products, about 17 litres are returned to the bloodstream through the veins, but the remaining 3 litres seep through the capillaries and into the tissues. The lymphatic system collects this excess fluid, now called lymph, and returns it to the bloodstream via lymphatic vessels to the right and left (also called the thoracic) lymphatic ducts. These ducts connect to the subclavian vein, below the collarbone, which returns lymph to the bloodstream and helps to maintain normal blood volume and pressure. It also prevents the excess build-up of fluid around the tissues (oedema).

This balance of fluids is also linked to the kidneys, which filter fluids and are involved in the balance of electrolyte minerals (page 141), and the adrenals (on top of the kidneys: 'ad-renal'), which affect fluids via the steroid hormone aldosterone, which is why oedema can be related to stress. Oedema (fluid retention) is the key sign of inflammation – fluid movement helps to reintroduce natural flow between tissues and resolve inflammatory responses.

Lymphatic vessels operate like veins in that they work under very low pressure and have a series of valves to keep the fluid moving in one direction, but they don't have the pump of the heart, so they need movement. Where that isn't able to happen efficiently, fluid can pool into regions, and that becomes oedema or swelling. This might be seen in the lower body, where fluid pools with gravity, for example, the feet and ankles, unable to move back upwards. Lack of integrity within vessels or collagen fibres in the body can also cause fluid pooling.

Movement around the collarbone area, such as undulation into the thoracic spine and counter-rotations of the neck in twists (looking in the opposite direction to the rib cage), can help with this lymphatic emptying or drainage, as can dry brushing up to this area.

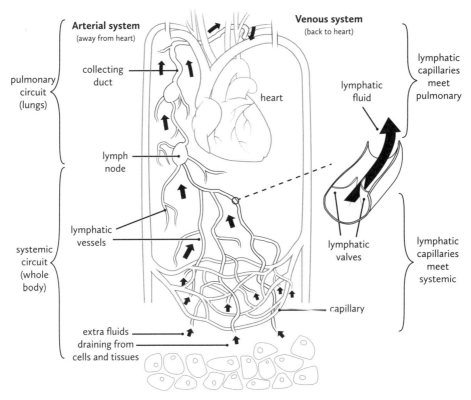

FIGURE 3D. LYMPHATIC FLOW

Fascia and lymphatics

The fascial organ is body-wide, a sensory organ. It is how we feel inwardly, our interoception, as well as how we sense outwardly, where we are in time and space, our proprioception. There is constant interplay between the interstitial fluid and the fascia. Tom Myers exlains: 'When tissue is squeezed – and it is squeezed through tension or compression, stretching or exercising, both do it – it is like wringing out your dishcloth at the end of the dishes. By wringing it out, you disperse all the dreck in the cloth and let new clean water in. It's the same with the tissue... Then the waste gets carried toward the liver by the lymph and vascular system, and the blood supplies new fluids to the tissue – whatever tissue it is.[4]

Fluid flows freely between lymph (when it's in the lymph vessels), to plasma (when it's part of blood), to cytosol (when it's inside a cell), to other specialties like cerebrospinal fluid (CSF), ovarian fluid, etc. The majority of water in the

---

4   Anatomy Trains (2017).

body is tied up in the fascia. This is where the fluid body and movement is really focusing into adaptive motion and hydration through the fascia.

The fluids in fascia are divided (controversially) into 'bound' and 'free'. Myers is among those who ascertain that 'free' fluids are those that are passing through fascia, while 'bound' water is that which is 'bound to the glycosaminoglycans (GAGS, mucous) part of the fascia, which binds water in the same way Jell-O binds water – to fern-like molecules that can bind a lot of water molecules (and affect millions more nearby)'.[5] Myers states that others consider all water in the body to be bound, but believes it is useful to distinguish between fluids that are 'free', moving through, and those that are bound in the tissues.

Hydration of fascia is vital, both by drinking plenty of water and eating that bound into plants, but also by squeezing or wringing old water out through the tension or compression of movement. This wringing out cleanses fascia and the waste is removed to the liver through the lymphatic and vascular systems. The movements we explore in this book, such as pulsing, compressing, squeezing, rocking – especially when close to the ground, not needing to hold ourselves up from gravity – are essentially more fluid; 'formless'. They promote fascial hydration, essential for our whole body's health.

Myers confirms the benefits of what we practise within somatic movements:

Make sure you're going through your body in a fairly systematic way – hence yoga asana routines, katas in martial arts, and workout routines in training, and all the exercises in a Pilates or Gyrotonics session. The other trick is get into unusual places in your body and make sure they are wrung out as well – which means varying your routine to find new places in your body that need a good squeeze. Bodyworkers and teachers can help you see the "forgotten" places if they are skilled, but you can also find them yourself by doing unusual things.[6]

Bonghan duct system

Within the fascia there is a vascular network independent of the lymphatic and blood pathways, called the Bonghan duct system, made of the same substance as fascia and believed to ease all body communication. This is currently being researched as potential for describing ancient meridian systems within the physical body.[7]

---

5   Anatomy Trains (2017).
6   Anatomy Trains (2017).
7   Soh (2009).

Fascial and interstitial hydration

A fluid body is an adaptable one; when brittle, dry, tense and rigid, we are left with poor shock dispersement and stress ripples through the organs. Fascia has shown to be responsive to change, undergoing continuous remodelling. For 'fascial hydration', a substance called hyaluronic acid (or hyaluronan) allows fascia to glide, locally or out into the whole system:

> Hyaluronan is produced by special connective tissue cells known as fasciacytes and can change its consistency from a thick gel to a watery lubricant. It therefore forms the synovial fluid – the substance that lubricates the joints in our knees, shoulders and hips, for example. Because hyaluronan is so effective at storing water, it also plays an important role in the proportion of fluid in the loose types of connective tissue. There are also high levels of this substance found in the spinal discs. Hyaluronan stores a lot of water between the collagen and elastic fibres in the skin, which is what gives faces that much sought-after plump, wrinkle-free complexion (which is why the substance is so popular in the cosmetics industry).[8]

Some researchers suggest that any change in this viscoelasticity – ability for fluid movement – activates pain receptors.[9] When tissues are dehydrated through lack or misdistribution of hyaluronic acid, the resulting viscosity can even become adhesive, altering the lines of forces within fascial layers. This has been offered as one of the causes of stiffness and pain on waking after sleep, more than joint issues that are often blamed. Matted fascia is an issue that increases with age:

> When the fascia matt up and stick together, it restricts our muscle function because the bundles of fibre are no longer able to slide past each other properly. This also interferes with the smooth transfer of energy from one muscle to the next, which in turn affects our coordination. This reduces the fluidity of our movements and uses up more energy. Our posture takes a hit too, as the reduced elasticity of the matted tissue makes us stiff. We now know that the majority of patients who suffer from back pain also have thickening and matting of the lumbar fascia.[10]

8   Schleip with Bayer (2021).
9   Stecco *et al.* (2013).
10 Schleip with Bayer (2021).

Tissue dehydration prevents proper removal of what are often termed 'toxins', but which are the by-products of respiration, energy production within each cell. These metabolites need to be removed efficiently for optimal function and could be equated with *ama* in Ayurveda, their build-up equated with states of disease. This accumulation has been shown to stimulate pain receptors and create a more acid environment within cells,[11] tightening fascia and creating a cycle of pain. This occurs alongside the release of inflammatory neuro-peptides, also associated with CFS/ME (chronic fatigue syndrome/myalgic encephalomyelitis).[12]

When tissues cannot slide, they show up as a fascial thickness under ultra-sound, linked to chronic pain that is not easily identified. This densification can eventually become fibrosis, the thickening and scarring of connective tissue, known to be caused by a chronically inflammatory environment, stress, trauma and immobility.[13] This pain and reduced slide-and-glide combination can also occur from scar tissue, operations, injury, inflammatory bowel disease (IBD) or other inflammatory disorders. Fluids can pool around these areas, as 'fluid retention' (oedema; page 143), but not hydrating fascia, only adding to pain and stiffness. To be released from continual cycles and to prevent their onset, we need fluidity, movement and the safety signals of a loose, pliable psoas.

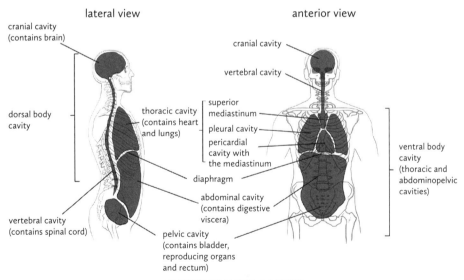

FIGURE 3E. BODY CAVITIES

Source: This illustration first appeared in Yoga Therapy for Digestive Health *by Charlotte Watts*

---

11   Stecco *et al.* (2011).
12   Rowe, Fontaine and Violand (2013).
13   Stecco *et al.* (2014).

For respiratory health, fascial fluidity, hydration and movement in the pleural cavity and in relation to the heart in the pericardial cavity (see the heart nestling between the lungs in Figure 3e) is vital. The pulsing, rebounding and twisting of the primal somatic movements in this section, where compression and release flood through tissues, are key to fascial hydration.

Fascia and inflammation

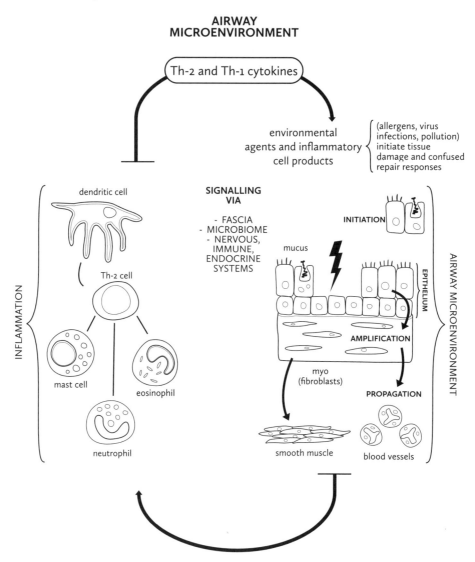

FIGURE 3F. INFLAMMATION CASCADE IN ASTHMA

In asthma, through inflammation, the bronchial fascia and epithelium become fragile and inflamed, which can include loss of the outermost epithelial layer.

Fascia is a crucial organ in relaying the coming down stages from the fight-or-flight response, and therefore immunity. Fascia conveys mechanical tension to help regulate inflammation that might be in response to injury or part of inflammatory conditions. Fascial fibroblasts activate the inflammation cascade via cytokines (see Figure 3f for an example in asthma); specific immune messengers (page 88) upregulated by stress: more inflammation relayed through the fascia in the presence of stress increases sympathetic action through lack of fascial glide – movement through the fascia – in protective 'bracing' responses. Sedentary behaviours tend to increase inflammation, having massive implications through the whole of our metabolism, switching on signals for inflammation. Sitting is said to be 'the new smoking' in terms of health implications.[14]

There is a ripple effect through the whole body's health when fascial tissue is affected by any of the following: visceral (from the organs and up through the enteric nervous system – our gut feelings); genetic predisposition; metabolic energy function; efficiency through the thyroid, the pancreas, blood sugar balance; vascular – through the whole circulatory system; and epigenetic issues (above or beyond genetic, so what happens in our lives that affects our body systems' expressions – lifestyle, diet, trauma).

Symptoms can show health deterioration beyond that which medical diagnostic methods would suggest. Often this is when people will get vague diagnoses for stress-related or idiopathic conditions, where there's no known cause, such as IBS, chronic fatigue, fibromyalgia or components of autoimmunity, where it's now being acknowledged that the fascial system is playing much more of a part than was previously acknowledged.

The *pancha kosha* model

This brings us to consider how the fluid body is seen in relation to yogic philosophy (and used as a cornerstone in yoga therapy[15]). This five-layered model (*pancha* = five, *kosha* = layer) describes layers of existence of the human experience. Looking at two of these sheaths can help us gain insight on our route into awareness via embodiment, within our context of the immune and respiratory systems. We can consider how the fascial and interstitial organs correlate to this view of the physical and subtle bodies.

14 Rodulfo (2019).
15 Finlayson and Hyland Robertson (2021).

The *koshas*
the five sheaths of human being

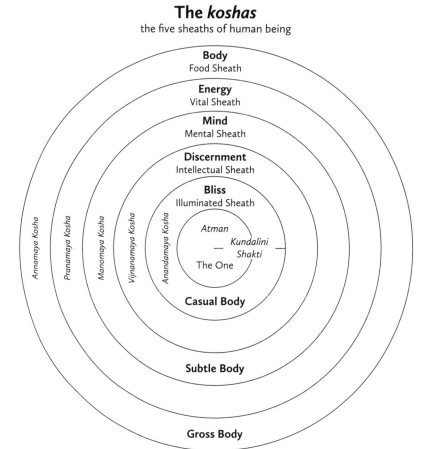

FIGURE 3G. THE *PANCHA KOSHA* MODEL

Current popular conceptions of the yogic body (from the *Taittirya Upanisad*) usually include that of the *sukshma sarira*, or subtle body, conceived as five *koshas*, or sheaths. These are the *annamaya kosha* (food sheath), *pranamaya kosha* (energy, life or vital sheath), *manomaya kosha* (mind sheath), *vijnanamaya kosha* (discernment sheath) and *anandamaya kosha* (bliss sheath).

Source: www.sahapedia.org; Mallinson and Singleton (2017)

Physical body: annamaya kosha

The material body, *annamaya kosha*, the 'physical matter' sheath, is where we most obviously push up against the external world. For many, this is mainly how they experience being themselves, rather than the more subtle, energetic sense of the fluid body. This is the more gross form of *prana* from food, water, air – it's easier to access.

Asana is the starting point in most modern yoga practices, accessing the physical. To access the deeper layers of the subtle body, we need to move beyond this physical (gross) body, to then recognise and move through our *samskaras*, our holding patterns (page 279).

Breath and fluid body: pranamaya kosha

Pranamaya kosha, the 'energy', 'life' or 'vital' sheath, where we meet the *pranic* or subtle body (where *prana* flows), is not just seen in this canon as the breath body but also as where the physical is fluid. This includes movement of blood, lymph, interstitial fluid and cerebrospinal fluid (CSF), in the skull-sacral tide throughout the spine (*sushumna*), digestive juices, menstrual flow and through fascia, which is where we might see meridians or *nadis* situated. And that pulse, that fluidity of breath and these constantly flowing vital fluids through the body are what gives physical matter shape and animation, the 'breath of life'. All this movement is what shapes the body; it is constantly moving and alive because of the constant flux of fluids.

The fluid body is connected to the five motor organs, to digestive function, which gives us our *agni* (fire); *bandhas* and *chakras*, where energy is coalesced and held, redirected; and the urino-genital, feet, hands, vocal organs and the excretory, what we literally let in and let pass. According to Indian scholar Sankarâchârya: 'Those who treat this vital force as divine experience excellent health and longevity because this energy is the source of physical life.'[16]

The more that we can recognise and tune into the spirit of inspiration (breath) and allow it to have space, the more we allow *prana* to flow with ease, not to be used up too quickly, promoting longevity.

The psycho-emotional realms of the mind (*manomaya kosha*) and the wisdom layer of discernment beneath the thinking mind (*vijnanamaya kosha*) are also part of the subtle body. Ultimately these are the route into awareness of the causal body (simply being, within the *anandamaya kosha*), that transports the essence of the individual from one life into the next reincarnation, through *samskara* and *karma*.

The polarity of fluidity and containment

Within the physical and breath/fluid states of being lies the polarity between fluidity and containment. Polarity may seem synonymous with opposite, but it is not either/or; rather, it is to recognise that you cannot have one without the other – you cannot have up without down, light without heavy. Viewing this through the *koshas*, within our breath practice, we might notice the containment of the physical body as the place that contains the movement of the breath, but not too rigidly; conversely, the breath animates the body. We want

---

16 Sankarâchârya (2018).

to feel that sense of expanse but, especially if there is trauma, to feel grounded through the physical, embodied – in the here and now.

This co-existent polarity is exemplified by the Taoist analogy of yin–yang, where the river doesn't exist without the yang of the banks and the yin of the water; one without the other is not a river, the balance between them continually changing and creating the next momentary outcome: 'The path of humanity is always coordinated with heaven and earth in the alternation of movement and stillness. Human energy is always in communion with heaven and earth in the alteration of exhalation and inhalation.'[17]

Different practices have different relationships between fluidity and containment. When we're lying on the ground, rolling in more somatic, fluid, practices, we're more formless, but then we need to come up from the ground to become more contained, more muscular, because this is how we move through the world. This containment can, however, become more rigid, brittle even, which doesn't allow us the more adaptive qualities of the fluid. This is when we can see patterns of sympathetic dominance and a greater tendency to inflammation and wearing out of body systems.

When we are overly contained (often from chronic stress, trauma or 'holding it all together'), this is revealed by movement (and thinking) that is less fluid. When we go into protective modes, we essentially become harder and smaller. Our outer shell can harden to protect us against the world, particularly if we're not fostering conscious awareness internally to allow release of these patterns.

Constriction for protection involves the body drawing everything in towards the centre, and can result in chronically restricted tissues and shrinking and bracing of structures overall. The diaphragm tightens and breath becomes shallow. Where there is trauma or chronic stress, hands and feet can be very cold as circulation is impaired with the body moving energy, oxygen and nutrients from the extremities back inward, towards the central nervous system and the core for protection.

Furthermore, strong tension can be felt at the base of the skull and bottom of the spine, interfering with cranial-sacral polarity, the tide of the spine, contributing to headaches, neck pain, jaw tension, holding around the temples and a bracing of the sacrum, which can interfere with full breathing, digestion and create lower back pain. We might see this manifest as people moving from the limbs rather than from the deep belly in a more integrated way, often with

---

17   Quoted in Cleary (2000).

accompanying shoulder and hip issues that don't allow reach out through the diagonals from the belly with ease.

These interruptions in the flow of *prana* may show up as lesions or adhesions in the fascia, where there is stickiness or disorganisation, experienced as movement, joint or organ dysfunction. In yogic terms, this is the physical manifestation of *granthis* (knots or doubts). The translation as 'doubt' highlights the somato-emotional connection, where something gets in the way of our own flow, as energetic as it is physical.

Granthi also translates as 'a difficult knot to untie',[18] which relates to *samskaras*, where we are entangled in preferences, desires and fears, our habits that get in our way, preventing us coming to our full potential, restricting spiritual as much as physical development. These are the barriers to freedom and liberation (*moksha*) that keep us entangled in our unconscious drivers, addictive cycles, fears, the sympathetic dominance of anxiety and rumination.

Knowledge and action are needed to unravel knots to consciousness and transcend their restrictions, noticing the physical blocks as an access to the more subtle levels of the fluid body; where we have the chance to resolve and dissolve deeply held patterns and habits. The *Hatha Yoga Pradipika*[19] instructs that these physical-emotional knots or blockages can be pierced by the practice of *bandhas*, which concentrate *prana* within the body.

Psycho-neuro-immunology

The modern way of looking at mind-body medicine starts to move past the more traditional medical perspective of 'mind over matter', which separates us out into the physical and emotional bodies. Psycho-neuro-immunology is a term that has been explored since the 1970s, of which the physician and trauma expert Dr Gabor Maté is a main proponent. His book *When the Body Says No*[20] explores the stress–disease connection, and *In the Realm of Hungry Ghosts*[21] he looks at the relationship between trauma and addiction. There is a focus on compassion as means of unravelling what we hold in the body as a result of trauma.

Dr Maté explains, 'Every emotion has a chemical correlate.'[22] We don't just emote and then the body has an experience over there, they are not separate entities. We feel emotions physically, and when we have a physical experience,

18   Swami Muktibodhananda (1998).
19   Swami Muktibodhananda (1998).
20   Maté (2019).
21   Maté (2018).
22   Maté (2019).

there is an emotional component. It may be that we don't access that, that we have become conditioned to think over feeling, which is how so many people make their way through life. Eventually we all have to listen to what is held in the unconscious, stored in the body. When the body stops functioning, this can be where there has been an absence of listening in, acknowledging the physical manifestation of emotions. This is particularly true of inflammatory and autoimmune conditions where deep listening and responsive rest are vital.

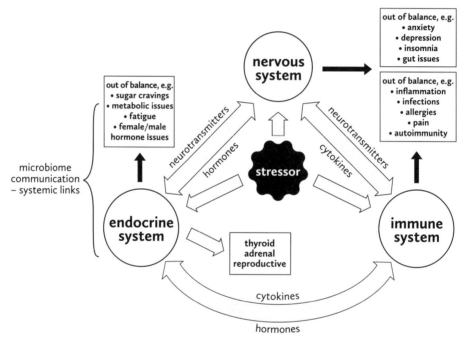

FIGURE 3H. PSYCHO-NEURO-IMMUNOLOGY

Connected systems

There is constant interplay between our psychological world, the nervous and immune systems, which is what gives us the term 'psycho-neuro-immunology'. Stress is always a part of the trauma response, where there is constant reliving of the original trauma as if it were in the present. This floods out into all systems: the under- or over-reactions of the immune system, seen as inflammation, infections, allergies or pain; anxiety, depression or sleep issues are the results of nervous system dysregulation – when inflammatory cytokines (page 88) get through the blood/brain barrier they have a very real and often depressive effect on our mood.[23] Their job there is to dampen down motivation

---

23   Liptan (2010).

(through lowering neurotransmitters such as dopamine) as a keen survival response; if the immune system is on such high alert, surely we need to slow down and recover?

The trouble is, we get stuck in this response and in low motivation, commonly seen with low-grade inflammation, where it is also a way to conserve energy as systems are running so high.

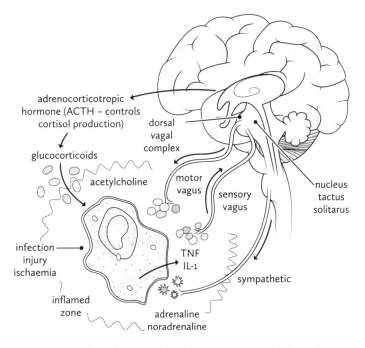

FIGURE 31. MODEL OF BRAIN IMMUNE INTERACTIONS
This shows how the nervous system responsively regulates inflammatory response to stress through constant, bi-directional communication between the autonomic, neuroendocrine and immune systems and the brain.[24]

Psycho-neuro-immunology view of the modern immune system

We evolved in nature, we are not separate from it, yet a lot of our modern evolution (the last 2000 years) has been about us dominating nature, largely separating us from the natural world. High psycho-social stress is linked to this reduced contact. Our microbiome (see Part 4) is predicated on this contact to the Earth and our immune system evolved to have contact with, to have constant assault – eustress, good stress – from our natural environment. The constantly changing elements of nature – cold, wind, weather, insects,

---

24 Cholinergic neurons are those of the parasympathetic nervous system (via the vagus nerve) and the neurotransmitter acetylcholine.

bacteria – are meant to challenge us at the periphery for healthy immune maintenance.[25] When we lack this relationship to the exterior (with cosseted warm clothes, houses and contained environments), stress tends to be directed into the gut and mind, often manifesting through the gut–brain axis.

The immune system can even stop seeing stuff at the periphery, for example a small cut on the finger that won't heal or skin issues that don't seem to resolve. This is why things like tapping, rubbing, pulling, squeezing, compressing, friction and touch are extremely important. Poor immune modulation or chronic fatigue can benefit from dry brushing the skin. Similarly in our somatic practices, where there is skin contact (touch and from the ground and our own limbs), this helps us to perceive the periphery again. Social engagement, where we touch others, brings down psycho-social stress, but positive self-touch can bridge the gap too (page 294).

Immune expression to emotion

Dr Maté equates many autoimmune issues with trauma, particularly where we were brought up not being able to say 'no', being unable to create a good sense of boundaries and self or autonomy: 'When we have been prevented from learning how to say no, our bodies may end up saying it for us.'[26] There is confusion in our sensing of boundaries that can manifest in the immune system left unable to distinguish 'self' from 'non-self'.

Dr Maté comments on how much of this is a reflection on how we treat disease in our society, our fractured social bonds, our lack of cohesion, highlighting how our social engagement is a huge part of our immune capacity:

> Our immune system does not exist in isolation from daily experience. For example, the immune defences that normally function in healthy young people have been shown to be suppressed in medical students under the pressure of final examinations. Of even greater implication for their future health and wellbeing, the loneliest students suffered the greatest negative impact on their immune systems. Loneliness has been similarly associated with diminished immune activity in a group of psychiatric inpatients.[27]

---

25   Pruimboom and Muskiet (2018).
26   Maté (2019).
27   Maté (2019).

Healing trauma in the nervous system

Following from Dr Maté's research, somatics offers an embodied response to held trauma in the body. Where the nervous system stays in a heightened and hyper-vigilant state, perceiving that a historic trauma is still current (as in post-traumatic stress disorder (PTSD)) or where everything is perceived as a threat, and there is no downregulation to calmer states, there can be huge overwhelm, which can manifest as inappropriate immune responses.

Childhood trauma (also see page 225) can manifest as structural dissociation, where the brain compartmentalises difficult experiences – the resulting inner fragmentation can create a dysregulated nervous system and conflicting senses of self. Cultivating compassionate awareness and presence, through repeated somatic and meditative practices over time, can bring a system back towards a regulated state.

In Somatic Experiencing®[28] (a body-oriented approach to the healing of trauma and other stress disorders, the life's work of Peter A. Levine, PhD), the concept of titration – slowly releasing energy – is explored, where repetition of rhythmic processes allows the participant to tune into internal sensations (contraction/expansion, pleasure/pain, warmth/cold) at a pace that allows the body-mind to build trust in its own safety. Slowly revealing the held beliefs or patterns that underlie habitual behaviour can be accessed through somatic movements, which continually bring us into the present.

Our sensory experiences are how we map our worlds. The olfactory nerve is the shortest of the cranial nerves, running from the nose to the forebrain. It conveys information relating to smell and is involved in the limbic system and memories. The olfactory nerve can trigger trauma – research has revealed that the olfactory system in the brain is biologically and structurally more sensitive to trauma cues than previously thought.[29] This exemplifies how complex our physical connection to emotional trauma can be, and how patiently we must approach releasing long-held trauma from the subconscious mind, stored deep in the physical body.

CASE STUDY: STRESS, SOCIAL INTEGRATION
AND VIRAL RESPIRATORY DISEASES
Dr Sheldon Cohen is professor of psychology at the Carnegie Mellon University in Pittsburgh, US, and has spent over three decades studying the

28 Payne, Levine and Crane-Godreau (2015).
29 Gottfried (2010).

connection between psychological stress and its impact on viral respiratory diseases.[30]

His research involves a thorough psychological assessment of his volunteers before they are placed in quarantine and exposed to viruses causing influenza or the common cold. The severity of the symptoms suffered by each individual is measured and compared with their pre-infection status.

Professor Cohen consistently finds that:

- People with the highest levels of long-term stress suffer more extreme symptoms than those with low stress levels.
- Smoking and low vitamin levels are linked to poor outcomes.

Factors associated with decreased risk include:

- Social integration: the degree to which an individual participates in a broad range of social relationships, generally defined in terms of the number of social roles one plays (for example spouse, parent, friend, fellow employee, volunteer, church member, etc.). This has been found to predict lesser mortality and lower risk for cardiovascular disease onset and progression. This is thought to be because social integration tends to boost positive psychological states that have beneficial effects on a range of disease-relevant physiology. Low levels of social integration – social isolation – is experienced as stressful.
- Social support: the amount of help received from family and friends, from practical help with basic chores, phone communication, to emotional support and more. This all improves our sense of self-worth by confirming that we are loved and cared for. Social interactions are vital to our humanity, and Professor Cohen's research shows they are vital for our immunity to disease.
- Physical activity.
- Adequate and efficient sleep.
- Moderate alcohol intake: interestingly, both teetotalism and excessive alcohol intake were both linked with worse outcomes. This may be because a drink or two tends to make us more relaxed and relieves stress for a time.

---

30   Cohen (2021).

The 'wandering' vagus nerve

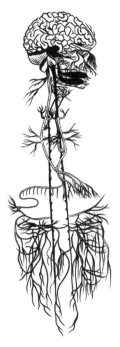

FIGURE 3J. VAGUS NERVE
Including brain and other cranial nerves.

Social engagement happens through the vagus nerve, which 'wanders' through the whole body, as its name means (the route of the word 'vagabond'). This is the 10th cranial nerve, part of the parasympathetic nervous system (PNS), innervated by the neurotransmitter acetylcholine. The vagus is the only cranial nerve to run out of the brainstem and down into the whole of the body, moving from the medulla (lower part of the brainstem) into the chest, the lungs, the heart, the diaphragm and the big bundle of nerves known as the solar plexus (see this within Figure 2a). It wraps around our heart and core areas, activating the PNS for the relaxation response and 'reset' after the stressor has passed, where we can drop back into the ventral (front) vagus, social engagement tones. This is 'putting on the brakes', allowing us to have the spaciousness and ease of reflection over impulse, open-mindedness.

In the brain, the vagus helps control anxiety and depression. In the heart, it controls heart rate and blood pressure. In the liver and pancreas, the vagus nerve helps control blood glucose balance. In the gallbladder, it helps release bile, which helps elimination and fat digestion. The vagus nerve promotes general kidney function and their localised release of dopamine. In the tongue, it helps to control taste and saliva; in the eyes, it helps to release tears; and it influences the release of oxytocin (page 294).

The vagus is our constant communication between the gut and the brain: this can be 'top-down', central nervous system (CNS) to enteric nervous system (ENS) in the belly via the vagus nerve, or 'bottom-up', gut to brain. Most of the communication, around 70 per cent, is bottom-up, highlighting the importance of listening to our gut feelings, the stuff of the unconscious, what is below the louder voices of the mind. We have the opportunity, listening in to those, to tune into the subtle body, the stuff of *samskaras*, through neuroplasticity. All the practices we're talking about offer us the potential to rewire that communication, although just like thoughts, some are the stuff of our conditioned survival responses; hence we listen in with compassion and discernment.

Soothing the vagus bundle

There is an extensive web of lymphatics all around the vagus at the base of the skull and also around the blood/brain barrier, the protective fascial casing around the spinal cord and brain. It is vital that fluids moving from the body into the brain don't take anything damaging along with them. Inflammation of the vagus nerve has implications in so many conditions, such as anxiety and panic, which are just starting to be uncovered, as explained in research by Schwager and Detmar: 'The lymphatic vasculature plays a crucial role in regulating the inflammatory response by influencing drainage of extravasated fluid, inflammatory mediators, and leukocytes.'[31]

We encourage healthy lymphatic and blood circulation around this area if when seated we lift up the back of the skull, also allowing our nose and mouth the optimal position to breathe nasally without strain, jaw soft. Either seated or lying, bringing our conscious attention to lifting the breastbone and dropping the chin to drop lightly towards this rise – *jalandhara bandha* (page 336) (with ease in the diaphragm and rib cage, softening around the eyes, jaw and front brain) – allows parasympathetic tone.

---

31 Schwager and Detmar (2019).

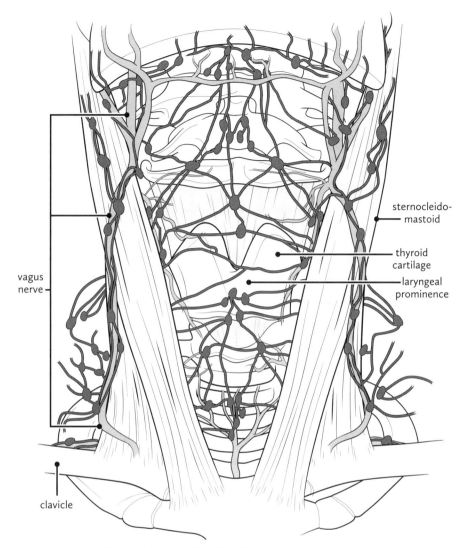

vagus
nerve

sternocleido-
mastoid

thyroid
cartilage

laryngeal
prominence

clavicle

FIGURE 3K. VAGAL LYMPHATICS AROUND THE THROAT

Polyvagal theory

Polyvagal theory was first suggested by Stephen Porges in 1994, and has changed the way in which we see the autonomic nervous system (ANS). It is a more useful model from which to elaborate the nervous system beyond the high of fight-or-flight or the low of rest-and-digest. This builds on the model of the triune brain (lower, mid and higher brain regions and function), which 1960s neuroscientist Paul MacLean had proposed as having evolved over time to control different functions of the body and nervous system.[32]

---

32   Roxo *et al.* (2011).

VVC (ventral vagus complex): social engagement system (facial expression and eye contact, *drishti*), presence, awe, wonder, creativity, connection, open-mindedness, healing – *sattva*.

SNS (sympathetic nervous system): fight-or-flight (doing mode, action with blood flow to muscles and brain via raised heartbeat), survival response, mobilisation, motivation, excitation, agitation, wearing down – *rajas*.

DVC (dorsal vagus complex): immobilisation, protective ancient freeze response via the viscera (gut feelings, absence of feelings), collapse or rigidity, check-out, dissociation, absentia, floaty – *tamas*.

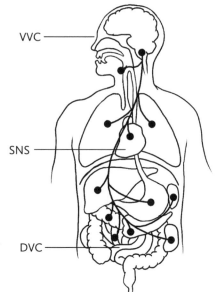

FIGURE 3L. POLYVAGAL ANATOMY
Source: This illustration first appeared in Yoga Therapy for Digestive Health *by Charlotte Watts*

Porges adds the importance of our social connection as pack mammals into the picture, replacing previous perceptions of the ANS. The ventral vagus complex (VVC) or the new vagus, at the front of the nerve, is more evolved, relating to social engagement – our first myelinated vagus parasympathetic circuit. In terms of the *gunas*, this is where we resolve things warmly, which we might equate with being more *sattvic* – aware, conscious and present, related to the eyes and seeing the world clearly and calmly. See the *gunas* related to polyvagal anatomy in Figure 3l, yoga therapist Marlysa Sullivan says: 'The relationship of the neural platforms and gunas helps to further a biopsychosocial framework for well-being'.[33]

If this approach fails, we devolve into a more primitive fight-or-flight response, where sympathetic circuits and adrenaline take over. This is more *rajasic*, related to the heart, that quickening of the pulse where we become more alert. It is active and fiery, and we need this to motivate us, feel enthusiasm and get up in the morning, but ideally, when it has been switched on by perceived danger, when we recognise that there is no real threat, we drop back into ventral vagus tone. Overactive sympathetic tone can be depleting and remove us from feeling able to be compassionate with ourselves or to others; we can have joy and excitement in life without depleting resources.

33   Sullivan *et al.* (2018).

Where there is prolonged distress, overwhelm or trauma, we can drop into our more primal, unmyelinated 'old' vagus circuit that causes immobilisation, freeze or dissociation. This state is *tamasic*, inert and listless, and is dorsal vagal mode. This is a protective state, related to the more curved shell of the back body, where we effectively 'check out', where animals play dead. Again, we need this quality in balance to come down from fight-or-flight, but if we live here, it can be the place of deep fatigue and disengaged states.

Note that this is not to be confused with 'spiritual bliss', referring to the high of the endorphin release we can receive in dissociated states. When meditative practices (still or moving) are ungrounded, out of body (particularly for those with trauma), this can create the delusion that dissociative experiences are connection, recognised by an 'out of body' quality. This can be a great place to hang out, as the dorsal vagal freeze response comes with a feel-good endorphin release. As Steve Haines says:

> One of the challenges with dissociation is that we simply don't recognise it – and this is especially true for people working within certain spiritual frameworks. This is because dissociation is an endorphin state, so it can actually feel amazing. We don't notice how disconnected we are because we have these chemicals inside of us that actually feel warm and floaty, and can be misinterpreted as transcendental, expansive experiences. Authentic experiences of growth and transformation include the body. Authentic flow states include the body, they aren't a separation from the body. And, luckily, the body is always available to return to.[34]

Cultivating our practice around real presence within the ventral vagus is also a route out towards post-traumatic growth. Recognising in life what triggers feelings of separation from feeling our feet, the ground, for instance, can allow us to consciously use practices that earth us, bring us back into the body and the real and attuned presence of ventral vagal tone.

Vagal tone – fluidity as adaptability in life and response

Vagal tone is really what we want to foster, to be able to drop back into ventral vagal mode often and easily, so that we have fluid, adaptive capacity – the smooth transition that those with chronic stress, trauma or sensory processing issues can have trouble accessing.

---

34   Haines (2021).

Vagal tone is inferred by measuring heart rate variability (HRV; page 132): heart rate speeds up a little on the inhalation, associated with the sympathetic nervous system (SNS); heart rate slows down a little on the exhalation, PNS tone. The bigger the difference between inhalation and exhalation heart rate, the higher the vagal tone, the more range we have, moving between states without jarring. The quality of transitions and the in-between spaces are vital within our practice, really occupying those liminal spaces, being present within the quality of transition:

- High vagal tone: within that relaxation after stress, we have better blood glucose regulation, reducing the likelihood of metabolic diabetes, stroke and cardiovascular disease, all of those bound up in ANS responses. It also relates to better mood, less anxiety, more stress resilience and adaptive capacity, so if something knocks us off course we can reroute quite easily, we have that emotional resilience. Studies have shown that high vagal tone is associated with greater closeness to others and more altruistic behaviour, because all of this comes from compassion. Our ability to recognise our own need for compassion is also affected.
- Low vagal tone: this is conversely associated with the diseases where we don't have adaptative capacities, such as cardiovascular conditions, strokes, depression, diabetes, chronic fatigue syndrome (CFS) and cognitive impairment. With low vagal tone there can be much higher rates of inflammation and autoimmune responses, showing as compromised immune modulation and conditions like rheumatoid arthritis, inflammatory bowel disease (IBD), endometriosis, autoimmune thyroid conditions, lupus, etc. People with fatigue, food sensitivities, anxiety and gut problems usually have lower vagal tones, reflecting where the vagus nerve is not able to perform its functions or adapt and drop back into social engagement. Connection with those we trust can help guide us back to regulation.

VAGAL TONERS

- Yoga, meditation, mindfulness.
- Humming, chanting, singing, speaking, gargling – vibration around the throat where the vagus comes back up into the brain. Speaking in

socially engaged tones helps us and others coregulate vagal tone (see 'Physical Practice' in Part 6).

- Nasal, abdominal and diaphragmatic breathing.
- Social interaction, touch, laughter, joy – we need this as pack mammals to give us a sense of safety, survival of the species.
- Massage – positive touch promotes vagal tone.
- Warm baths – womb-like support coaxes the nervous system to a place of safety.
- Cold (spritz showers, wild swimming), drinking cold water – stimulating the periphery, helps to promote immunity and regulate autoimmune disorders.
- Fasting – ketogenesis (a challenge for the body) eustress (positive stress; pages 101 and 155).
- Probiotics – to support immune signalling back to the vagus from the gut wall (see Part 4 on the microbiome).

APPLICATIONS OF VAGUS NERVE STIMULATION

Scientific research into the wide-reaching applications of vagus nerve stimulation is just beginning. Experiments in bioelectronic medicine are exploring how the vagus nerve can be stimulated with electrical currents to reduce inflammation – the 'inflammatory reflex' – with potential applications for autoimmune, metabolic and cardiovascular diseases.[35] In 2017, a patient was brought out of a vegetative state after 15 years through vagal nerve stimulation,[36] and there is evidence that stimulating the vagus nerve after a stroke can recover motor function.[37] Implants of electrical nodes that work as an artificial vagal nerve (stimulating vagal tone) have been effective for people suffering from anxiety, depression and autoimmune diseases.[38]

Breath and fluidity

Nasal breathing is supportive for vagal tone as it is more parasympathetic (see Part 1).

---

35 Pavlov and Tracey (2012).
36 Corazzol *et al.* (2017).
37 Engineer *et al.* (2019).
38 Liu *et al.* (2020).

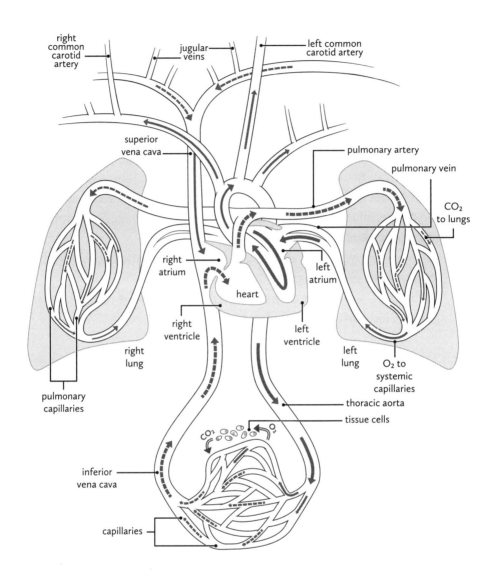

right
common
carotid
artery

jugular
veins

left common
carotid artery

superior
vena cava

pulmonary artery

pulmonary vein

CO_2
to lungs

right
atrium

left
atrium

heart

right
ventricle

left
ventricle

right
lung

left
lung

O_2 to
systemic
capillaries

pulmonary
capillaries

thoracic aorta

tissue cells

CO_2

O_2

inferior
vena cava

capillaries

veins bring CO_2 back to heart and lungs ----------
arteries deliver O_2 from lungs and heart to all cells and tissues ————

FIGURE 3M. HEART AND LUNGS

Nasal breathing – oxygenation benefits

Breathing through the nose is more oxygenating through higher nitric oxide production (page 44), as opposed to the mouth, which is much more about taking on food. Nasal breathing drives oxygen into the lower lobes of the lungs where there are more parasympathetic receptors and more pooled blood because of gravity, so better carbon dioxide exchange and release. Breathing nasally also uses less exertion (Borg Scale[39]), so is more oxygen-efficient, and this translates in exercise as better performance and shorter recovery time.

Physical benefits of nasal breathing

Nasal breathing involves engagement of the whole physical breathing apparatus: more diaphragmatic movement, the lower lungs and the entire rib cage moving to massage the heart and lungs. Full rib activation acts as a pump to pull lymph from the lower body up to the chest cavity and heart, promoting better circulation and immune protection. This is all crucial for a full range of motion and flexibility through the spine, head, neck and lower back, and if we have that capacity for flexibility that supports our breathing mechanisms, it supports our posture, allowing more nasal breathing. Like many things in our health, this function is cyclical: the nasal breathing supports how we move to support nasal breathing itself, and if any of these factors are interrupted, we can get caught in vicious cycles of immune and respiratory imbalances.

Nervous system pros of nasal breathing

The benefits of nasal breathing are profound for the nervous system, increasing alpha brainwave activity. Of the five levels of brain waves, alpha is related more to peaceful, conscious mindful or meditative states (not the very deep meditative, theta, state that we might go in after 20–25 minutes or might access through transcendental meditation), the place of creativity and mood elevation (page 348). GABA (gamma-aminobutyric acid), is a calming neurotransmitter that works within the PNS and blocks or inhibits certain brain signals, decreasing nervous system activity and regulating cytokines.

There is a wealth of research showing that yoga and mindfulness meditation practices increase GABA levels in the body,[40] and that nasal breathing increases brainwave coherence: more calm mind states, integrated, effective thinking and behaviour; our ability to get along with others and to see different sides, to switch ways of thinking; intelligence, creativity, learning ability, emotional stability and self-confidence are supported. Nasal breathing is said to be related to a significant reduction in sympathetic states and high limbic (vigilant) brain states, so is hugely impactive on our immune and respiratory health.[41]

---

39 Hallani, Wheatley and Amis (2008).
40 Streeter *et al.* (2012).
41 Zaccaro *et al.* (2018).

Mouth-breathing issues

Mouth breathing bypasses all the important stages in the breathing process. It is injurious to the tissues lining the respiratory tract and the oral cavity, bringing cold, dry, dirty air and pollutants in the air in through the mouth, which doesn't have the capacity of the nasal cavity to protect us. The mouth's mucous linings need to stay moist – saliva is a huge immune component in the mouth, but this is dried out by mouth breathing. This can result in sleep apnoea and possibly misdiagnosis of attention-deficit hyperactivity disorder (ADHD), as mouth breathing can keep us stuck in sympathetic dominance. Prolonged mouth breathing has also been related to changes in the musculoskeletal structure of the face and the teeth.[42]

Many of the roots of mouth-breathing issues are postural: when the head is habitually pushed forward of the spine and the chin juts out, this causes a lot more tension in the throat and less room for the air to flow freely into the nasal cavities, creating a feeling of gasping for air through the mouth. This can derive from nasal issues such as a deviated septum or broken nose, anything to do with excess mucus (which can be nutrition related, such as dairy or other intolerances, and dehydration, which tends to produce more mucus and is inflammatory because it tends to set off a histamine cascade), as well as things like colds, polyps, enlarged tonsils and adenoids (lymphatic nodes in inflammation or overload), inflammation and poor immune modulation seen around the nasal and upper respiratory area, manifesting as hay fever, sinusitis, rhinitis, asthma and allergies.

Habit is also a factor in mouth breathing: where we get used to things as we have been doing and it can be hard to unravel, especially when that is laid down in our fascial and muscular patterns. Mouth breathing can be a habit formed around keeping things in sympathetic dominance, constantly doing, alert, where we get used to living in that tone of the nervous system; it is familiar and we can therefore register it as feeling more 'safe', with rest states feeling less so. Many avoid rest, slower forms of yoga or meditation for this reason.

---

42 Lieberman (2014).

The posture of fluidity or inflexibility

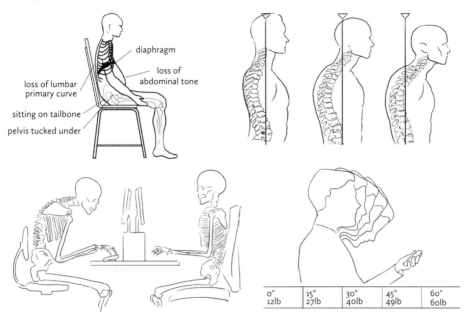

FIGURE 3N. MODERN POSTURAL HABITS

Head tending to shunt forward of the shoulders and neck: 'tech neck' with rounded upper back,
collapsed chest and loss of easeful abdominal support – note that compensation via repetitious 'core
work' contracting the abdominal muscles may further exacerbate difficulty lifting up through the
front body and allowing the head to 'float up' above the rib cage.

Source: This illustration first appeared in Yoga Therapy for Digestive Health *by Charlotte Watts*

In Figure 3n we can see postural issues that come from slumping on chairs: a
loss of abdominal tone, less diaphragmatic movement and less natural lifting of
the chest. In the bottom left-hand corner of the diagram, the skeleton hunching
over the computer has to lift the chin to see the screen, to be front facing, which
then makes mouth breathing more likely to get air in through the collapsed
airways and chest (as well as compression at the base of the skull – where the
brain stem and vagus nerve are housed).

The 'tech neck' of the bottom-right diagram shows that when the ears aren't
calibrated up above the shoulders – as they are designed in order to hold the
weight of a heavy head – the more the head drops forward (often to look at a
device), the more weight is put on the cervical spine. In the most acute angle,
the one that's most pushed forward and down at about 60 degrees, an extra
60 pounds of weight is pushing onto the back of the neck, a recipe for tension
and headaches. As Tias Little states:

Given the fragility and highly sensitive nature of its vessels, glands, and nerves, the neck and throat together are a common repository for strain. Veritably, this area is a potential perfect storm, for not only is it prone to musculoskeletal strain but due to its proximity to the brain it is vulnerable to the high winds of psychological tension. It is common for emotional turbulence including worry, anxiety, and fear to constrict the throat. Traditional yoga practices make us aware that the throat chakra is a critical conjunction of energetic forces, and only by unbottling the neck can prāna in the subtle body flow unconstrained.[43]

The ideal posture that you see as the first of the three side views at the top right of the diagram makes it easier for the shoulders and chest to lift easily with freedom through the throat and nasal passageways. The fluidity this allows for the breath will correlate with greater fluidity, flow, in all parts of the body, including the nervous system: 'Changes in posture can affect the resting length of the diaphragm, which is corrected through increases in both diaphragm and abdominal muscle activity. Furthermore, postural alterations can diminish airway patency, which must be compensated for through increases in firing of particular upper airway muscles.'[44]

43   Little (2016).
44   Yates *et al.* (2002).

PHYSICAL PRACTICE: PRIMAL MOTIONS – LUNGING, STEPPING AND SQUATTING

Somatic movement follows natural gestures, patterns and the range of motion that we need for basic and optimal function. It also looks to unravel patterns of holding, stress, trauma, tension and forgetting (absence) in the tissues by taking us back to before that story imprinted and took over as 'normal'. In meeting our default setting as a functionally moving human being, we have the opportunity to relearn patterns held deep in our personal and species evolutionary programming. This is where we can access neuroplasticity and the flexible adaptation that is the creative, open-minded and playful tone of the ventral vagus mode.

As Bessel van der Kolk says in *The Body Keeps the Score*; 'In order to change, people need to become aware of their sensations and the way that their bodies interact with the world around them. Physical self-awareness is the first step in releasing the tyranny of the past.'[45]

In terms of natural movement patterns, as modern humans we are often (if not mostly) in postural habits that have wandered far from our original design and function. The word 'primal' is used to describe movement, diet and lifestyle that is considered to be 'the original' in terms of either our individual or species evolution. This can relate to how we evolved from fish, to reptiles, to four-legged mammals, through to primates, and still have these animals' types of motions within our range. We move through these same patterns from our foetal shape within the womb to the full expression of upright human within our own lifetime.[46] Life experiences, stresses, traumas, criticisms, judgements, comparisons and other conditionings can support or interrupt how we stand upright; how we may need to protect ourselves or keep ourselves small can affect our whole-body expression. A common trauma (and shame) pattern held in body tissues, for example, can be collapse in the chest and hunched posture.

Body psychotherapist Stanley Keleman[47] explains: 'Human uprightness is a genetic urge, yet it requires a social and interpersonal network to be realised. Put another way, what nature intended as the development and expression of human form is influenced by personal emotional history.' If movement is how

---

45   van der Kolk (2015).
46   Valentini *et al.* (2019).
47   Keleman (1985).

we make our way through life rather than something we do, we can view it more as gesture than mechanical form. This helps us break away from moving in tight, hard and limited motion ranges that can be far removed from the reaching, pulsing, spiralling, shimmying, shaking, swaying, pushing and pulling gestures of natural motion. If we sit rigidly on chairs all day and then limit our movements to similar, set exercises at the gym or activities such as running and cycling, we are limiting our potential tissue adaptability, leaving us more prone to injury: 'We are built to contradict the force of gravity, but also to perform a broad spectrum of different movements. If one of or both of these elements is missing in our lives, our bodies respond with degeneration and illness.'[48]

Even following similar patterns in movement systems such as tai chi, yoga or pilates, we may become literally set in our ways, shapes and capabilities. Changing body movement habits and including all animalistic forms in our evolution supports basic functions; cardiovascular, immune, respiratory and nervous systems and endocrine (hormone) balance and optimal health.

Primal movement as pleasure and play

There is little evidence specifically on primal movement; most results are anecdotal, from those who have trained for years and found that shifting movement patterns from more mechanically based (and focused on specific body parts or regions), to more fluid and primal, reduces injury, increases body awareness and relation to self. This means that rather than viewing our bodies as separate to 'us', as we are conditioned to, we can feel our whole being ('body-mind' or 'mind-body') from the inside.

This extends into our body relationship. When we are children, we simply move and play, with no specific purpose beyond exploring, reaching, expressing and responding to our present-moment experience in ways that give us joy and a sense of freedom. Play is creative and not limited to a specific endpoint or goal; we shut down this spectrum of possibility as our movement and 'games' lessons at school become about the specific rules, competing and getting the 'form' right for best performance.[49] Many follow this into fitness regimes that target specific areas to fix what is perceived as 'wrong'.

More playful and responsiveness activities, such as climbing, explorative yoga (for example, Scaravelli), watersports and rough terrain hiking, involve

---

48   Schleip with Bayer (2021).
49   Tortora (2019).

the whole body and myriad shapes, responding moment to moment. Stepping away from counting and fixating on numbers of steps, calories, minutes and repetitions helps shift our viewpoint from what we 'should' be doing to how to listen in and respond. It is not bad *per se* to want to walk a certain number of miles or feel more physically able in a yoga pose, but if that takes over as the primary focus, it can create a relationship that we must punish our bodies towards body ideals or comparison with others.

Play is bouncy and elastically responsive in quality, as Robert Schleip says: 'Exercises that effectively train the elastic storage capacity of fascia not only make our movements springier, but also restore springiness in the architecture of our fascial tissue.'[50]

Imposing our will on our bodies to simply make them do more (often with pain and injury) can also be the relationship we expect from fitness professionals. We can be accustomed to being told what to do and doing it even if it doesn't feel right, because surely they know best? But no one can feel the experience within our body for us. When we trust our instincts (primal messages), we can move in ways that are playful and curious instead, without pushing beyond our healthy (or current) range of motion – parts that have felt previously stiff, sore, painful or shut-down can begin to loosen, open up and soothe signals of distress. Playful movement is known to promote adaptability, injury prevention, strength, balance, agility, coordination, speed, skill and mental focus, and a little can go a long way.

Daryl Edwards, who developed the Primal Play™[51] methodology to help people unravel from rigid movement patterns, says: 'Primal people danced, celebrated, competed, hunted, walked, dealt with nature – and played. In incredibly creative and fascinating ways. You can still see our human past in what we do today. Music, drumming, hiking, camping, fishing, swimming, gardening, sports, laughter, even dancing in dance clubs, all tap into the primal part of us.'

Dance and group games are often the most accessible modes of play for adults, where embodiment, fun, joy and laughter are involved to include the release of feel-good chemicals such as beta-endorphins and other endogenous (self-produced) opioids. According to the somatic therapist Jim Feil:

Life makes shapes. These shapes are part of an organizing process that embodies

---

50 Schleip with Bayer (2021).
51 www.primalplay.com

emotions, thoughts and experiences into a structure. This structure, in turn, orders the events of existence.[52]

We produce our own cannabidiol (CBD, the chemical in cannabis that has medical properties) in the form of endocannabinoids (precursors to endorphins) that are released during and after physical activity. Endorphins are like a natural analgesic and block pain signals. Interestingly, endorphins are elevated even more when playing, and even more when playing with someone else. These increase our feelings of wellbeing and social inclusion, and are known to relieve depression, anxiety and stress-related symptoms such as inflammation and chronic pain.[53,54,55] Indeed, as George Bernard Shaw said, 'We do not stop playing because we grow old; we grow old because we stop playing.'

Crawling

Four-legged, mammal-like motions from crawling, gathering strength, drawing the limbs underneath the hips and shoulders, allow us to lift off the ground and look around, involving the more emotional brain – moving towards and away from that we deem safe or unsafe. The cross-lateral (across the centre, different on each side) nature of crawling develops the bridge (the corpus callosum) between right-brain and left-brain hemispheres and left–right mastery of the limbs. There is new, conscious use of the skeletal muscles, and we can revisit crawling motions (especially with pandiculations; pages 56 and 290) to rewind back to when we laid down these patterns. If crawling was dysfunctional, we can find new, conscious function, and if any dysfunction occurred after our crawling phase, we can reset back to when we had this ease.

Squatting

In primate-like motions such as sitting and squatting, head upright from the ground, we can rest and stay alert. For primates, this means retaining the use of the hands, and for humans, our opposable thumbs. Squatting is a primal position for stability on the ground through the feet and weight of the pelvis, and needs a range of motion through the ankles, knees and hips – we can regain this motion through somatic practices where the weight is not on these areas, and then build up weight bearing there through other primal sitting

---

52 Quoted in Walsh (2019).
53 Balsevich, Petrie and Hill (2017).
54 Mechoulam and Parker (2013).
55 Kaur, Ambwani and Singh (2016).

postures, such as 'z-legs' (page 119) and '4-sit' (page 176). These positions (not chair-sitting) are our most natural arrangement.

Walking

Walking is the fruition of movement for humans – all of our movement patterns self-organise to reach this point and calibrate through our spinal curves up from the ground. Gravity is a continual force pushing down on us, and our ability to lift up against it relies on ground reaction force. This is the force the ground exerts upwards, away from the Earth's core, and is stronger through the body when we are still. Movement lessens this strain and relieves compressive transmission forces through the body, especially through the spine as the structure that supports vertical positioning. Somatic practices can help us feel how to move with most ease with the forces that move through us and our organisation with them.

Back to his seminal book on how trauma is stored in the body, *The Body Keeps the Score*, Bessel van der Kolk says: 'As I often tell my students, the two most important phrases in therapy, as in yoga, are "Notice that" and "What happens next?" Once you start approaching your body with curiosity rather than with fear, everything shifts.'[56]

Primal movement from the fluid body

It is the inherent fluidity of the interstitium (page 142) that allows such movements. Interstitium is said to have the following qualities:[57]

- Viscosity – dissipates sudden forces, minimising tissue damage in shock or injury.
- Elasticity – allows tissues to change shape and then reform as needed.
- Plasticity – allows remodelling after changes, for example, gravitational forces in posture, or scarring from a wound.

These are fluid responses we can explore and even reorganise in practice, as we shift our weight and shape in relation to gravity and the ground.

---

56   van der Kolk (2015).
57   Myers (2018).

4-sit shape stepping into lunge

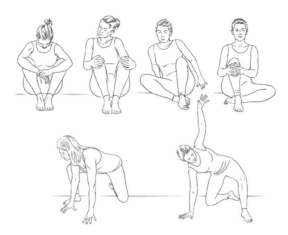

The movement of stepping is preparation for the physical patterns of walking, which sets off pumping actions through the fascial and interstitial organs. Getting down to the ground, moving through squatting positions towards lunges, is in our natural functional design, unlike the collapse, rigidity or stagnation of many hours sitting on chairs or slumped on sofas.

The uplift and movement through the lymphatics and around the diaphragm is much freer in these more primal movements than nearer to the ground – where we start to feel out the space around us and up towards the sky as we realise, recognise and organise our shifting weight in relation to gravity.

1. Start in an upright foetal position; take your time to arrive into your seat and feet, a bind around the front of the knees to allow the head to drop towards the cave of the belly, connecting to your breath there with soft jaw and eyes. This is a very passive squat, more dorsal, where we don't need to lift the front of the spine. Dropping into a protective stance cues the parasympathetic nervous system and draws our focus inwards. Allow the noise of the mind to settle into the tide of the breath, down towards the belly.
2. Gently rocking this side to side, begin to play with a sense of movement, waking up nerve endings where we connect to the ground. Hold the knees and rotate the ribs around to create pliability around the diaphragm area, rolling the shoulder blades, undulating through the shoulders. Release the tongue, jaw and face in any expressive way you feel.

3. Sit in a '4-sit' shape, one leg bent on the floor, the other foot crossed over on the ground, knee up. Swap side to side, rocking back to take the feet up as we shift easefully, fluidity in the breath. Feel the circularity of the sitting bones to encourage fluid movement upwards, trusting your body to find its way over these 'heels' of your seat.

4. Start stepping the foot further away and shifting your weight forward towards a natural lunge. Again, move this forward and back, side to side, in a creeping forwards and backwards movement. This brings a more fluid, formless exploration to how we shift weight in relation to the ground – there is no need to line up in any specific way; each shape might be quite different, a sense of curious play.

5. As you come forwards bring up the same arm to the front leg, turning through the belly and the chest. Keep this moving side to side and play with different foot and arm positions, feeling pliability in the psoas here.

6. Returning to the foetal position, notice the rise of *prana* as electricity or tingles in the body after movement.

Shoulder, upper back and neck release

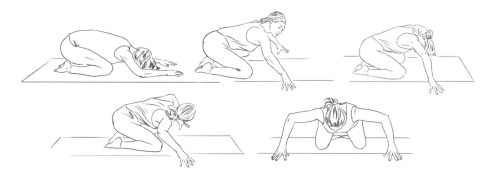

When we can hold such deep patterns of stress in the shoulders, neck and jaw, this reptilian stance in the upper body offers a responsive stage to meet and enquire into these. Fingertips on the ground both enlivens the hands (*hasta bandha*, gathering up through the palms) and provides a playful platform where you are free to move up from a responsive relationship through the arms, open across the collarbone, front and back chest areas.

From there you can recognise, and gently exaggerate, stress and protective holding patterns – for example, squeezing into tight shoulders, frowning or clenching the jaw – to remind tissues to go full circle and release from stuck tensions. Feel into any places where there may be *granthis* (knots), where you might pulse a little, roll into, shake or move through, including the tongue, lips, nose, cheek, sinuses and around the eyes.

1. Come to *balasana* (child's pose) as another soft squat, or foetal position, with the legs wide enough to drop the ribs in the cradle of the thighs in a womb-like way. Feel the fluid pulse of the breath.
2. Gather the belly of the spine up just high enough to take your arms out from the shoulders, out wider than a yoga mat, a long line, elbow to elbow. Come up onto the fingertips to feel *hasta bandha* (gathering up through the palms), where there is a sense of play (place hands higher onto a chair seat if needed) and connection with active fingers.
3. Move in any way that allows exploration of the shoulder girdle, the neck, base of the skull and tongue, even bringing in *simha pranayama* (lion's breath; page 369).
4. Come higher on the fingers and hammock the chest between the shoulders, releasing the head down.

All-fours – freeing up body tissues

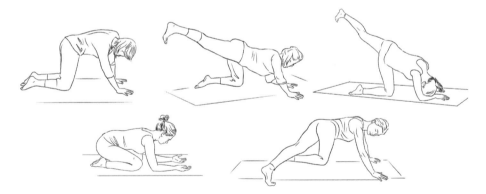

The mammalian position – all-fours, limbs stacked under their major joints of hips and shoulders – mimics the belly, heart and throat protection that most mammals (apart from us!) come to in survival mode, even when they can stand up on two feet.

Expanding movements from the belly out through the hips to the legs goes through the same journey we humans do from the ground, a chance to come to new stories rather than be governed by the routes we took in the past. With curiosity as our guide, we can explore the myriad ways we can unform and reform even within a particular starting position. When we adapt to each moment, we can find the agency where there is no 'right or wrong'; rather, feeling what the body needs moment to moment, without attaching to any end point, or needing to get anywhere.

1. From all-fours, move in any way that feels good through the shoulders, hips, neck and ribs, into the face, neck, jaw and eyes, releasing any sighs, yawns, noise or other expressions of nervous system release. Rotate the tailbone in each direction, feeling how this loosens tissues in the pelvic floor, diaphragm, throat and back of the skull (page 128).
2. Feel free to crawl around in all directions to integrate all parts, squeezing and opening to pandiculate any time that feels organic.
3. Lift each leg in turn for free movement, letting the elbows bend as needed, to be able to move through all planes available from the places you are rooted.
4. Bend the elbows as the leg extends, countering the weight of the head and the pelvis. Activate the postural muscles at the front of the leg, reaching through the psoas, or any response that spontaneously arises as you listen in to your body.
5. Rest into *balasana* (child's pose) onto the forearms to rest the wrists between sides, lengthening between the breastbone and the pubic bone with the arms supporting here, in a squatting motion.
6. Step one leg back and across the body to lengthen the whole side, including the neck, as to look around to see the foot. Also feel the side movement into the spine, releasing tension as you step this out side to side, before resting back at the midline.

Lunging to foot-walking action

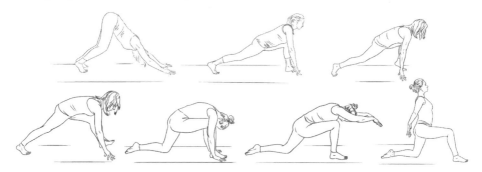

Deep squatting is vital for healthy digestion (and therefore the gut microbiome) as it relieves abdominal and anal tissue strain (when we sit up on a toilet seat, rather than squat to defecate, the puborectalis muscles choke the rectum, causing congestion). Leaning the torso forward, while bending the knees to drop the hips, is a deeper angle than most people reach. Refamiliarising the body with this motion through lunges can encourage the muscular actions needed for bowel movements; engaging lower abdominal muscles massages the colon, reminding it to get going where constipation is an issue or creates an awareness of containment where loose bowels occur – supporting our ability to hold back or let go, as appropriate.[58]

Here, we also play with ankle pliability – so important for deep bends in the hips and knees, but also for ease in the nervous system from the ground up. Shifts in body weight distribution through the feet encourage responsiveness and tension release in the tissues stacking up from the feet when we come to upright positions and movements.

1. Coming into *adho mukha svanasana* (down-face dog), explore with fluidity before settling into a still place, letting go of any focus to 'get the heels down', rather feeling space between the pubic bone and the breastbone, and letting the legs arrange themselves and play.

2. Inhale one knee in towards the chest and exhale to step the foot between the hands (or through all-fours), feet hip-width apart, front foot facing forward, coming up onto fingertips (or hands onto blocks); you can bring the back knee down if you need. Move back and forwards through the hips, exploring a 'walking' motion on the

58   Watts (2018).

front foot – lifting the heel as the hips come forward and shifting onto the ball of the foot, moving onto the heel (front foot raising) as the hips move back. Keep a deep bend in the knee to explore the ankle pliability required for the important natural movement of squatting and lunging.

3. Drop the back knee, softening the hands, upper body over the front thigh, head released. Tune into inner rhythms as you feel the shifts and adaptations of a gentle balance.

4. On an exhale reach the arms forward, leading with the wrists to open into the back body.

5. Inhale to draw the arms back (with fingers expressive) and open the front body, with arms about 45 degrees out to the side, so their length and weight naturally open across the collarbone. This is a helpful position to encourage the inner edge of the shoulder blades to draw down the back and find easeful opening of the front heart space.

Low *vinyasa* salutation

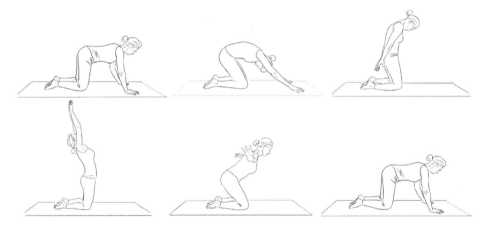

This low and soft salutation creates a rippling movement through all body tissues up from the knees, centring and grounding as we alternate extension and flexion (as undulation), naturally stretching and massaging the region around the diaphragm and stomach junction.

This sequence can be used as an alternative to the usual *vinyasa*, sparing shoulder, wrist and neck tension that can easily build if going into *chaturanga dandasana* (low plank) and *urdhva mukha svanasana* (up-face dog) on top of the postural effects of secondary breathing and psycho-social stress. It can also pre-pare for these stronger sequences, offering a similar skull–sacrum connectivity.

1. From all-fours, folded blanket under the knees if needed, wriggle the hips and shoulders to loosen the joints. Feel the belly area between the hip bones and lower ribs, where movement will be initiated.

2. Drawing the belly into the spine, drop backwards, rounding the back to drop the head and draw the weight off the hands.

3. Continue drawing the belly back and up, to raise up onto the knees, up through the inner legs, spine and neck, taking the arms out and up, rolling up the front body, looking up just to where the neck is comfortable.

4. Bend at the hips and drop the bottom back, spine lengthening tail-bone to crown, arms back out and down. Engage the 'square' of the belly between the hip bones and lower ribs to support the lower back and bring the hands down onto all-fours.

5. Continue the sequence at an easeful pace, staying to hold and breathe fully in any position that needs exploration or opening.

Twisting the viscera

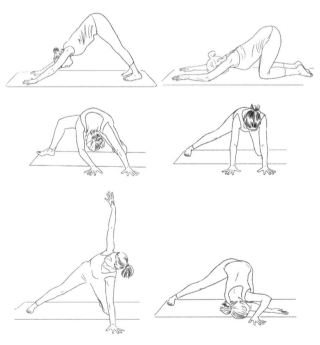

The resting pose here, with the centre of the forehead to the ground, activates the trigeminal nerve there. This cranial nerve has ophthalmic (eye), maxillary (upper jaw) and mandibular (lower jaw) branches as well as autonomic fibres and activation of the vagus nerve. You can rock the head side to side to further stimulate parasympathetic activity, ensuring it is possible via space at the base of the skull and between the back teeth.

This is a useful place to orient back to between movements that open us out to the world and may create strong feelings as we engage the inner legs, hips and take weight on to a knee. Time to soothe any heightened experience can help weave adaptation and resilience into our neural landscape, offering modulation to breath and immunity.

1. Come back to a playful exploration of *adho mukha svanasana* (down-face dog), listening in to respond and play through the fascia.

2. Drop down to the knees and forearms, forehead to the ground, dropping into the area between the shoulder blades, decompressing the lower spine through this inversion, softening the heart, allowing lymphatics to move from the lower body to the torso with the ease of gravity.

3. Gather back up to all-fours and take the right leg out to the side, front toes in line with the knee, left thigh bone angled in. Lift the right heel and explore rolling over the ball of the foot between an open lunge and squatting, rotating in and out through the thigh bone within a comfortable range of motion. From there you can move in any way at all, feeling out different positions with the foot, hip and anywhere that ripples out from here.

4. With the right leg outstretched (gathering up through the instep and inner leg, outside of that foot parallel to the edge of the mat), lift up through the right side of the body, unfurling the arm, keeping the chin in line with the breastbone. Thread the right arm through, under the left armpit, allowing the left arm to bend to drop down. Continue the movement, unfurling up on the inhale, exhaling to furl down. Check the neck is not moving independently of the shoulders – chin a little drawn in towards the chest, length from the pubis to the breastbone. Soften the eyes, steady the *drishti* (gaze) as the position of the face moves. Come through bridging at the midline (that feels appropriate for your energy) before repeating on the other side.

Prasarita padottanasana (wide-legged forward standing fold)

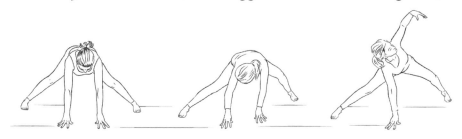

Drawing up from the insteps (*pada bandha*, foot lock or gathering) wakes up the inner channels of the legs up into the soft spaces of the pelvic floor and psoas–diaphragm matrix area. You can innervate there by lifting and spreading the toes, playing with the weight onto the fronts of the heels, so hand contact stays light. Coming to a raised (half) version of this wide-stride forward bend, we have the room to explore subtle shifts and allow for the evolution through whole-body movements.

1. Place your fingertips onto the ground or a chair (under your shoulders) with feet parallel, as wide as comfortable for your knees, exploring the length between the pubic bone and the breastbone.
2. Explore shifting weight side to side and deeply bending one leg, lifting that heel, allowing the heels to move, walking the hands further into a deep squat to each side.
3. Twist towards the knee that is bending deeply, lifting the same arm as the bent leg, reaching with a bent arm for ease through the shoulder, moving side to side, pumping the heart, but not registering as a sympathetic response, staying easeful.
4. Reorganise around the midline on the return to centre.

Parivrtta parsvakonasana (revolved side-angle pose)

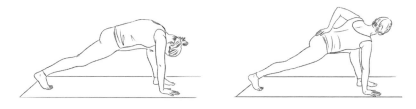

Back leg strong, front leg balanced allows support for the upper back and head to release down. Feeling the support of a three-point contact with the ground, we can drop our attention more inwards towards the breath in the spine. Lifting the head can then evolve as we feel the length of the body awaken from the outstretched heel towards the crown of the head, to twist around this axis.

1. Move one leg forward, the opposite arm under the shoulder, supported on the floor or a block if you need. The same arm as front leg resting on that shin to allow yourself to settle into the support of strong legs; the back knee can be down if you need. Let the head drop to settle and stay, adapting to the changes in breath needed to find easeful sustainability throughout your whole body and being.
2. Keep anchoring through the back leg, rotate from the belly towards the inside of the front thigh, top hand resting on the back of the pelvis (to open the top shoulder and collarbone for lymphatic drainage), allowing the body to turn easefully from the belly, neck without strain. Lengthen the whole body – back heel to crown of the head – to allow expansion of the breath, inhaling up the body, exhaling down.

Malasana (garland)

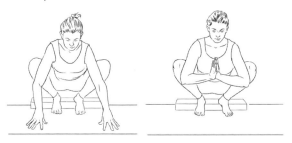

Squatting is a key primal movement for fascial hydration, the free flow of lymphatic and other fluids, compression and flooding into organs for their circulation, etc. Squats allow full digestive elimination for the health of the gut, microbiome and immune system by easing the passage of toxins out. Previous practices helped prepare for squats, including *adho mukha svanasana* (down-face dog), as a place with space to explore this deep bend of the legs with length in the front body (space for diaphragmatic movement). This was room to explore fascial fluidity without dropping our weight down into the hips and pelvis as we do when fully squatting.

Squats tap into the downward-flowing energy of *apana vayu*, particularly in the pelvis, so including some that move in and out before settling connect to this flow. They strengthen the whole lower body for earthing, grounding and lower *chakra* connection.

1. Come into a squat, if necessary supporting under the heels or taking the feet wider, thighs rotated out, so the knees are wider than the hips (or both). In this wider stance, the neck of the femur is less likely to impinge on the acetabulum (hip socket) or the anterior superior iliac spine (hip bone) to come into compression with the top of the thighs. Find a place where the seat is happy and can be sustained with ease to breathe into responses in the belly. Feet can be together or apart.

   Note: This is not an issue of improving flexibility, but rather, accepting individual bone shapes; bone-to-bone compression is not something we can change. Supporting ways to bring the floor up to us (for example, heels on blocks) rather than fixating on 'how far down' offers more space to lift up through the front spine to surrender inwards.

2. Fingertips can be on the ground to lift the breastbone or hands together, elbows meeting the inner legs to raise the breastbone. Surrender the eyes and the forebrain in towards the heart, breathing to find ease through the spine, squeezing of the dorsal to allow opening of the ventral body.

3. This then prepares for a seated meditation or *savasana* (corpse pose) to complete the sequence.

WHERE SQUATTING IS IMPINGED

- Sit on a chair and lift one leg at a time into the chest to emulate this motion.
- Like squats, lunges are a 'primal' movement. The two go hand in hand as motions that keep our basic knees-into-chest pattern supple. In lunges, one leg is back in the opposite motion; that length allows the psoas the pliability it needs (particularly after release in CRP; page 55) for postural ease and full diaphragmatic motion.
- Rotating ankles and pointing and flexing the feet help re-introduce elasticity and pliability around the ankles (like

lunge motions; see above). Increasing the range of motion in the feet, ankles and lower legs also determines what happens above in our posture, and here, our ability to squat. Ankles are designed to quickly absorb force as part of ground stability, then quickly shift and stabilise weight for the next movement, which happens faster than thought. We rely on learned motor patterns and reactions to be able to trust these responses. When we cannot (for example, in injury or the effects of a lifetime of little movement there, in old age) there is a jarring in the platforms above; knees, hips and into a protective tautness in the viscera; less fluid adaptation and more stress as our body awareness registers we are less able to reroute and protect ourselves quickly.

- Fascial fluidity between the 26 feet bones determines this range of motion and the angle we can personally flex our feet (dorsiflexion), but this does not set our squatting range alone. The average range of dorsiflexion with knees bent is 32 to 46 degrees, nicely within the range needed for squatting, but this can lessen when we don't do much of this primal action. We actually come to maximum dorsiflexion about halfway down into a squat; resistance coming in may be limited by hip flexion, but also tightness in the calves and Achilles tendons (back of the heels).

- Foetal positions nurture this shape passively, so that ultimately we can bring strength to the lifting up through the anterior spine required in squats.

SUBTLE PRACTICES: HEART FOCUS

Heart *mudras*

Mudra translates as 'seal' or 'gesture' that within yoga, Buddhism and other meditation practices tune into the sensitivity of our fingers to concentrate focus. In Hatha yoga, they are often practised within *pranayama* (page 307) to guide the flow of *prana*. This may be to stimulate different parts of the physical or subtle body, or to gather consciousness there.

Mudras are also attributed to certain symbology and health benefits (through *marma* points, the Ayurvedic equivalent of acupressure points), and those used here have a heart-based or compassion focus. You can tune into the deeper meaning or simply feel your attention taken up by the refinement of sensation in the fingers and hands. These *mudras* hold the hands in different positions around and at the heart space, focusing into this place that is not simply symbolic of compassion; our heart–brain axis is an extremely responsive route for the autonomic nervous system to be able to settle, soothe and regulate breath and immunity (page 342). Bringing focus to the heart helps us come into ventral vagal tone and lay down paths to be able to go there more quickly, that is, adapt to stressors and find routes to calm and equanimity more directly.

Atmanjali mudra (honouring the true self)

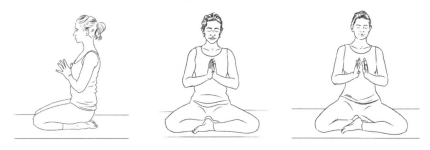

A gesture of reverence and connection to something greater – bringing that into our heart at the centre of ourselves (*atman* means 'self'). Held into the heart, it is linked to the spiritual/divine within us (whatever that might mean for us individually), where the true self is said to reside in the heart. When we bring our attention into the heart, holding this space with a hand gesture, we have a focus point to foster compassionate presence.

1. Sit lightly, with support, to connect to the fluid nature of the breath, and tune into the echoes and ripples of the physical practice (that had a strong lymphatic pumping effect) assimilating *prana*, allowing diffusion through the tissues. Slowly take *atmanjali mudra*, palms together at the heart, thumbs resting along the breastbone.
2. Slowly open a space between the palms to notice any subtle sensations available to you, without interpretation, just feeling. Observe the space in front of the heart, the pulsing of the breath and the heartbeat; mimicking our interoception with external gesture.
3. From here, keeping your eyes closed, let the conduits of your fingers find each other again, into any of the other heart *mudras* below, as you intuit this through proprioception (pages 232, 266 and 297), experiencing the lightness of touch and the space between hands and body.

Padma (lotus) *mudra/vajrapradama mudra/hakini mudra*

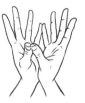 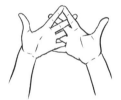 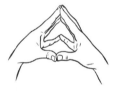

You can use these *mudras* within the meditation as guided, or bring them into your own meditations or gestures of support whenever you need – experiment with how they feel and resonate. They can be brought to the heart area for a self-compassion focus, or to any other centre or area that you feel drawn to bring kind attention and soothing towards. This might also be a place to explore an in-road towards sensing the interior – a space inwards for the tides of the fluid body and ease in the breath, setting the scene for nasal breathing.

1. *Padma mudra*, from *atmanjali mudra* – open out the fingers and palms, keeping the thumbs and little fingers connected. The lotus is a symbol of purity, light and beauty in many cultures – it sits on the surface of the pond, opening to the sun as its roots remain deeply embedded into the muddy waters, often equated with our murky unconsciousness. The *mudra* symbolises the clarity that can be borne from this place through meditation.

2. *Vajrapradama mudra* – this *mudra* of 'unshakeable trust' interweaves our fingers into a protective basket over the heart (elbows dropping, thumbs opening out), to cultivate self-confidence, inner strength and restore faith in and connection to something greater than ourselves; this might be of a spiritual nature, but could be as simple as community. Feel the breath underneath the hands.

3. *Hakini mudra* – named after the Hindu goddess, who represents intuition. *Hakini* means 'power' or 'rule', so the practice encourages the practitioner to channel *prana*, developing focus, 'gaining power' over the racing mind, stimulating calm, connecting right and left hemispheres of the brain and enhancing clarity. Palms apart, facing, bring the finger and thumb tips into light contact, breathing into awareness at this 'cradle' representing a holding of your heart, or towards any other body area where it feels supportive to settle.

Self-enquiry questions

1. What does 'the fluid body' mean to you as you move inward and sense your breath in your body?
2. When you transition between breaths, movements and postures, how do you feel your adaptive capacity with these shifts?
3. How do the more primal movements affect your emotional body and states?
4. How do postural shifts to support nasal breathing affect the rest of your body and mind?
5. How does a focus on the heart affect the quality of breath at your diaphragm?

Further resources

Steve Haines and Sophie Standing (2015) *Trauma is Really Strange*. London and Philadelphia, PA: Singing Dragon.

Gabor Maté (2019) *When the Body Says No: The Cost of Hidden Stress*. London: Vermilion.

Stephen Porges (2017) *The Pocket Guide to the Polyvagal Theory: The Transformative Power of Feeling Safe*. New York: W.W. Norton & Company.

Robert Schleip with Johanna Bayer (2021) *Fascial Fitness: Practical Exercises to Stay Flexible, Active and Pain Free in Just 20 Minutes a Week*, 2nd edn. Chichester: Lotus Publishing.

John Stirk (2015) *The Original Body: Primal Movement for Yoga Teachers*. Pencaitland: Handspring Publishing Ltd.

References

Anatomy Trains (2017) 'Q&A with Tom: Hydration in the fascial matrix.' 24 July. Available at: www. anatomytrains.com/blog/2017/07/24/q-tom-hydration-fascial-matrix

Balsevich, G., Petrie, G.N. and Hill, M.N. (2017) 'Endocannabinoids: Effectors of glucocorticoid signaling.' *Frontiers in Neuroendocrinology 47*, 86–108. Available at: https://pubmed.ncbi.nlm.nih.gov/28739508

Cenaj, O., Allison, D.H.R., Imam, R., Zeck, B., *et al.* (2021) 'Evidence for continuity of interstitial spaces across tissue and organ boundaries in humans.' *Communications Biology 4*(1), 436. Available at: https:// pubmed.ncbi.nlm.nih.gov/33790388

Cleary, T. (2000) *Taoist Meditation.* Boulder, CO: Shambhala Publications.

Cohen, S. (2021) 'Psychosocial vulnerabilities to upper respiratory infectious illness: Implications for susceptibility to coronavirus disease 2019 (COVID-19).' *Perspectives on Psychological Science 16*(1), 161–174. Available at: https://pubmed.ncbi.nlm.nih.gov/32640177

Corazzol, M., Lio, G., Lefevre, A., Deiana, G., *et al.* (2017) 'Restoring consciousness with vagus nerve stimulation.' *Current Biology 27*(18), R994–R996. Available at: https://pubmed.ncbi.nlm.nih.gov/28950091

Engineer, N.D., Kimberley, T.J., Prudente, C.N., Dawson, J., Tarver, W.B. and Hays, S.A. (2019) 'Targeted vagus nerve stimulation for rehabilitation after stroke.' *Frontiers in Neuroscience 13*, 280. Available at: https://pubmed.ncbi.nlm.nih.gov/30983963

Finlayson, D. and Hyland Robertson, L. (eds) (2021) *Yoga Therapy Foundations, Tools, and Practice: A Comprehensive Textbook.* Philadelphia, PA and London: Singing Dragon.

Gottfried, J.A. (2010) 'Central mechanisms of odour object perception.' *Nature Reviews. Neuroscience 11*(9), 628–641. Available at: www.ncbi.nlm.nih.gov/pmc/articles/PMC3722866

Haines, S. (2021) 'The hidden mystery of trauma.' Body College, 12 November. Available at: https:// bodycollege.net/the-hidden-mystery-of-trauma

Hallani, M., Wheatley, J.R. and Amis, T.C. (2008) 'Enforced mouth breathing decreases lung function in mild asthmatics.' *Respirology 13*(4), 553–558. Available at: https://pubmed.ncbi.nlm.nih.gov/18494947

Kaur, R., Ambwani, S.R. and Singh, S. (2016) 'Endocannabinoid system: A multi-facet therapeutic target.' *Current Clinical Pharmacology 11*(2), 110–117. Available at: https://pubmed.ncbi.nlm.nih.gov/27086601

Keleman, S. (1985) *Emotional Anatomy: The Structure of Experience.* Berkeley, CA: Center Press.

Lieberman, D. (2014) *The Story of the Human Body.* London: Penguin.

Liptan, G.L. (2010) 'Fascia: A missing link in our understanding of the pathology of fibromyalgia.' *Journal of Bodywork and Movement Therapies 14*(1), 3–12. Available at: https://pubmed.ncbi.nlm.nih.gov/20006283

Little, T. (2010) *Meditations on a Dewdrop: Poems and Teachings on the Flow of Presence.* Santa Fe, NM: Prajna Yoga.

Little, T. (2016) *Yoga of the Subtle Body: A Guide to the Physical and Energetic Anatomy of Yoga.* Boulder, CO: Shambhala Publications.

Liu, C.-H., Yang, M.-H., Zhang, G.-Z., Wang, X.-X., *et al.* (2020) 'Neural networks and the anti-inflammatory effect of transcutaneous auricular vagus nerve stimulation in depression.' *Journal of Neuroinflammation 17*(1), 54. Available at: https://pubmed.ncbi.nlm.nih.gov/32050990

Mallinson, J. and Singleton, M. (2017) 'The Yogic Body.' In J. Mallinson and M. Singleton, *The Roots of Yoga* (Chapter 5). London: Penguin.

Maté, G. (2018) *In the Realm of Hungry Ghosts: Close Encounters with Addiction.* London: Vermilion.

Maté, G. (2019) *When the Body Says No: The Cost of Hidden Stress.* London: Vermilion.

Mechoulam, R. and Parker, L.A. (2013) 'The endocannabinoid system and the brain.' *Annual Review of Psychology 64*, 21–47. Available at: https://pubmed.ncbi.nlm.nih.gov/22804774

Myers, T. (2018) 'Interstitium: A Statement from Tom Myers' Anatomy Trains. March 29. Available at: https://www.anatomytrains.com/blog/2018/03/29/interstitium-statement-tom-myers

Pavlov, V.A. and Tracey, K.J. (2012) 'The vagus nerve and the inflammatory reflex – Linking immunity and metabolism.' *Nature Reviews. Endocrinology 8*(12), 743–754. Available at: https://pubmed.ncbi. nlm.nih.gov/23169440

Payne, P., Levine, P.A. and Crane-Godreau, M.A. (2015) 'Somatic experiencing: Using interoception and proprioception as core elements of trauma therapy.' *Frontiers in Psychology 6*, 93. Available at: https:// pubmed.ncbi.nlm.nih.gov/25699005

Pruimboom, L. and Muskiet, F.A.J. (2018) 'Intermittent living; the use of ancient challenges as a vaccine against the deleterious effects of modern life – A hypothesis.' *Medical Hypotheses 120*, 28–42. Available at: https://pubmed.ncbi.nlm.nih.gov/30220336

Rodulfo, I.J.A. (2019) 'Sedentary lifestyle a disease from xxi century.' *Clinica e investigacion en arteriosclerosis 31*(5), 233–240. Available at: https://pubmed.ncbi.nlm.nih.gov/31221536

Rowe, P.C., Fontaine, K.R. and Violand, R.L. (2013) 'Neuromuscular strain as a contributor to cognitive and other symptoms in chronic fatigue syndrome: Hypothesis and conceptual model.' *Frontiers in Physiology 4*, 115. Available at: www.ncbi.nlm.nih.gov/pmc/articles/PMC3655286

Roxo, M.R., Franceshini, P.R., Zubaran, C., Kleber, F.D. and Sander, J.W. (2011) 'The limbic system conception and its historical evolution.' *The Scientific World Journal 11*, 2428–2441. Available at: www.ncbi.nlm.nih.gov/pmc/articles/PMC3236374

Sankarâchârya (2018) *The Taittirîya Upanishad: With the Commentaries of Sankarâchârya, Suresvarâchârya and Sâyana (Vidyârya)* (Classic Reprint). London: Forgotten Books.

Schleip, R. with Bayer, J. (2021) *Fascial Fitness: Practical Exercises to Stay Flexible, Active and Pain Free in Just 20 Minutes a Week*, 2nd edn. Chichester: Lotus Publishing.

Schwager, S. and Detmar, M. (2019) 'Inflammation and lymphatic function.' *Frontiers in Immunology 10*, 308. Available at: www.ncbi.nlm.nih.gov/pmc/articles/PMC6399417

Soh, K.-S. (2009) 'Bonghan circulatory system as an extension of acupuncture meridians.' Review Article. *Journal of Acupuncture and Meridian Studies 2*(2), 93–106. Available at: www.sciencedirect.com/science/article/pii/S2005290109600418

Stecco, A., Gesi, M., Stecco, C. and Stern, R. (2013) 'Fascial components of the myofascial pain syndrome.' *Current Pain and Headache Reports 17*(8), 352. Available at: https://pubmed.ncbi.nlm.nih.gov/23801005

Stecco, A., Meneghini, A., Stern, R., Stecco, C. and Imamura, M. (2014) 'Ultrasonography in myofascial neck pain: Randomized clinical trial for diagnosis and follow-up.' *Surgical and Radiologic Anatomy 36*(3), 243–253. Available at: www.blackroll.ch/wp-content/uploads/2016/02/Stecco_myofascial_neck_pain.pdf

Stecco, C., Stern, R., Porzionato, A., Macchi, V., *et al.* (2011) 'Hyaluronan within fascia in the etiology of myofascial pain.' *Surgical and Radiologic Anatomy 33*(10), 891–896. Available at: https://pubmed.ncbi.nlm.nih.gov/21964857

Streeter, C.C., Gerbarg, P.L., Saper, R.B., Ciraulo, D.A. and Brown, R.P. (2012) 'Effects of yoga on the autonomic nervous system, gamma-aminobutyric-acid, and allostasis in epilepsy, depression, and post-traumatic stress disorder.' *Medical Hypotheses 78*(5), 571–579. Available at: https://pubmed.ncbi.nlm.nih.gov/22365651

Sullivan, M.B., Erb, M., Schmalzl, L., Moonaz, S., et al. (2018) 'Yoga therapy and polyvagal theory: The convergence of traditional wisdom and contemporary neuroscience for self-regulation and resilience.' *Frontiers in Human Neuroscience 12*, 67. Available at: www.ncbi.nlm.nih.gov/pmc/articles/PMC5835127

Swami Muktibodhananda (1998) *Hatha Yoga Pradipika*, 4th reprint edn. India: Bihar School of Yoga.

Tortora, S. (2019) 'Children are born to dance! Pediatric medical dance/movement therapy: The view from integrative pediatric oncology.' *Children (Basel) 6*(1), 14. Available at: https://pubmed.ncbi.nlm.nih.gov/30669668

Tracey, K.J. (2002) 'The inflammatory reflex.' *Nature 420*(6917), 853–859. Available at: https://pubmed.ncbi.nlm.nih.gov/12490958

Valentini, N.C., Pereira, K.R.G., Chiquetti, E.M.D.S., Formiga, C.K.M.R. and Linhares, M.B.M. (2019) 'Motor trajectories of preterm and full-term infants in the first year of life.' *Pediatrics International 61*(10), 967–977. Available at: https://pubmed.ncbi.nlm.nih.gov/31293014

van der Kolk, B.A. (2015) *The Body Keeps the Score: Brain, Mind, and Body in the Healing of Trauma*. London: Penguin.

Walsh, M. (Host). (2019). 194. Formative Embodiment – With James Feil [Audio podcast episode.] In *The Embodiment Podcast*. https://embodiedfacilitator.com/194-formative-embodiment-with-james-feil

Watts, C. (2018) *Yoga Therapy for Digestive Health*. London and Philadelphia, PA: Singing Dragon.

Yates, B.J., Billig, I., Cotter, C.A., Mori, R.L. and Card, J.P. (2002) 'Role of the vestibular system in regulating respiratory muscle activity during movement.' *Clinical and Experimental Pharmacology & Physiology 29*(1–2), 112–117. Available at: https://pubmed.ncbi.nlm.nih.gov/11906468

Yi, S.-R., Man, Q.-W., Gao, X., Lin, H., *et al.* (2021) 'Tissue-derived extracellular vesicles in cancers and non-cancer diseases: Present and future.' *Journal of Extracellular Vesicles 10*(14), e12175.

Zaccaro, A., Piarulli, A., Laurino, M., Garbella, E., *et al.* (2018) 'How Breath-Control Can Change Your Life: A Systematic Review on Psycho-Physiological Correlates of Slow Breathing.' *Frontiers in Human Neuroscience 12*, 353. Available at: https://www.ncbi.nlm.nih.gov/pmc/articles/PMC6137615

PART 4

MINDFUL BOUNDARIES

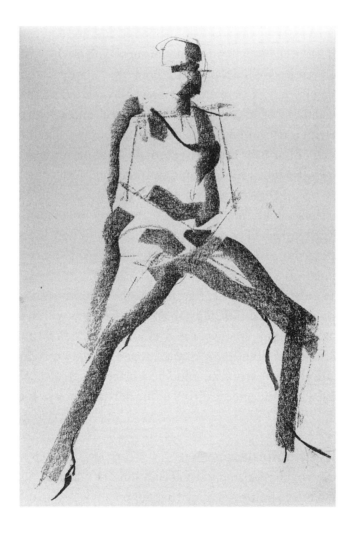

Discovering how we create appropriate containment for body fluids alongside our sense of cohesion and safety through the sanctuary of our physical form – into which we can breathe fully, through clear distinction between our internal and external worlds, for healthy boundaries and self-protection.

There is no separation between our physical, emotional and mental boundaries; we are constantly sensing where we are in time and space – the inside in relation to the outside and how that registers through the nervous system. We can feel this through a whole host of sensations, emotions, thoughts and feelings about thoughts. Although we can focus on specific parts – for example the skin – ultimately, all parts and aspects of ourselves are intertwined in terms of their responses.

Where the voluntary meets the involuntary (autonomic) is also a boundary, although when we start to observe the autonomic, to some degree this becomes voluntary as it has been brought into consciousness. This is why, when we start to have mindful awareness of the tones of the body, the nervous system, the breath, we begin to have greater participation in our whole experience. This can offer us greater understanding of where inner and outer meet, and we can participate at this junction with touch and moving different parts of our skin on the ground.

When much of our lives is either externally loud or our inner experience is dominated by thoughts, refining our awareness to notice the subtleties of mental processes and emotions that affect us means dropping beneath the more obvious noise. It is here that we can register a boundary before the point it has already been pushed past, the quiet voice of 'enough' before we barely noticed reaching 'more than enough', as many people experience within burnout or inflammation.

Healthy boundaries are neither rigid and stressed, nor too relaxed – we need both contraction and relaxation, tension and release – it is within this full cycle that we find stabilisation. We need the containment of being tonified against the ground or another point of resistance, that boundary which allows us to move with ease through space. It could be a place of support, of grounding, really knowing where our physicality is in the here and now.

The polarity of boundaries

Within the realm of physical, mental and emotional boundaries, our autonomic nervous system is constantly tracking what our breath is doing, subconsciously monitoring whether we approach or withdraw. We approach if we feel safe or withdraw if we are uncertain or feel danger. There is an allowance or resistance (desire or aversion). We need to feel the whole spectrum of open and close, fluidity and containment. The inhale and the exhale have these polarities too, and our innate immunity is constantly monitoring what we let in and what we keep out or even destroy.

On a psycho-emotional level, we absorb what feels safe – including ideas or social dynamics – or keep out ideas, people or situations we do not feel safe or comfortable with. It is the welcome, as in inviting someone into our homes (more ventral vagus), or attack, stay out (more sympathetic). There is a constant interplay of approach or withdraw that we may not be consciously aware of but can explore within practice where we tune into our boundaries and the pulsation of coming in and out as feels appropriate.

This can follow through in body states: held in ease (*sukha*, feeling that something is opening) or dis-ease (*dukkha*, suffering, unhappiness, pain, unsatisfactoriness or stress) – relating to disruption to *prana* (page 278).

Counterwill and healthy resistance

It is not simply a bad thing or a difficulty to push back against something that is coming to our world that we have a choice to resist. Counterwill is the instinctive reaction to resist being controlled.

It is healthy to be able to resist where someone or something invades our personal space or when someone is pushing into our autonomy, for example dominating physical adjustments from a teacher in a yoga class. Our resistance is healthy when we are able to express clearly and non-aggressively in ventral vagus mode, rather than jumping into the reactivity of fight-or-flight, or the check-out of dorsal vagus immobilisation (and even overcompliance). When we can recognise that we are present and something does not feel safe, we can respond consciously. When we react from a defensive stance, this can show up as aggressive opposition, negativism, apathy, noncompliance, disrespect, lack of motivation, belligerence, incorrigibility, even antisocial attitudes and actions – we may not be able to tolerate a different opinion to our own, or feel we shouldn't 'rock the boat'.

Inner narrative

When we are really listening to our own voices, we can have healthy counterwill. When we hear ourselves say things like 'we are not enough' or 'not right' – derogatory phrases that we have internalised from external influences, conditioning – we can push back internally, protecting ourselves against ourselves.

Healthy boundaries can be disrupted if we have learned from an early age that we have no agency or that we are unheard, or abused, not knowing or trusting where these edges between our inner states and the world beyond them lie. Similarly, physically, when what the body feels is diligently overridden with interoceptively suppressing phrases such as 'push on through' or 'no pain, no gain', where we are not listening to the voice of 'that's enough', injury is more likely to occur. 'You are not enough' or 'you do not have enough' is the inherent message of capitalism, the inherent conditioning that makes it possible to sell us stuff – messaging that is designed to erode our boundaries. Recognising that resources are found within and numbing with yet more stuff is not the answer means having a relationship with our vulnerability, the stronger choice. As Brené Brown says: 'Daring to set boundaries is about having the courage to love ourselves even when we risk disappointing others.'[1]

This is where we can meet gentleness, kindness and the safety of being listened to and our needs heard and met. When this is overridden, perhaps through the disconnect of trauma (page 157), pain can shout out to be heard instead.

The immune system is constantly tracking what is safe or unsafe, and much of its work happens on our physical boundaries within the body, which are always responding within the ANS. Bessel van der Kolk states: 'The role of our emotions is boundary integrity. To keep out what is unhealthy and let in what is enriching. The job of the immune system has similar roles.'[2]

The enteric nervous system

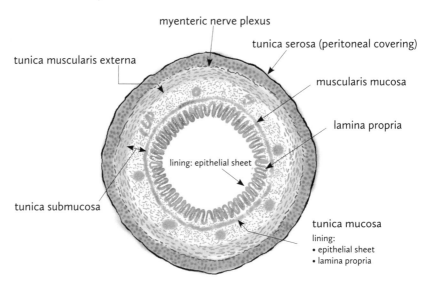

FIGURE 4A. THE ENTERIC NERVOUS SYSTEM
Cross-section of the gastrointestinal tract (gut) – shown at the small intestine,
where the finger-like villi can be seen on the inner lining.
Source: This illustration first appeared in Yoga Therapy for Digestive Health by Charlotte Watts

---

1   Brown (2015).
2   van der Kolk (2015).

The enteric nervous system (ENS) is part of the autonomic nervous system (ANS; page 78), considered the 'second brain', cited as having as many nerve endings as a cat's brain.[3] It lies throughout the whole gut tube at the inner and middle layers and acts autonomously – it needs no communication from the brain (central nervous system (CNS)). The CNS can override ENS function, however, shutting it down as part of a stress response, interrupting our gut feelings as well as digestive function. The ENS is in constant communication bottom-up (towards the brain) via the vagus nerve (see the connections shown in Figure 2a; page 79), sending information about chemical and food states (including immune signals).

It also relays 'gut feelings' – impressions of what is and is not safe – that we have laid down in the gut, messages that come up to guide us, to be listened to, played back by the ENS when we encounter an association or trigger with a similar situation, sight, sound or smell. In neuroscience, it is theorised that an impression has been made on the CNS by our gut feelings, as somatic markers.[4] We might equate these to *samskaras* within yoga philosophy (page 279), the subtle mental impressions left by all the thoughts, intentions and actions that we experience, and the habits these create.

Tuning in consciously to the nuances of this inner landscape is the route to liberation of *samskaras* and responding in ways that feel true to ourselves and offer us the choice to rewrite associations – liberation. Chronic stress and trauma can shut down this interoception. Just like thoughts, gut feelings can be true, the stuff of intuition and awareness, but can also be the playing out of triggers from previous experience, shutting us down because of associations, somatic markers of perceived threat. Learning these subtle differences is bringing our unconscious drivers to consciousness; self-study or *svadhyaya*.

Physical boundaries

To orient inwards, we need to know where the edges lie. We have many of these external physical boundaries: the skin, the cavities in the mouth, the ears, the anus and the genitalia – the external and the internal places where the world comes to meet us. The structural components of our innate immune system[5] are also physical barriers, such as:

---

3   ScienceDaily (2021).
4   Damasio (2000).
5   Bush and Cummings (2021).

- Cells lining the intestines
- Stomach acid
- Cells lining the airway
- Blood–brain barrier
- Tight junctions (regions of cell membranes where the cells are joined to one another).

Dendritic cells are located in tissues of our bodies that have direct contact with the outside world, most obviously on the skin, but also where air meets the lungs and food meets the gut wall. These identify foreign material and act as messengers alerting the rest of the immune system.

The integumentary system, aka skin

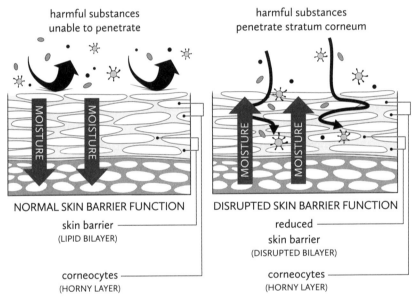

FIGURE 4B. SKIN BARRIER

The integumentary system, more simply the skin, is both a boundary and a contact surface, a sensory organ: 'It plays a major protective role against pathogens as physical barrier, as site of first recognition, and as orchestrator of consecutive immune responses.'[6]

Where the gut interface is around 98.4 square feet, the skin is 328 square feet. Every inch of the skin contains over 2.5 million bacteria: 'Complex

---

6   Skabytska *et al.* (2016).

communities of bacteria, fungi, and viruses thrive on our skin. The composition of these communities depends on skin characteristics, such as sebaceous gland concentration, moisture content, and temperature, as well as on host genetics and exogenous environmental factors.'[7]

The makeup of the skin microbiome (page 219) varies greatly depending on the individual as well as the area of the skin, influenced by:[8]

- Physiology: sex hormones, age and site
- Environment: climate and geographical location
- Immune system: previous exposures and inflammation
- Genotype: susceptibility genes such as filaggrin
- Lifestyle: occupation, hygiene (harsh chemicals erode)
- Pathology: underlying conditions, for example diabetes, atopic conditions (page 99).

Skin is constantly sensing what we come up against and assessing how we feel about it. The casing of our skin is part of our embodiment, how we move in relation to the external physical world, how we relate to others and the emotional tones we then process internally. This is a reason to practise yoga in bare feet, or we are stepping away from the sensory relationship with the potential to ground, to connect to what is coming up from our environment. As discussed on pages 112 and 232, a large part of our psyche is related to how we evolve upwards towards bipedal standing. In the practices in this part we explore that grounding relationship with soles of the feet earthwards.

Dysbiosis (bacterial imbalance) in the skin microbiome is similar to leaky gut syndrome (gut permeability), where the gut's surface allows substances into the bloodstream between cells, rather than going through them. This means things that shouldn't enter or undigested food particles enter the body, a common route for intolerance that is related to compromised healing (and often inflammation) at this gut boundary. In the skin (or via the gut) this permeability can show up as issues such as acne, dermatitis, eczema and rosacea, even premature wrinkles, a result of inflammation where the protective barrier is disrupted and substances penetrate through. Toxins, stress, processed sugar (which feed unhealthy bacteria), too much alcohol and harsh sanitising products can all affect the skin microbiome and how it functions as a healthy boundary.[9]

---

7   Chen and Tsao (2013).
8   Grice and Segre (2011).
9   Barnard and Li (2017).

The lymphatic system and dermatomes

A dermatome is an area of skin – a peripheral nerve field and key sensory boundary – mainly supplied by nerve fibres reaching from a single dorsal root of spinal nerve. There are eight cervical (C1 an exception, with no dermatome), 12 thoracic, five lumbar and five sacral nerves. Each relays sensation (including pain) from a particular region of skin to the brain. Although the general pattern seen making up the contours of our human map is similar in everyone, the precise areas of activation are as unique as a fingerprint.

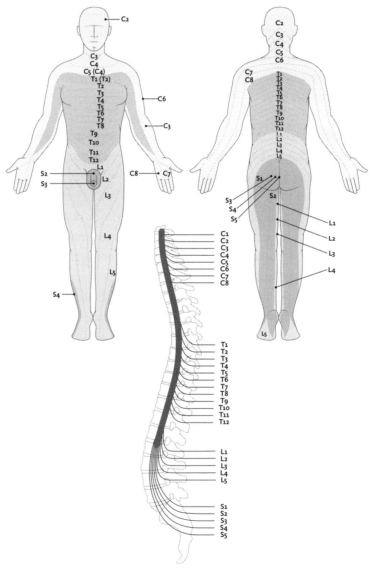

FIGURE 4C. DERMATOMES

Our relationship to the outside world via skin contact feeds back into our centre via the somatic nervous system and into the CNS. In somatic practices, rubbing, rolling and changing pressures onto our external body help the process of making sense of the outer world by creating clear sensory feedback that we can consciously affect and play with. This sensing of the periphery links back into our immune responses.[10,11] We can also have referred pain out to the periphery in the mix, rooted more in the conscious perception of sensations in areas other than their original location.

The ventral, front body and the aspects of the superficial lymphatic system closest to our surface are wider boundaries where we meet the world. Our skin is fed by the lymphatics, congregating in places that are often soft and vulnerable: sides of the throat, armpits, groin and top of the cheekbones. These lymphatic ducts drain into the upper chest, the outside of the collarbone and back to the blood pumping via the pulmonary circuit; moving into these areas supports this flow.

The torso, front and back, and the ventral, soft part of the inner arms relates to T1–T12, the whole of the thoracic spine. Whether we're rubbing the ground or receiving touch, we are moving through nerve endings into the thoracic spine.

The lymphatic system is constantly moving in and out, the interior to the exterior, coming out to feel the world, feeling it in internally and then coming back out to relate to the world, to others. Where blood is always being pumped out from the heart to the periphery of the body, lymph moves inward. It can't move unless we do, so sedentary habits can lead to stagnation and, ultimately, compromised immunity.

---

10 Skabytska *et al.* (2016).
11 Pruimboom and Muskiet (2018).

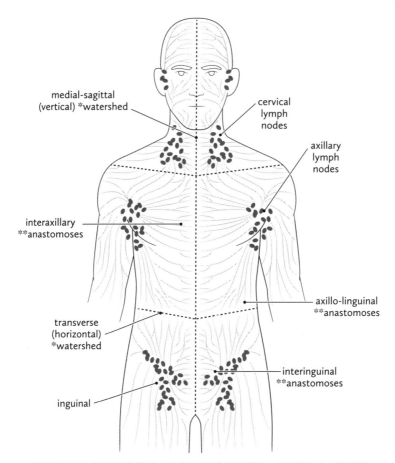

medial-sagittal
(vertical) *watershed

cervical
lymph
nodes

axillary
lymph
nodes

interaxillary
**anastomoses

axillo-linguinal
**anastomoses

transverse
(horizontal)
*watershed

interinguinal
**anastomoses

inguinal

FIGURE 4D. SUPERFICIAL LYMPHATIC SYSTEM – VENTRAL ASPECT

Vertical watershed – area of lymph drainage along the skin in the midline,
both on the ventral and the dorsal aspect of the neck and head.

Horizontal watershed – area along the clavicle, which continues posteriorly to the midline. This
drains above to superficial cervical lymph nodes and below to parasternal nodes or axillary nodes.

* Watershed areas, where networks of lymph capillaries communicate, particularly where
there is more than one direction of venous discharge – also at lines of fusion including
the midline where lymph vessels from each side communicate extensively across it.

** An anastomosis is a connection or opening between two things that are normally diverging or
branching, such as between blood vessels, leaf veins or streams – here the flow of lymphatics.

Source: Adapted from www.klosetraining.com

Compromised lymphatic system function and flow can show up in a number
of ways that can be supported by massage, kind touch and movement:

- Enlarged lymph nodes – throat, groin, armpits.
- Skin conditions.
- Arthritis – inflammation around the joints.
- Unexplained injuries, such as blockages into fascia or interstitial

organs (page 142), which reduce inflammatory potential from the body. Lymphatic flow is interrupted, as well as electrolyte (page 141) movement around the body and injury repair.

- Excess weight or cellulite, where fluids pool or become affected metabolically by poor flow.
- Headaches (may also be linked to 'leaky brain'; page 210), which can show up around the shoulders and up into the jaw, where drainage to the collarbone is not flowing well.
- Chronic fatigue, in relation to the fascia as well as compromised liver clearance of toxins – pathological detoxification.
- Sinus infections.
- Digestive disorders.

Lymphatics of the head and neck

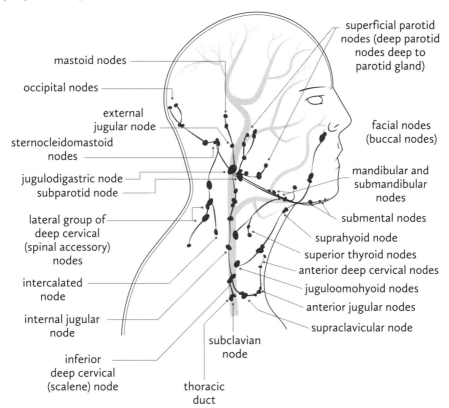

FIGURE 4E. LYMPHATICS OF THE HEAD AND NECK

Where the lymphatic system meets all the nodes in the head and neck – the tonsils, thyroids, adenoids – lie vital immune boundaries, designed to stay moist. When we mouth breathe, these areas become more exterior and then dry out through direct contact with air. When we come more into ventral vagal, soft parasympathetic tone, nasal breathing is easier and we salivate more, so these boundaries are better hydrated and protective.

Surface of the lungs

The tree-like branches of the lungs that become ever more delicate – trachea to bronchioles to alveoli (gas exchange) – are boundaried by the pleural sacs containing pleural fluid. With issues like pleurisy (inflammation of the pleura, accumulation of fluid in the pleural cavity), there is catching, friction at the fluid boundary. The lungs' surface area is about 2400 kilometres (1500 miles) of airways; where air comes in, carbon dioxide seeps out. Many organs (including the gut) rely on the largest possible boundary surface to function fully.

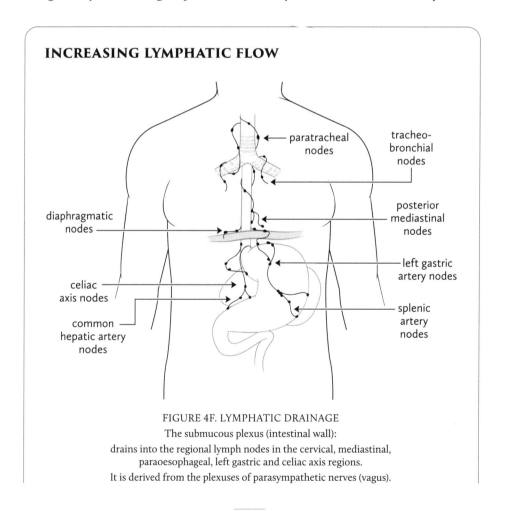

INCREASING LYMPHATIC FLOW

FIGURE 4F. LYMPHATIC DRAINAGE
The submucous plexus (intestinal wall):
drains into the regional lymph nodes in the cervical, mediastinal, paraoesophageal, left gastric and celiac axis regions.
It is derived from the plexuses of parasympathetic nerves (vagus).

When we move around as nature designed, the lymphatic system moves out to the periphery, giving a quality of 'glow'. When someone is experiencing chronic stress, trauma or fatigue, fluid flow can be trapped inward as bracing towards the centre in self-protection (page 152). We can often see illness, exhaustion or stress in another as a loss of lustre; vitality showing through healthy lymphatic flow just below the skin.

We can support the lymphatics through massage or dry brushing, which increases this circulation and provides eustress – good stress at the outer layers – letting the immune system know where the outer boundary is (pages 101 and 155). The lymphatics often need some help going back to the heart. The direction of movement is away from nodules at the armpits, the groin and the backs of the knees to improve circulation.

Lower abdominal lymphatics

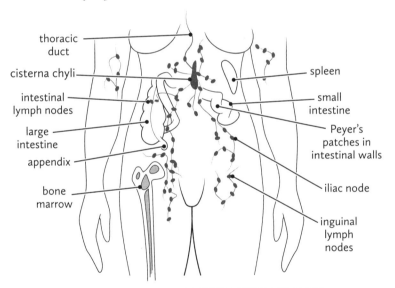

FIGURE 4G. LYMPHATIC SITES IN THE ABDOMEN

Lymphatics around the abdomen are vital, 70 per cent of the immune system being housed on the gut wall (page 41) in gut-associated lymphoid tissue (GALT). This plays into our anti-inflammatory potential, related to our microbiome gut bacteria in the gut wall (page 208). This feeds out into intestinal lymph nodes to take out anything harmful in the gut. Movement around this area – undulating, side to side, forward and back, twisting – is essential to get the lymphatics moving and support the barrier of the gut wall.

Epithelium

Epithelial cells, collectively known as the epithelium, are one of four basic types of animal tissue, along with connective, muscle and nervous tissues. Epithelial tissues line outer surfaces of the whole body, from the epidermis, the outermost skin layer, to organs and blood vessels throughout the body, as well as the inner surfaces of cavities in many internal organs: sinuses, intestines, lungs, vaginal tract and bladder. Hollow spaces can quickly prevent barrier breach (when injured or not healing) with inflammation as a first-line innate response.[12]

Functions of epithelial cells include:

- Secretion, vital for boundaries to be moist, malleable, hydrated and responsive.
- Microbiome, which lives here (page 208).
- Selective absorption – it is porous, permeable, letting things in through cell walls (not between them; 'leaky'), so there is a direct relationship between what is coming in as a physical barrier.
- Transcellular transport and sensing – the whole body has sensory capacity; 'sense making'.

Epithelial layers have nerves but no supply. We are not generally conscious of this level – our blood supply or our gut working – but sometimes we get a sense of a story of pain from here, where there is no known cause. These boundaries must receive nourishment via diffusion of substances from the underlying connective tissue, through the basement membrane (that provides cell and tissue support and acts as a platform for complex signalling). When we get tight or stressed, when trauma holds tissue in protective armouring, that nourishment supply can be compromised. There can be skin issues, numbness, lack of both circulation and healing – often relayed as pain.

The epithelium of the gut wall is a living, responsive boundary:

The epithelium impacts microbial communities... In addition, bacteria provide, as by-products of their metabolism, various compounds (essential vitamins, antioxidants, short-chain fatty acids [SCFA] etc.) that impact host homeostasis...dietary intake can also have significant impact on both the gut epithelial barrier and the bacterial communities.[13]

---

12 Hedberg (2020).
13 Guzman, Conlin and Jobin (2013).

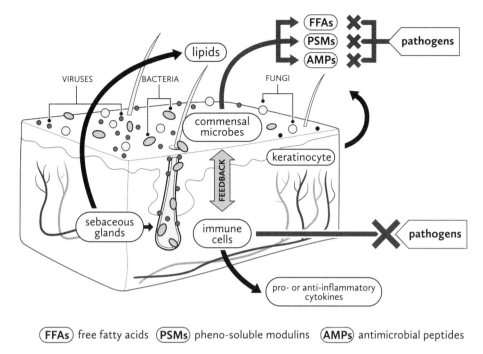

(FFAs) free fatty acids   (PSMs) pheno-soluble modulins   (AMPs) antimicrobial peptides

FIGURE 4H. MICROBIOME AND SKIN IMMUNOLOGY
Source: Adapted from Chen and Tsao (2013)

Form, function and orchestration of the epithelium and our microbiome are completely intertwined, affecting immunity and overall gut health.[14] The epithelial cells in the lungs are similarly complicit in our immune responses.[15] Various studies have revealed the beneficial effect of aerobic exercise on chronic allergic airway inflammation, for example asthma.[16] Futhermore, 'Lung epithelial cells are increasingly recognized as active effectors of microbial defence, contributing to both innate and adaptive immune function in the lower respiratory tract.'[17]

Inflammation of the airways and bacterial dysbiosis are also associated with COPD (chronic obstructive pulmonary disease; page 102). Ongoing studies are providing further insight into understanding the relationship between microbiome alteration and host inflammatory response.[18] This further validates the effectiveness of movement around the rib cage, nasal breathing, freeing the thoracic spine, diaphragm, channel of the throat, collarbone – all supporting

14   Solis *et al.* (2020).
15   Bartlett, Fischer and McCray (2008).
16   Hansen *et al.* (2020).
17   Invernizzi, Lloyd and Molyneaux (2020).
18   Ramsheh *et al.* (2021).

posture for creating volume and increased surface area of the lungs on the inhalation.

The microbiome

As explained in an article for *The Lancet* during the COVID-19 pandemic:

> During this most extreme collapse of human health in our history, we have made a startling discovery: human cells are not at the center of human health. Instead, it's the cells within our microbiome, functioning as the life-giving soil within our gut and internal organs, which is at the core. The microbiome guides human health and is one of the most important contributors to the functioning of our immune system.[19]

Our microbiome is microbes living inside us, that we evolved with, and which outnumber our body's own cells. The gut microbiome weighs about 2 kilograms (more than the 1.4kg human brain), and may have just as much influence over our bodies:

> The colonization of the intestine begins at birth and has been shown to be influenced by vaginal or C-section birth. However, the microbiota changes with exposure to various environmental factors during maturation. Much like a genetic imprint of an individual, each individual has a unique microbiota, though approximately one-third of the species are common across most humans.[20]

The boundary of our own body – where we meet the outer world and its own microbiome – communicates with, is influenced by and needed for our microbiome to flourish. This is one way our diet affects us epigenetically (page 92):

> The immune systems of plants have to respond to stress they are exposed in response to changes in the environment. A plant cannot run away or hide, but rather responds to the stress by turning on genes that regulate their immune response to the challenges. When these genes are turned on in response to the changing environment it results in the production of specific phytochemical

---

19   Bush and Cummings (2021).
20   Taneja (2017).

compounds. These compounds when ingested by people in turn modify how the genes that regulate the function of their immune systems are influenced.[21]

VASCULAR/ENDOTHELIAL HEALTH

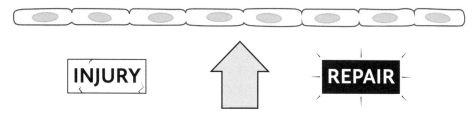

INJURY   REPAIR

nitric oxide production and bioavailability
types and amount of interleukins (inflammation response and resolution)
relative, endogenous, anticoagulant activity

MICROBIOTA

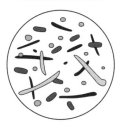

FIGURE 41. MICROBIOME AND ENDOTHELIAL FUNCTION
This diagram shows the importance of nitric oxide (page 44) and nasal
breathing to link microbiome/biota with endothelial health.
Source: Leslie and Annex (2018)

Outsourcing to the microbiome – the 'second human genome'

Thousands of species of microbes – not only bacteria, but also fungi and archaea (single-celled organisms important in the gut, mouth and on the skin), with as many as 20 million genes among them (a human being has just 20,000 genes) – mean that our gut bacteria can make and use nutrients and other molecules in ways the human body cannot. Arguably, viruses play a part in our microbiome too (page 219).

Our microbiome is an important part of our innate immunity, a mechanical barrier (endothelial system; page 30). Often referred to as the structural components of the innate immune system, these barriers include the skin and membranes that line our mouths, nose, airways, urinary tracts and gastrointestinal

21   Dr Jeffrey Bland, quoted in Hyman (2022).

organs. When intact with a healthy microbiome, they provide a physical barrier against the entry of toxins and harmful organisms, and replenish the linings of the gut and skin, replacing damaged and dying cells with new ones. Unless things have been assimilated through the gut barrier, they are still considered to be outside of us: that intact sweet corn in the toilet bowl never entered your body via the gut wall!

Of the total numbers of microorganisms within our gut, a healthy level of microbiome is considered to be 80 per cent. According to research by Yong: 'The immune system is not innately hardwired to tell the difference between a harmless symbiont and a threatening pathogen...it's the microbe that makes that distinction clear.'[22] Probiotic means working for the organism within you, a symbiotic relationship, the bacteria in our gut that are 'good'. These are our first lines of immune defence on the gut wall barrier, with many other functions:

- Produce lactase – for milk digestion.
- Produce vitamins B and K.
- Create fuel for the colon – keeping our gut boundaries integrated.
- Lower colon pH – maintaining the best environment for gut bacteria.
- Enhance peristalsis – how we move things through.
- Support liver function – essential for elimination and detoxification.

Kayama and Takeda state that: 'In intestinal mucosa, abnormal activation of innate immunity, which directs adaptive immune responses, causes the onset and/or progression of inflammatory bowel diseases. Thus, innate immunity is finely regulated in the gut.'[23]

Blood–brain barrier
The membrane around the whole of the brain and the spinal cord is key to immune function there, keeping the CNS safe. Cytokines – immune messengers, some of which can set off the inflammatory cascade (page 88) – can cross the blood–brain barrier, where they can have a depressive effect, by lowering dopamine levels (the neurotransmitter associated with reward-motivated behaviour). Flooding of inflammation (within the sympathetic response) requires a very high energetic response, so the drop in dopamine imposes a parasympathetic state for recovery and energy conservation – it literally stops

22 Yong (2016).
23 Kayama and Takeda (2016).

us running around doing things so we can heal. When we feel less motivated, there is more energy for the immune system, that feeling at the beginning of an illness, that's to be listened to rather than subscribing to the 'no pain no gain', 'keep pushing on' mentality that never allows us to fully replenish resources.[24]

Acute stress increases the permeability of the blood–brain barrier, meaning that substances move between cells rather than through them as they do with a healthy barrier. This means they escape identification or being denied entry. This has shown up in research on Alzheimer's,[25] and also, multiple sclerosis as an autoimmune condition has shown this breaching of the blood–brain barrier and attacking of self.[26] This is much like the loss of integrity at the gut wall referred to as 'leaky gut' or intestinal permeability. At the blood–brain barrier, 'leaky brain' is associated with brain fog, chronic fatigue, motor delay or clumsiness, anxiety, depression and personality changes. Supporting the gut and microbiome supports the blood–brain barrier.

Cerebrospinal fluid (CSF) and interstitial fluid (page 142) drain from the CNS to regional lymph nodes, so we still have crossing of fluids at this internal boundary.

Spine undulations for blood–brain barrier health

Spine undulations (page 112) support the rich vascular, lymphatic and immune presence at the blood–brain barrier. They foster opening this area at the base of the skull that becomes compressed in modern, postural habits (page 169) and their motion has a squeeze-release, soaking effect into the epithelium there.

They also support jaw and neck release to help untense tissues in the whole head area for improved circulation and oxygenation. See the jaw release in CRP (page 117) to lead into easeful and conscious movement around the occiput.

---

24   Montiel-Castro *et al.* (2013).
25   Zenaro, Piacentino and Constantin (2017).
26   Nishihara and Engelhardt (2020).

The 'psychobiome' – gut bacteria and the brain

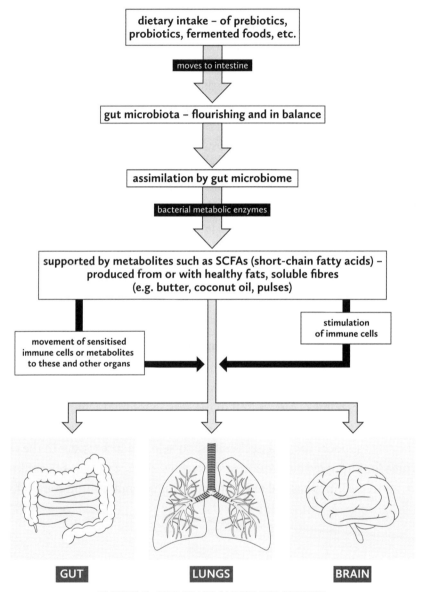

FIGURE 4J. GUT–BRAIN–LUNG MICROBIOME

The 'psychobiome' is a term that refers to the role that gut bacteria play in our mental health – our thoughts, feelings and how we act. We now know that probiotic bacteria can cross the blood–brain barrier[27] as part of our emotional landscape, including those gut feelings from the ENS (page 196).

---

27 Braniste *et al.* (2014).

There are many ways in which gut microbes are thought to affect the brain that are key to appropriate immune responses. Development of microbial therapies is a hot topic – they mostly fall under probiotic rather than drug standards regulations, but are hoped to have powerful psychobiotic effects. Research has been maximising on the evolution of the microbial and human brain connection: 'Epidemiological researchers have turned up intriguing connections between gut and brain disorders. For example, many people with irritable bowel syndrome are also depressed, people on the autism spectrum tend to have digestive problems, and people with Parkinson's are prone to constipation.'[28]

Where some gut microbes secrete messenger molecules that travel through the blood to the brain, other bacteria may relay signals to the vagus through cells in the gut lining. Inflammation may also be a key factor in disorders such as depression[29] and autism.[30] Gut bacteria are key to proper immune system development and maintenance, and microbial imbalances can promote inflammation and affect hormones.[31]

The gut–immune–stress connection

The main anti-inflammatory part of our immune system sits in the mucous linings of the digestive, respiratory and urinary tracts. These link directly to the lymphatic system, the route by which lymphatic fluid delivers foreign and toxic agents to these sites, where they are killed and destroyed. Protection at these barriers, particularly at the gut and lungs, is the first-line, generalised innate immunity defence. We need specific (acquired) immunity developed against particular invaders (such as COVID-19 or influenza), but our ability to fight these off and how severe (or even fatal) these can be are dependent on the health of the linings (epithelia; page 206) of our internal passageways.

It is the beneficial bacterial colonisation – microbiome, probiotics – at the gut and lungs that determine the quality of our immune responses, and also affect our mood, energy, appetite and more. In the gut, a healthy microbiome can contain 7lb of probiotic bacteria, heavier than all of our skin cells. These good bacteria are altered or lowered by stress, sugar, alcohol, antibiotics and

---

28 Pennisi (2022).
29 Maeng and Hong (2019).
30 Prata *et al.* (2019).
31 de Punder and Pruimboom (2015).

pharmaceutical medications[32,33,34,35,36] in ways that may contribute to irritable bowel syndrome (IBS).[37]

Immunity on the gut wall is regulated by secretory antibodies (sIgA), low levels of which can evoke poor signalling from the gut that result in inappropriate immune responses (such as reacting to 'self' in autoimmune diseases) or overreaction contributing to inflammatory conditions (eczema, asthma, hay fever, migraines, arthritis, psoriasis). The gut–lung axis describes the constant communication via the gut microbiome with the respiratory system, with recent research recognising the link between lowered healthy gut bacteria and the lungs: 'Gut dysbacteriosis might result in chronic inflammatory respiratory disorders, particularly asthma.'[38]

Continual and chronic stress has shown to reduce levels of probiotic bacteria and sIgA, resulting in tendencies to an inflammatory cytokine response.[39] Cytokines have come to public consciousness recently in relation to the more severe cases and deaths of COVID-19 (page 103): 'We know from many studies that the gut microbiome has important immunological functions. The microbiome could be contributing to the immune system's overreaction to the virus – the so-called cytokine storm that overwhelms the lungs and is the main cause of death in patients with COVID-19.'[40]

Analyses of the gut microbiome before and after people's COVID-19 exposure could help predict which patients with the infection are likely to experience a cytokine storm, and engender preventative strategies. This is an interesting direction, given the findings of a recent study that discussed the evidence that ageing alone alters the gut microbiome and likely contributes to age-related inflammation, 'inflammaging' (page 103). The authors concluded that the microbiome could be modified to positively impact outcomes from age-related diseases, which could now, of course, include higher age-related vulnerability to COVID-19.[41]

---

32 Engen *et al.* (2015).
33 Payne, Chassard and Lacroix (2012).
34 Foster, Rinaman and Cryan (2017).
35 Becattini, Taur and Pamer (2016).
36 Walsh *et al.* (2018).
37 Kennedy *et al.* (2014).
38 Frati *et al.* (2019).
39 Mackos, Maltz and Bailey (2017).
40 Albert Einstein College of Medicine (2020).
41 Spychala *et al.* (2018).

Immune antibodies on the gut wall

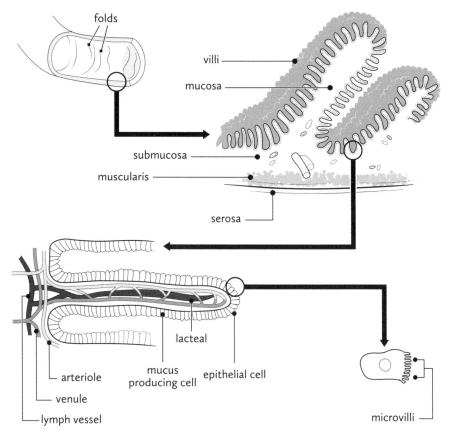

FIGURE 4K. THE GUT WALL

Our sIgA immune antibodies on the gut wall are the main anti-inflammatory part of our immune system, responsible for appropriate immune response modulation (page 26) – not too much, otherwise we wander into the territory of allergies or autoimmunity; not too little, so we can fight off infection or the proliferation of cancer cells. These are found in the following places:

- Respiratory epithelium, the boundaries of the lungs
- Tears, saliva, sweat and colostrum – the first nourishment that babies receive before breast milk comes in
- Genitourinary tract secretions
- Gastrointestinal tract
- Prostate.

Stress reduces levels of probiotic bacteria and sIgA, meaning stress can increase inflammatory cytokine responses at these sites if there is a compromise specifically in a topical part of the epithelium. Inflammation sets up a vicious cycle; as well as the links mentioned on page 213, research has observed:

- Probiotic supplementation relieves stress itself, including improving cognitive function, alleviating negative emotions and reducing abnormal behaviours.[42]
- Antibiotics increase depression – but not antiviral or antifungal medications that leave gut bacteria unharmed.[43]
- Upper respiratory symptoms are related to a breakdown in the homeostatic regulation of the mucosal immune system of the airways.[44]

These symptoms bring us back to the importance of nasal breathing and being in parasympathetic tone: 'Yoga (as a mind-body therapy) has shown effective in reducing inflammatory cytokines, through the resulting alterations in neuroendocrine, neural, and psychological and behavioural processes.'[45]

The gut–brain axis

The gut–brain axis is crucial. It is gut–brain not brain–gut, as 70–80 per cent of information – from the gut to the ENS to the CNS to the brain – travels upwards. We can only think our way to feeling safe to a small degree. If we haven't really dealt with truly feeling safe from the gut, there will always be an underlying feeling of doubt from below. This is where embodiment and somatic practices have become part of psychotherapy – affecting our gut motility, secretions, immune system, microbial balance on the gut wall – also signalling back up to the brain to support regulation of stress levels, mood, behaviour, movement and socialisation.

---

42 Zhang *et al.* (2019).
43 Pennisi (2022).
44 Colbey *et al.* (2018).
45 Bower and Irwin (2016).

CASE STUDY: ALZHEIMER'S AND THE MICROBIOME[46]

The research lab of neurologist Giovanni Frisoni[47] has been working for several years on the potential influence of the gut microbiota on the brain and, more particularly, neurodegenerative diseases. Frisoni states: 'The gut microbiota composition in patients with Alzheimer's disease was altered, compared to people who do not suffer from such disorders... We have also discovered an association between inflammatory phenomenon detected in the blood, certain intestinal bacteria and Alzheimer's disease.'[48,49]

Intestinal bacteria can influence the functioning of the brain and promote neurodegeneration, through several pathways; they can influence the regulation of the immune system and, consequently, can modify the reaction between the immune and nervous systems. Lipopolysaccharides, proteins located in the membrane of bacteria with pro-inflammatory properties, have been found in amyloid plaques and around vessels in the brains of people with Alzheimer's. In addition, the intestinal microbiota produces metabolites which, having neuro-protective and anti-inflammatory properties, directly or indirectly affect brain function.

Immune signalling axes

We don't just have a gut–brain axis; we also have lung–brain, gut–lung, gut–skin, heart–brain axes, talking back to each other via microbiome in the gut and lungs (Figures 4j and 6j) in ways we are only just beginning to understand.

The bidirectional (two-way) gut–brain–microbiota axis (GBMA) is how the brain regulates the gut and its microbiota via neuroanatomic, immunological and neuroendocrine-hypothalamic-pituitary-adrenal (HPA) axis pathways, communicating via neurotransmitters, neuropeptides or microbial-derived products affecting gut microbiota. In the opposite direction, the gut microbiota influences the brain.[50,51]

The microbiome as a microcosm

Although the microbiome may seem separate to our own, larger self, there is a parallel between the microbiome's relationship with the body and the yogic

---

46   Marizzoni *et al.* (2020).
47   Dr Giovanni Frisoni is director of the HUG Memory Centre and professor at the Department of Rehabilitation and Geriatrics of the UNIGE Facility of Medicine. See www.j-alz.com/content/link-between-alzheimers-disease-and-gut-microbiota-confirmed
48   Zhao *et al.* (2018).
49   Painold *et al.* (2019).
50   Zhao *et al.* (2018).
51   Painold *et al.* (2019).

connection of the individual self with the larger consciousness (*samadhi*), reweaving our innate place within, not separate to, the natural world as 'other'. We evolved with our microbiome, symbiotically. The consequences of our increased separation from nature, exacerbated by factors such as stress, sugar excess and over-washing, impact negatively on our microbiome.

We can see from Figures 4j, 4l and 4m how the larger biome in the natural world around us is part of communication with our outer surface microbiome and reaching inwards via that in our immune system.

Yoga practices that foster embodied awareness bring us back to soma – first-person, phenomenological experience – rather than third-person, 'what's wrong, let's fix it' – and allow us to retune into that symbiosis with which we evolved. Yoga helps us modulate and adapt to stress, positively affecting inflammatory markers as we have seen (page 101).

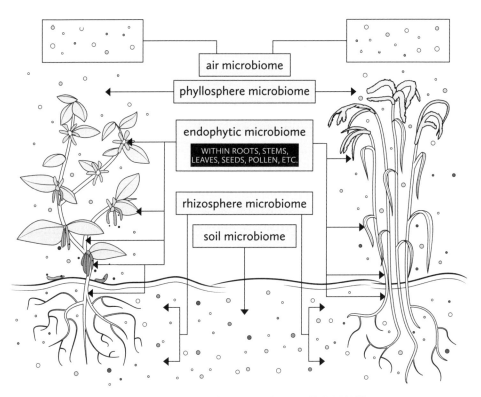

FIGURE 4L. THE LARGER ENVIRONMENTAL BIOME

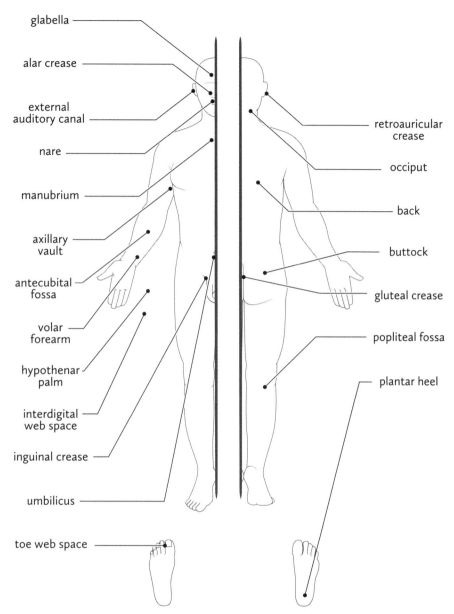

FIGURE 4M. TOPICAL DISTRIBUTION OF SKIN BIOME

The virome

In conversation with Charles Eisenstein, Zach Bush refutes the idea that viruses are part of our microbiome; rather that:

> The virome, which is a description of this global genetic information that's coursing out of biology – is the machinery of adaptation, and it's the language

of adaptation within life. And without the virome we would never have had the first bacteria or the first human cell. We've been built literally by the compilation and insertion of genetic information by these viruses into life forms around the planet for billions of years. The first viruses can be found in the fossil record some three and a half billion years ago. And so that's fascinating to me that this genetic information has been really the building block by which we now have life.[52]

Bush expresses that greater stressors in our environment and lack of biodiversity (from monocropping to over-sanitised environments, antibiotics and pesticides) increase our vulnerability as a population to genomic 'upgrades' coming into our bodies from connection with community:

> What looks like virally spread disease is happening for two reasons. One is that we are facing so many stressors, we need so many updates, we need to get these updates and it can be difficult to integrate that information. Added to that is that we have destroyed much of our ability to even receive those updates, through the decimation of the microbiome.[53]

So rather than being part of a 'biome', viruses may have a different role within the symbology of our organisms. Shifting our viewpoint from demonising them as the enemy, we might see them as essential to our evolution, communication beyond the self across community. This is where germ theory – the concept of battling against invaders to health – comes up against terrain theory, where the emphasis is placed on prevention rather than cure, exploring and treating the environment from which pathogens come rather than the illness caused by the pathogen.[54]

Breaching the barriers

The body's barriers prevent microorganisms from entering, but if these barriers are crossed, microorganisms are destroyed by innate immunity (page 27). Antibodies – part of acquired immunity (page 33) – inactivate microorganisms not destroyed by the innate immune system, also 'priming' cells so that subsequent responses are faster and more efficient (this is the basis of vaccination). Regulation of immune and inflammatory responses depends

---

52 Zach Bush, quoted in Eisenstein (2020).
53 Ibid.
54 Ayoade (2017).

on communication between cells' cytokines (page 88), which have a tightly regulated, transient action.[55]

The microbiome may be negatively affected by environmental factors, including:[56]

- Chronic stress
- Artificial sweeteners
- High-fat diet
- Caesarean section and formula milk – our gut microbiome is influenced by what we receive during vaginal birth and in the first six weeks of life from our mother and through breast milk (acquired immunity).
- Antimicrobials – in drinking water
- Arsenic – in farmed rice
- Pathogens
- Harsh laundry products, antibacterial washes – these target the skin and oral microbiome[57] (page 340)
- Pesticides
- Ultrafine particles – present in air pollution.

Mindful eating

How we eat can have as much of an impact on the microbiome and gut health as the food itself. Thoroughly chewed food has the best chance of complete digestion and brings less harmful agents into the body. Our saliva contains multiple immune components, a first line of immune defence that we can miss when gulping quickly. This isn't just important to absorb nutrients, but also to ensure that partially digested food doesn't hang around, when it can putrefy and create gas and bloating. This debris at the gut wall prevents full digestion and immune function and can lead to symptoms such as constipation, diarrhoea and food intolerances.

Habitually eating 'little and often' may also strain digestive health. Grazing may support short-term energy levels, but continually putting food into our mouths sets us up to become fixated on eating constantly and confuses our relationship with hunger. Eating a fuller meal with the requisite protein and healthy fats creates a sense of satisfaction from the gut to the brain (via

55 Galley and Webster (1996).
56 National Institute of Environmental Health Services (2022).
57 Acharya (no date).

neuropeptide messengers in the stomach) that can create a whole-body calming effect – we can relax from the primal imperative to need to seek out more food, at least for a while.

Our digestive tract needs periods where each section can rest and heal. Constantly having to digest food as we start the process from the beginning again demands vast energy. It takes an average of 40 hours for food to travel from mouth to anus, and each time we put something else into our mouths, we start up the whole process over again.

Mindful eating during meals has been shown to naturally regulate portion size and create the satisfaction that lowers food cravings later. Chewing also stimulates the thymus gland to produce T cells, a major part of the protective immune system.

Rest and renewal

Regularly allowing full rest and good quality sleep allows the energy that the gut needs to repair. Thinking, moving and even just standing to eat directs fuel, circulation and nutrients to our muscles and brain. When you consider that the most recent approximation of gut surface marks it the size of half a badminton court and each cell is renewed every four to five days, it's easy to see how our digestive health can suffer without adequate rest. Sleep disruption has been shown to alter the gut microbiome and increase inflammatory tendencies and metabolic disruption.[58]

Visceral tissue health and movement

When functioning optimally, viscera (organs) have space between for ease of movement. Visceral *mobility* is the ability of organs to rub against and move alongside other organs and tissues. Adhesions that stick visceral tissues together can cause obstructions in the fascia, for example parts of the bowel fused together or to other organs, or any part of the digestive tract stuck to the wall of the abdominal cavity. We might feel these as internal 'pulls' or related to reproductive, pelvic, diaphragmatic or lower back issues, as connective tissue in the fascia unites these and other areas as a continual web. An osteopath who works viscerally as well as structurally can help feel and ease such tensions.

Visceral *motility* is the movement that happens within organs, for example peristalsis within the digestive tract. This can also be affected by mobility issues. Efficient visceral motility allows ease and regulation of bowel movements, and supports immune modulation via the microbiome.

---

58 Poroyko *et al.* (2016).

Regular movement creates the fascial 'slide and glide' that supports gut motility as well as full physical mobility and reduces fascial lesions that interfere with full digestion. We need to keep hydrated and pliable in the mid-torso area that can become stuck and rigid through sitting, and accrue more weight there as we grow older. Movement systems such as yoga, dance, belly-dancing, tai chi and qi gong, where there are differing patterns, fluid and twisting motions through the abdominal area and an emphasis on freeing up diaphragmatic movement and breath, keep this mid-section pliable and rotational.

Getting out into nature and having contact with a biodiverse environment (as we evolved) is an important component of gut health, often missing from those living in urban areas.[59] Taking our movement patterns and exercise into the countryside is beneficial on many levels; we humans need wonder and beauty to access the nervous system mode (ventral vagus) that allows gut healing, digestive support through stress reduction and bringing down inflammatory tendencies.[60]

For optimum fascial fitness, these cover the full range of essential human movement:

- Squatting
- Lunging
- Bending at the hips
- Twisting
- Gait – walking, running, carrying
- Arms – pushing, pulling, swinging, throwing
- Dance and spontaneous shifts within play.[61]

WAYS TO ENCOURAGE A FLOURISHING GUT MICROBIOME[62]

- Fibre: 40g of fibre per day can reduce cardiac issues, cancers and weight gain. We derive this from plant fibres in vegetables, fruit, pulses, wholegrain, nuts and seeds. Artichokes, leeks,

59   Hanski *et al.* (2012).
60   Komegae *et al.* (2018).
61   Schleip with Bayer (2021).
62   Spector (2020).

onions and garlic contain high levels of prebiotic (which feeds probiotics) fibre inulin.

- Varied seasonal fruit and vegetables: the different nutrients and fibres each support our variety of microbial species. Eating diverse seasonal vegetables is more beneficial than taking food supplements.
- Polyphenols: antioxidants that fuel microbes, found in seeds, berries, green tea, olive oil, brassicas and coffee.
- Snack less: greater intervals between eating allow gut healing and microbial replenishment. Occasional skipping of meals or fasting can also be beneficial.
- Fermented foods: kefir, raw milk cheeses, sauerkraut, kimchi and soybean products contain live microbes.
- Alcohol: gut diversity is improved by small amounts of alcohol, but destroyed by too much.
- Artificial sweeteners and processed foods: reduce gut diversity and disrupt microbial metabolism, and can cause obesity and diabetes.
- Terrain: gardening, outdoor activities and spending time with animals increases our gut diversity.
- Antibiotics and non-essential medicines: 'good' and 'bad' microbes are destroyed by antibiotics,[63] and even paracetamol (acetaminophen)[64] and nonsteroidal anti-inflammatory drugs (NSAIDs)[65] such as ibuprofen and antacids (proton pump inhibitors)[66] can disrupt microbial function.
- Hygiene: over-washing or use of antibacterial products can damage our gut microbiome; soap is the most effective at reducing pathogen exposure and leaves the microbiome intact.
- Vitamin D: getting out into nature and absorbing sunshine plays a pivotal role in maintaining microbial gut homeostasis.[67]
- Exercise: gut microbiota are positively affected by exercise, but this may also be linked to healthy eating.[68]

63 Lange *et al.* (2016).
64 Clayton *et al.* (2009).
65 Maseda and Ricciotti (2020).
66 Vila *et al.* (2020).
67 Fakhoury *et al.* (2020).
68 Clarke *et al.* (2014).

Adverse childhood experiences (ACEs) – developmental trauma

We've talked about the trauma patterns and the related inflammatory responses (Part 3) that can compromise our barriers, fluidity and access to calm states. One of the most important things we can do for our gut-immune-neuro-respiratory health is to recognise the responses (*samskaras*) we circle round and meet these stories as part of our whole being (and so often, our present) with kindness, friendliness and generosity to ourselves.

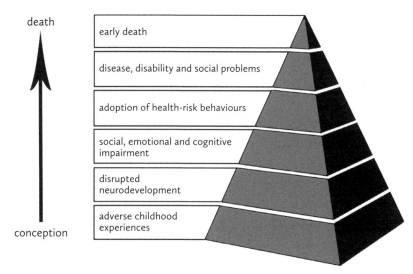

FIGURE 4N. MECHANISMS BY WHICH ADVERSE CHILDHOOD EXPERIENCES
INFLUENCE HEALTH AND WELLBEING THROUGHOUT THE LIFESPAN
Source: Adapted from the Adverse Childhood Experiences (ACE) study (Felitti et al. 1998)

Much research has been examined around physical and mental health (as well as addictions) in relation to early life trauma. This is particularly true for respiratory conditions, where breath tends to recreate the stress states being relived, keeping secondary breathing (sympathetic) as the norm and low-grade inflammation running in the background.

The Adverse Childhood Experiences (ACE) study in 1999[69] (Figure 4n) examined a huge body of data to clearly link early life (developmental) trauma to chronic degenerative or inflammatory conditions, the stuff of Western civilisation and increased stress. Impaired cognitive, social and emotional function is also observed, which is not surprising when we have seen that disruption of the ANS and microbiome are at the heart of poor immune modulation.

Developmental trauma (ACEs) may be something distinct such as abuse or

---

69 Felitti *et al.* (1998).

neglect, but can also be more subtle, such as attachment or attunement issues. We are social animals and flourish most in social engagement (ventral vagus) mode, needing strong and healthy attachments to caregivers, especially as we are so dependent when young. Our nervous systems are primed through social contact, and if this is lacking when we are developing, there is disruption to the ANS, to the CNS and the gut, creating disrupted neurodevelopment, the basic default of 'not safe'. Being seen for who we are (attunement) is another ingredient for us to be able to register safety – everything is okay. Lack of eye contact (or the 'not present' of being on a smartphone), or not feeling heard or understood is detrimental to growing nervous systems and minds.

This isn't a case of blame, often lack of attachment or attunement ripples down the generations; we pass on our survival styles, and we are all just doing our best. This leads us back to the great need for awareness and compassion. If we add in isolation and loneliness on top of adverse childhood experiences, the impact on immune, respiratory and all other body systems is enormous.

The ACE study looked at how the more challenging experiences or lack of connection a child had, the more likelihood of issues with socio-emotional and cognitive development. The study showed that these issues made it more difficult for the child to relate to others, and could lead to more risk-taking behaviours and less ability to self-care, ultimately to disease, disability and social problems, even early death. When we also consider that much trauma can also be intergenerational, inherited or cultural – factors that we have been conditioned with, but don't necessarily serve us well – we can choose to tune into our own current needs, by fostering a relationship with what is true right now.

Developmental trauma is commonly seen with freeze, immobilisation and dissociation, a checking out (see dorsal vagus mode, page 162), particularly if there hasn't been a safe holding by someone in a child's younger years. If we grew up in an angry household, the need to stay quiet and small, or not rock the boat, could mean we minimise our existence with this check-out mode. These stress responses can be deeply held in the body from a time when we were unable to protect our self or run away.

In many trauma therapies, strong work with the legs can be used to repattern where we have been physically unable to run away, retraining the subconscious to literally stand our ground (such as the standing practices in this part). Much of this work is now being moved through into police and social care, with the understanding that antisocial behavioural patterns can be linked to early or developmental trauma.

Examples of unhealthy energetic boundaries

In their book *Healing Developmental Trauma*, Laurence Heller and Aline Lapierre[70] discuss boundaries as expressions of nervous system regulation, and explore different ages, from babyhood to the teenage years. This is the stuff of the intuitive, subtle body, beyond the physical or the emotional. We need a sense of cohesion and safety within the boundaries of our skin. When we don't have this (often through trauma), we can have:

- Self-protective 'tough outer shell' – the opposite to feeling vulnerability.
- Extreme sensitivity to another's emotions – not having a filter.
- Oversensitivity to touch – it is important for bodywork teachers to gain consent to touch students.
- A raw feeling of walking around without 'skin' – no autonomy.
- Energetic merging with other people, animals and the environment – this can be wonderful in terms of sensitivity, but there needs to be healthy boundaries of protection, back within one's own skin.
- Sensing danger – on alert can come from anywhere at any time.
- Hyper- and/or hypovigilance – in general or in specific directional vectors such as from behind. Sensory experience can be felt as pain that needs to be relieved immediately; for example, responding in a heightened way to a drop in temperature, the 'danger' seems imperative.
- Environmental sensitivities and allergies.
- Social discomfort – in groups or crowds, where there is no filtering out one person's voice above the sea of noise, an indicator of adrenal fatigue, chronic stress or trauma.
- Agoraphobia – needing social isolation where there is overwhelm.

Examples of healthy energetic boundaries

In *Healing Developmental Trauma*, Heller and Lapierre[71] describe examples of healthy energetic boundaries as having:

- Comfort in one's own body.
- Feeling safe in the world.

---

70   Heller and Lapierre (2012).
71   Heller and Lapierre (2012).

- Differentiation – a clear sense of self and other.
- Setting parameters – being able to say 'no' and set limits, as well as saying 'yes'.

Gabor Maté expounds: 'Most chronic illness is the body saying no when the person suppressed their no to fit in. When illness comes on, we can look upon it as a nuisance to get rid of or an enemy to fight or we can say, "OK, it's here now, what's the teaching?"'[72]

Boundaries can be skewed further through isolation in modern society, which was especially exacerbated by lockdown during COVID-19 restrictions and continues with much contact on screens. This is what we can reset within our practices, embodied realities where we feel our feet on the ground. We can explore in somatic practices where we meet our 'edges', and define our own boundaries to stand up to the world. Understanding embodied awareness in terms of the unravelling of trauma is explored famously in Bessel van der Kolk's *The Body Keeps the Score*, where he says: 'The single most important issue for traumatized people is to find a sense of safety in their own bodies.'[73]

Humans have neuroplasticity – change and post-traumatic growth are always possible.

The role of the yoga teacher
Healthy boundaries can be re-established within the context of a yoga class by including:

- Skin contact (only when appropriate from a teacher (with consent) or from self): rub, pull, squeeze, compress, friction, touch. Incorporating eustress – positive stress (pages 101 and 155) – as a resource rather than something to react to – comes from feeling safe and the relief of being present. The chemical release from safe touch has profound effects: 'Oxytocin modulates immunostatus, metabolic state and gut microbiome.'[74]
- Grounding: feeling a full, physical sense of where we are, in the present, including our relationship to the Earth that holds us up and gravity that pushes us down – the basis of trust in ourselves. A yoga

72 Maté (2021).
73 van der Kolk (2015).
74 Park *et al.* (2020).

practice that reinforces embodied awareness (explored in Part 5) helps create new pathways of safety that allow processing feelings with space, rather than re-traumatisation. Grounding is one of the most important guides in allowing us to have this journey.

- Orientation: sensing fully where we are in time and space (proprio-ception), as well as registering our inner world (interoception) such as navigating back to the midline. *Drishti*, where we consciously orien-tate gaze (focused attention, soft around the edges), turning the head while lying on the ground, mimics the hypervigilant looking around for danger but in a conscious, calm way, to register we are looking out for ourselves.

- Social engagement: eye contact, smiling, being open and human, but with good boundaries ourselves. Coregulation from a teacher is there to help a student find their own capacity for self-regulation; much of this is through voice tones – clear enough to hear, with soothing tones. Directing *drishti* regularly can help students orient back into the space, held as a clear boundary for when attention invariably wanders. If they appear to dissociate, drawing attention to something in the room offers a real place to come back to. Ask them to feel their body, themselves, in the present moment.

- Agency: moving beyond unhelpful *samskaras* into healthy boundaries requires a teacher to step back from a more traditional role and allow students agency. This means giving them permission to follow their own needs, for exploration in a practice, facilitating inner process – autonomy. By encouraging deep inner listening and appropriate response (or abstention), we can guide students to trust decisions from their own bodies over an instruction of what is 'right' when it may not be right for them. Praising students can reinforce patterns of wanting to please others rather than listening to real need; we can support with compassion instead.

- Time and space: our own grounding as teachers supports us to 'hold space' for others. This means having the courage to let invitational instruction to land, be acknowledged, then felt and maybe responded to. Rather than imposing our idea of a practice or what another person may need, we can step back and allow them to have their own unfolding journey.

- Allowing for unknown trauma: in somatic and meditative practices we need to be aware that traumatic experiences can be accessed, even though we are not diagnosing. We don't even need to mention the word 'trauma'; just recognise its prevalence and that practices that may seem gentler can reach much deeper spots as they access vulnerability. Unless you are specifically trained in verbal therapy, the embodiment that is the route back from trauma doesn't need to get into the story of the situation or events. This is about meeting ourselves, where we are, and recognising we need different things at different times, and these need to be listened to.

PHYSICAL PRACTICE: STANDING INTO FULL BREATHING AND PROTECTIVE SUPPORT

Standing poses offer the possibility of transformation for those with chronic stress or trauma as they provide a firm, physical rooting, grounding and earthing through the feet. If practised with awareness and space to cool and come back to the breath between, they can create a 'good' stress (eustress) that challenges without wearing out. Holding to find the balanced *guna* (page 274) of *sattva* (wisdom, balance) via the breath can help create the resilience and adaptation that prevents lurching from 'highs to lows' – fluctuating between a continual see-saw of *rajas* (motion and activity) and *tamas* (inertia, inactivity), that within the polyvagal model (page 161) we can view as getting stuck between the extremes of hypervigilance (*rajas*) and dissociation (*tamas*).

Becoming aware of when (and where in the body) we might overwork or underwork can help us find *sattva* – equanimity, grace under pressure and the middle way.

The *Sutra sthira-sukha-asanam* (posture should be steady and comfortable)[75] becomes clear as a guide for this moment-to-moment observance of balance between the containment needed to hold a stronger pose and the *sukha* to occupy it with openness and equanimity.

Focusing on strengthening through the legs encourages *apana vayu* (the winds in the body that govern digestion and elimination; page 286), that can diminish as we grow older, from being sedentary or chronic stress, and add to loss of vitality. We do not need to rattle through endless standing poses to 'build heat' (*agni*); most people in the 21st century are pretty overheated from constant stimulus already, which can show up as inflammation and sympathetic dominance (page 88). Neither is it more 'advanced' to speed up: to be able to stay, hold and be with the experience of the pose unfolding is to drop beneath the habitual mind's want to drive forward and do more; to slow down to feel and meet the deeper unconscious realms.

When we back away from attachment to extremes, we can move towards functionality within our natural range of motion (as in the primal motions in Part 3, and opening here) – that which has the most chance of taking us through

---

75   Bryant (2009).

231

physical and movement health into elderhood. Walking is the basic fruitional function for the human being – all of our movement patterns self-organise to reach this point and calibrate through our spinal curves up from the ground.

Gravity is a continual force pushing down on us, and our ability to lift up against it relies on ground reaction force: the upwards force from the Earth's core that is stronger through the body when we are still. Movement lessens this strain and relieves compressive transmission forces through the body, especially through the spine as the structure that supports vertical positioning.

TWISTING TO WALK

When we effortlessly walk and swing our arms with our stride, we are occupying our spiral lines (page 114) to their full expression. They meet the erector spinae muscles, holding us up the spine, and the abdominal fascia, drawing us up through the front body. This allows us to continually shift our posture, rotate and compensate for any weight changes, while lifting upright from the ground. When we walk, forces are transferred from one sacroiliac joint (where the lumbar spine sits into the pelvis) to the other side, and if our spiral lines are free, this can feel less jarring in the lower back, hips and abdominal and pelvic organs.

Somatic practices can help us feel how to move with most ease, with the forces that move through us and our organisation with them. These forces are boundaries we encounter as we come to standing, literally meeting the world. Proprioception is how we sense these boundaries and allows us to foster interoception, the inner processing of what we meet and with others without triggering fear states (unless appropriate!). There is constant communication through our lymphatics, epithelium and therefore microbiome as we experience our environment.

Following from Keleman's quote on page 171, 'Human uprightness is a genetic urge...'[76] we can compare our physical relationship to the Earth – in particular, the biological ground from where we originate, its microbiome being symbiotic to our own, where the grounding we develop in safe attachments as a child are like the strong roots needed for a tree to develop. Bipedalism in itself, however, is unstable. Keleman again: 'It was when man stood up that his

---

76   Keleman (1985).

relationship with the earth became insecure. And that state of unsureness and instability serves as the foundation of human consciousness.[77]

This is why we come back to the ground in our yoga and somatic practices, returning to 'dependency and helplessness' to undo physical and emotional patterns laid down by consciousness, so that the return to the vertical may bring transformational insight. Intelligent work is needed in the feet to feel effortless coming up to support the weight bearing on the knees when they bend. We began this journey in the primal motions of Part 3, leading into the standing movements in this sequence. We explore this through the vertical axis, with fascially fluid movements here great preparation for any other standing practices.

Standing practices bring a sense of agency, ability and the strength of stable legs. Liz Koch states: 'putting one's foot down is a powerful biological gesture.'[78]

Research has shown that more active practices followed by relaxing ones can lead to more deep release than relaxing practices alone. This is referred to as cyclic meditation (CM) in some schools, and helps regulate the ANS:

> In CM, the period of practicing yoga postures constitutes the "awakening" practices, while periods of supine rest comprise "calming practices". An essential part of the practice of CM is being aware of sensations arising in the body. This supports the idea that a combination of stimulating and calming techniques practiced with a background of relaxation and awareness (during CM) may reduce psycho physiological arousal more than resting in a supine posture for the same duration.[79]

Free crawling to *balasana* (child's pose)

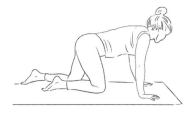 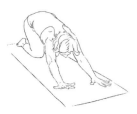

---

77 Keleman (1985).
78 Koch (2019).
79 Subramanya and Telles (2009).

- Crawling creates motion across the 'diagonals' of the torso. This is where we 'move out from the centre', fostering integrated movement. When we crawl on all-fours, we can feel any movement in response to intuitive need. The pelvis is not pinned to the ground, so we don't tend to pull into the sacroiliac joint (SI) as we move in multiple directions.
- Moving away from the confines of the mat, we can also come out of any boxes of 'right' or 'wrong' our conditioned minds might be bringing along for the ride. You can explore sideways, backwards or any other angle or direction for a full range of motion and the brain coherence of marrying up both sides of the brain hemispheres.

1. Crawl around (pages 174 and 362), occupying space around you (even off the mat!), meeting the ground – bringing attention and sensitivity to connection there.
2. Start to feel into and around the diaphragm, rolling between the ribs and seeing what movements that might prompt up into the shoulders, neck, head and jaw – preparing to calibrate vertically up from the ground.
3. Roll into rotations of the tailbone, almost like a small, soft *nauli* (page 128). Feel the rippling up, freeing fascia between the organs, encouraging interoception.
4. Feeling the boundaries of the floor, explore the fluid body without looking for issues to fix, but rather listening and responding to nuance and organic movement, without an agenda.
5. In *balasana*, extend and move through the fingers, expanding out through the spaces between, especially releasing after time spent on devices – habitual 'tech fingers' create tension in the diaphragm.

Vajrapradama mudra (unshakeable trust) in *vajrasana* (diamond pose)

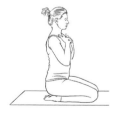

- Interlinked fingers draw together both sides of the brain hemispheres and the polarity of *ida* (moon, left-hand side of the body and right-hand side of the brain) and *pingala* (sun, right-hand side of the body and right-hand side of the brain) around the central axis of *sushumna nadi*.

- Offering the trust we can tune into via the balance of *sattva* at the heart, noticing the autonomic nervous system soothing this can bring via the heart–brain axis (page 342).

1. Support the knees or come up on the knees if sitting back in *vajrasana* isn't easeful.
2. Interlink the fingers and bring the palms over the top of the chest.
3. Come to the focus of *vajrapradama mudra* (unshakeable trust; page 190), tuning into support at the heart, the rise and fall of the breath.

Vinyasa as low salutation into *adho mukha svanasana* (down-face dog pose)

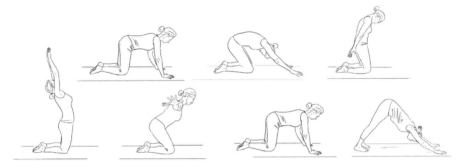

- This sequence has similarities to some versions of a moon salutation (*chandra namaskar*) as it stays lower to the ground, and is thus more cooling than the heat of a sun salutation (*surya namaskar*).
- Punctuating movement with this short *vinyasa*, exploring movement up away from the floor, we are expanding the boundaries of the body in a smooth, steady, spacious way, drawing back towards the floor. Finding fascial flow, noticing what it is to move in this way, how the mind may try to plan and organise, but how we can drop beneath those habitual voices and trust into the body and breath finding their stride of ease, *sukha*.

1. See instructions on page 181.
2. Add a *adho mukha svanasana* (down-face dog) in after coming back down to all-fours whenever it feels appropriate for the energy, tone and breath within the movement.

3. Then feel out the 'right' amount of time to stay in each *adho mukha svanasana* (not too little, not too much) before moving into the salutation, where you might inhale to rise up, exhale to drop back down towards the earth.

Rising from foetal squat

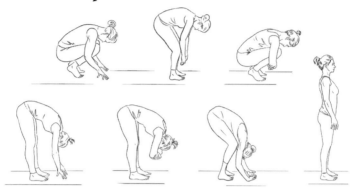

- To calibrate the upper body with the natural curves of the spine, we roll up and down to finally find ears above the shoulders, above the top of the thigh bones, above the ankles – rising up through the front body and settling the shoulders on top of the volume of the rib cage. Growing up from the ground, with awareness of the feet, allows the most effortless organisation upwards.
- As you finally arrive into standing, reorientate with the eyes soft, noticing the breath. Sway slowly without planning, noticing the natural wave of the body, noticing the point where the body tonifies at the boundary of gravity to come back to centre. It is okay if there is uncertainty or instability; simply notice.
- Feel the rise of *prana vayu*, lifting up the front body, *apana vayu*, dropping down the back of the body – supporting spaciousness between the ventral and dorsal.

1. Come into a foetal squat; chest curled, heels up, head released. Finger-tips can be lightly on the ground, or the arms bound around the legs in the paradox of a nurturing but vertical foetal position, combined with the activity of the squat; breathing with any twitch in the ankles.
2. Bring the heels down and hands off the ground to draw up the legs. Come up and down several times, feet hip-width apart.

3. Drop the weight of the head to settle into a soft forward bend, looking between the legs rather than down to the ground, the weight dropping to the front of the heels. Back away from any forceful forward fold, simply letting the spine decompress.

4. Take hold of opposite elbows, allowing the upper body to hang. Toes spread, draw up the insteps – vital fascial slings of the feet that influence and innervate up through the inner legs – in *pada bandha*, translated as foot lock but 'insteps gathering' a more sensitive description.

5. Bend the knees deeply, dropping the upper body completely over the thighs, arms like a rag doll, releasing any doing. Feel the compression of the diaphragm into the thighs, trusting the strong support of the legs in this upright version of a child's pose.

6. Uncurl up with knees bent. Notice any point where you have a habit of pushing the pelvis forward or tucking the tailbone under and retrace back. Come to the point before up by raising the thigh bones above the ankles and letting the lower back have its natural curve, while gathering up through the belly. Roll up and down with bent knees, allowing your lower back and body above to organise themselves, ribcage above the pelvis, head floating over the ribs.

Standing twists

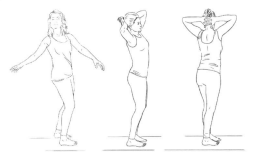

- Small, repetitive twists (such as swinging arms around the body) help open the intercostal muscles between the ribs and create fluidity in the breath. This mimics the freedom and ease through the rib cage we have when walking – how this most natural of our movements is linked to optimal breathing and lymphatic movement.
- Revolving around the ribs and the diaphragm opens front, back,

sides and all of the nooks and crannies in the upper body, which then radiate out to the whole.

1. With soft knees, swing the arms round the central axis to loosen tissues around the central body and diaphragm, feeling the movement come from the belly, hands like weights at the ends of the arms as ropes. Allow the head to turn naturally, in line with the spine. Come back to this periodically throughout the practice. Feel here how the outer boundaries become more alive, aware, possibly softening defensive barriers.

2. Explore your head position above the shoulders when standing by clasping the bottom of the skull, feeling the back of the head dropping into the hands to support postural information. Feel the back of the skull rising above the heels, rather than the head pushing forward of the shoulders and midlinc (see 'tech neck', page 169).

3. With the hands still supporting the head, twist side to side from the belly, calibrating the head above the ribs, dropping away from second- ary breathing in the shoulders down into the diaphragm and the belly.

4. Rotate around the diaphragm and the ribs, breathing fully 'through the armpits' and feeling the turn coming from the belly rather than the shoulders, soft eyes following the positioning of the face in line with the breastbone.

Shoulder rolls to sensing the belly

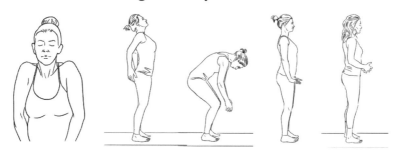

- Feel the support of *pada bandha* (gathering up instep), connection through all four corners of the feet, to explore awareness of the space between the boundaries of the ventral (front) and dorsal (back) body.
- Bring awareness into the belly, up from the legs into the root of the spine, around the pelvis, tailbone and lower abdomen, the inner

channel (core sheath) from the feet through the inner legs, the psoas, the diaphragm and into the base of the skull.

- Through standing spine undulations, we can feel the presence of boundaries. The polarity between where we rise from the ground and meet the world (where we also digest life's experience, lay down our impressions and feel into our true relation to any moment) on the inhalation, and come back into rest, rejuvenation and touching base with the exhalation.

1. With the knees bent, inhale the shoulders forward and right up to the ears, then back and down with the exhalation, allowing the full range through the shoulder girdle and reminding us where lifted is, and also where not lifted lies. Notice any habitual holding patterns and rigid boundaries of self-protection loosening their grip.
2. Reverse the roll: inhale the shoulders back and up, exhale forward and down. Allow a dropping down to bent knees on the exhale, opening the full front body on the inhale.
3. Ground down into the feet. Draw fingers up, palms facing the ground, pressing down to lift the back of the skull.
4. Bring the hands to hold the space in front of the belly or *hara* (Daoist *dantien*), tuning into subtle body space around the *annamaya kosha* (physical body, page 150).

Standing rib cage roll and spinal undulation

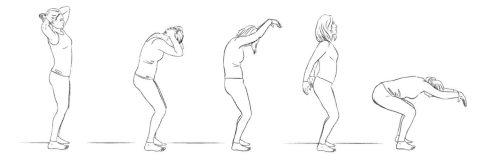

- These motions moving through the rib cage, diaphragm and organs encourage lymphatic drainage around the collarbone and pliability in the respiratory area. Support up from responsive feet and legs allows uplift through the spine, through the centre.

- Allow the natural pause at the end of the exhale (*kumbhaka*) before moving back up through the inhale, letting the breath lead, body follow, mind observe.
- These arm movements can also be done within a low lunge or kneeling position for different effects within the pelvis.

1. Clasp hands behind the head again and circle the upper body, around the ribs, solar plexus and diaphragm. One direction and then the other.
2. Release the arms, then, from standing with knees bent, exhale to curl in to the front body, reaching the arms forward with soft wrists, knees bent to allow responsive movement.
3. Inhale to turn the hands over (palms up) to draw the arms back past the hips and open the front body, arms about 45 degrees out to open across the collarbone with their weight.
4. On the exhale, find pliability through the ankles by repeating the curl in, squatting down lower if comfortable in the knees.

Moving *vrksasana* (tree pose)

The motion is like somatic practices on the ground where we arrive in to attune to the feelings of our 'emotional muscle', the psoas. On standing, we can feel how easefully – or not – we rise up from the legs to the spine. If this feels interrupted (or we walk from the thighs rather than the spine) this might suggest tightness in this muscle region where we can lay down self-protective habits in tension. As its relationship to the diaphragm affects how we stand up and how we breathe, softening here can ripple release into the whole mind-body.

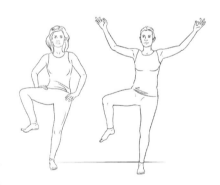

- In this loosening movement (great before stronger standing postures or holding *vrksasana*), we invite malleability into the psoas of the raised leg while extending the psoas on the standing leg, feeling the proprioception of the standing leg grounding.

- Arms raised may seem more effortful, but it allows balance as a responsive counter to the shifts in the lower body below.

1. From standing, keeping the gaze steady, lift one leg, knee bent. Feel the innervation in the standing leg from the ground up, hip gathering in, rising up the inner leg through the spine, jaw soft (see more on balance on page 268).
2. Circle the raised leg from the hip, out and up from the centre (touching your big toe to the ground each time, if you need). Hands can be on the hips or arms raised, hands in *chin mudra*, finger to thumb tips, in a gesture of receptivity and expansion.
3. Clear the space of expectation before changing to the other side.

Utkata konasana (intense angle pose) explorations 1

- From feet alive with *pada bandha* (gathering instep), we can find the pelvic positioning where the *chakras* rise from the root; this position (aka wide horse stance in martial arts) allows us to explore this via the stronger sensations offered up through the legs. There can be a tendency here to 'over-tuck' the tailbone where engagement is lost in the inner thighs, and the other excess is to let the belly contents spill forward – common if the psoas is tight.
- The middle way is where we retain the natural curve of the lower back and also find stability – bringing the sitting bones forward and letting the tailbone simply be. Then, gathering the belly in and up, we can sit into the pose with knees easily pointing in the direction of the toes, breathing fully to meet sensations up the central channel from the inner legs.

1. Step legs out to the side, protecting the knees by keeping the feet in line with the knees. Move side to side, feeling the weight shift between the feet.
2. Bending the legs, lengthen the inner thighs so knees stay pointing in the direction of the toes, balanced inner and outer. Only come

down to a comfortable degree and lift the insteps to stabilise and not collapse into the inner feet; lift and spread toes to help this.

3. Clasp the hands to the back of the skull to tune into the lift through the spinal curves.

Utkata konasana (intense angle pose) explorations 2

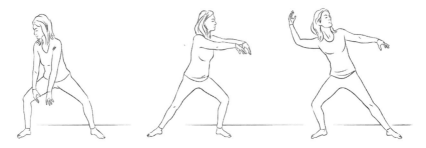

- Arm movements within this posture allow us to move the hips within a whole-body motion and explore shifting weight between feet and knees. We can sweep the arms as here, or explore other movements such as figure-of-eights, or inhaling up, exhaling down, in various configurations.
- In this continuous motion, we draw the arm back in a protective circle around the head as we shift weight onto the same knee bending. That side of the body creates an elastic loading in the fascia. This is where energy is built within fascia to be released as effortless movement, and here, it then takes us back the way we came with a rebounding feeling to the movement.

1. From the wide stance, begin by sweeping both hands in semi-circles side to side, as far as shoulder height. Feel the motion from the feet, fostering support through the legs as the knees bend towards the direction the arms are reaching.
2. Then, as you sweep, open the arm furthest forward up and over the head, like a bow, holding the space around the ear. Sweep it back and then both arms all the way to the other side and open there, moving side to side in continual motion, opening the heart and lung space.

Utthita trikonasana (extended triangle pose) to *virabhadrasana II* (warrior II pose)

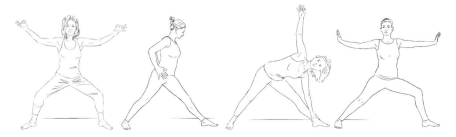

- The triangle is a potent female or divine symbol in many cultures, and feeling the stability of its angles from the ground helps us connect with others in the body, such as the triangle within the sitting bones and pubic bone that contain the pelvic and abdominal contents. Moving through the triangles of our feet upwards, we can have an alive relationship with stability.
- Warrior poses empower up into the third *chakra* as we inhabit our bodies fully and reach out into the world. *Virabhadrasana II* (warrior II pose) reaches the arms out in both directions, sitting into the centre with the courage to be present.
- In *trikonasana* (triangle pose) and *virabhadrasana II*, turn the back hip in strongly, to allow ease throughout the pelvis and viscera, as well as a non-forceful alignment from heel–knee–sitting bone through both legs, where the lower back can find its most comfortable place.

1. Back in centre, take *chin mudra* with the arms raised, continually soften the jaw and loosen the shoulder blades down the back to lift the arms from the belly rather than the shoulders, finding how to support their weight (through the breath) without strain or stress. Gather up through the belly from the insteps and inner legs.
2. Turn the left foot in, right foot out, where the pelvis and lower back are comfortable rather than an overly prescribed 'one size fits all' alignment. Reach the bottom arm to come into *trikonasana*, as far as it comes, while still able to revolve the belly and chest upwards with ease. Draw the rib cage around as the top arm lifts, so this becomes more of a twist between the hips turning down and the upper chest opening. If the top shoulder lifting does not create space, the top hand can rest on the top hip or back of the pelvis to open the area

between the shoulder capsule and the ribs, providing space to open across the chest and lengthen the spine and neck. *Trikonasana* can be a particularly useful pose for exploring our relationship with the heel and the ground, up to the belly.

3. From *trikonasana*, ripple the arms up towards *virabhadrasana II*. Fingers lift as we reach through the arms and wrist to explore the world beyond our boundaries to meet a sense of embodiment, safe and strong within our physical form.

4. Inhaling, bring the arms together above the head, legs straight, and exhale down into *virabhadrasana II*. A flowing movement with the breath here can focus both the attention and connection with the midline and bring awareness to the shoulders. Move with each breath for continual awareness of dropping down through the midline (rib cage above pelvis), lengthening the inner thigh of the front leg and drawing up the inner knee of the back one for resistance to drop down with grace. Then we can settle into both feet and our breath, softening the shoulders, jaw and eyes to find *sattva*.

5. Move through *utkata konasana* (intense angle pose) with arms raised before moving to the other side.

Utkata konasana (intense angle pose) explorations 3

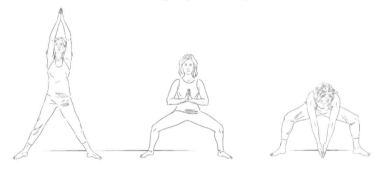

When we consider the midline in terms of mouth-to-anus tube, the gut–brain axis, spine and *sushumna*, it is within a physical practice that we hone a conscious relationship with this place of gathering in and reaching out from. With our asymmetrically arranged torso contents, finding our way back to 'even' is never quite complete, but it does offer the mind the chance to drop back into the tidal rhythm of the breath and cerebrospinal fluid (CSF) pulse.

This can be felt as 'coming home', connecting with our most primal rhythms and within rest. Noticing how we move out from, twist around, curl in, open up and then come home to the midline is to feel our existence in the world, our very essence. This melding of interoception and proprioception is the space for 'listening and responding' within an embodied movement practice.

1. Come back to the midline after the asymmetry of *trikonasana* (triangle pose) and *virabhadrasana* (warrior pose II). Stand with feet apart and turned out 90 degrees from one another, in a wide *vatayanasana* (horse face pose). Bend the knees to a comfortable height. Inhale to lift the arms out and round, to above your head, as the legs straighten.
2. Exhale to bend again, and bring the hands down the midline to the heart.
3. If room is available to you, with happy knees, follow the exhale movement of the downwards trajectory to drop the upper body and touch the fingertips to the floor.
4. Continue this movement, inhaling to sweep the arms back, round and up, exhaling down the centre line.

Utkata konasana (intense angle pose) undulation

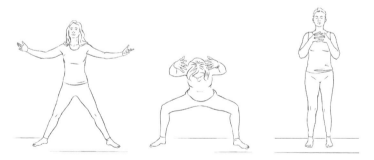

Moving undulations up from the ground in ever-stronger ways can help bring the nervous system balancing effects into the more active tones of mobilisation. This helps how we shift between states of high and low with less jarring or reactivity within life, that is, better adaptation that affects immune and respiratory health.

Similarly, coming back to the right–left brain integration of *vajrapradama mudra* at the resting meditative position of *tadasana* (mountain pose) gathers back in towards self-regulation capacity. If we work with one *mudra* within a practice session (as a punctuation), bringing it into different positions and planes, we can come back to its meaning or qualities as a signpost along the way.

1. Legs wide, inhale to come up, as you open out your arms with the inner edge of the shoulder blades dropping. Exhale to lean your torso forward, long, taking your arms in the shape of a large ball around the head, creating a boundary for the head. Engage the belly, lengthening the tailbone away from the crown of the head. Move between the two, gathering up through the belly as you inhale back up.
2. Return to *tadasana* (mountain pose), with the hands interlinked across the upper chest (*vajrapradama mudra*; page 190) feeling the return inwards after reaching outwards.

Qi gong moving meditation

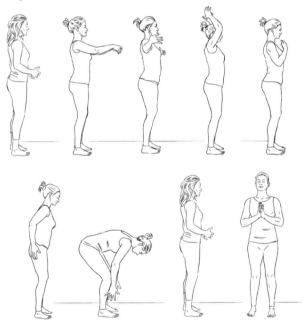

These patterns of movement from qi gong retrace the boundaries of the subtle body (about 12 fingers out from the skin), our peri-personal space. In this sequence, the hands trace around the outside of the body, feeling into the surrounding space and mapping our presence.

This is a wonderful meditation on its own, moving into a standing meditation at the end of a practice or to begin a fully standing sequence.

1. From *tadasana* (mountain pose) with soft knees, bring the hands up in front of the belly, the *hara* – the seat of awareness and intention.
2. Bring them up in front of the heart space, with a bowl-like holding of self-compassion there, elbows and shoulder blades soft.
3. Expand the arms to the side, shoulder height, opening to receive and offer a sense of community (this is great in group circles).
4. Raise the arms above the head, palms forward, reaching up to the sky, but still aware of the ground.
5. Slowly bring the hands down behind the protective carapace of the skull, following downwards around the front of the chest.
6. Skim the hands from in front of the belly around the hips, bending the knees softly, dropping the hands around the outside of the legs, over the tops of the feet.
7. Bring the hands, palms facing away from each other, up through the midline between the legs on the slow, curling ascent, palms coming back together at the belly, registering the safety there, taking in a sense of the entirety of the body.
8. Continue the sequence as a meditative continuum, staying at any position where you feel an intuitive need for offering yourself kindness, friendliness, generosity and compassion.

SUBTLE PRACTICES: INTERNAL SOOTHING

Ujjayi breath

Ujjayi, or 'victorious', breath slows the passage of breath with gentle constriction of the opening of the throat. The resistance to the passage of air creates a well-modulated and soothing sound, much like the sound of ocean waves rolling in and out. When practised with softness around the eyes, *ujjayi* breath has been shown to increase the baroreflex sensitivity shown to support parasympathetic action via blood pressure control.[80] See more on page 309.

1. Sitting (or lying), supported, comfortable and with the chest open and spine long, close the mouth and tune into breathing through the nose. Be mindful of holding tension around the mouth, jaw, throat and neck.
2. Sensitively, without gripping, bring awareness to the inner boundary of the throat and create a sense of drawing in so that the breath makes a rushing sound, almost like snoring, or waves rolling in and out.
3. Feel into the movement of the diaphragm, that the movement of the breath originates here, building up the practice from this sensitivity.
4. Find a sense of the equality between the inhale and the exhale and pressure creating the soft sound, how this balances – this may be equal between the two: *sama vritti* (equal ratio breathing) if it feels easeful, or letting your breath have its natural rhythm.

Autogenic release

This is regulated or produced (genic) by self (auto). In this technique, we respond to verbal cues, body sensations and visual images that lead to a state of deep relaxation. The repetition of words or phrases aims to reduce body tension and bring about an experience of relaxation.

Most studies looking at the effects of talking to ourselves in such ways have focused on anxiety reduction, where the results are significant. This reduces the fear-based response of the sympathetic nervous system on 'constant alert' that can create such dysregulation in immune, respiratory, digestive, endocrine, cardiovascular, lymphatic and other body systems.

---

80 Mason *et al.* (2013).

Although the phrase 'autogenic training' is attributed to the German psychiatrist Johannes Heinrich Schultz in 1932, such inner dialogue of self-soothing has been used historically by Buddhist teachers, for example, recently Thich Nhat Hanh: 'Breathing in, I calm body and mind. Breathing out, I smile. Dwelling in the present moment I know this is the only moment.'[81]

The specific autogenic training[82] works through a series of self-statements about heaviness and warmth in different parts of the body, relaying messages that we might relate to ease and parasympathetic activity.[83] These practices can help us to locate and feel the boundaries of the body as much as our energetic or emotional boundaries.

The first practice here covers such a script. Others are then offered as suggestive phrases that can be used within *savasana* (corpse pose), meditation and body scans.

Heavy and warm focus (autogenic training version)

1. Quietly say to yourself, 'I am completely calm.'
2. Focus attention on the arms. Quietly and slowly repeat six times, 'My arms are very heavy.' Then, 'I am completely calm.'
3. Refocus attention on your arms. Quietly and slowly repeat six times, 'My arms are very warm.' Then, 'I am completely calm.'
4. Focus attention on your legs. Quietly and slowly repeat six times, 'My legs are very heavy.' Then, 'I am completely calm.'
5. Refocus attention on your legs. Quietly and slowly repeat six times, 'My legs are very warm.' Then, 'I am completely calm.'
6. Quietly and slowly repeat six times, 'My heartbeat is calm and regular.' Then, 'I am completely calm.'
7. Quietly and slowly repeat six times, 'My breathing is calm and regular.' Then, 'I am completely calm.'
8. Quietly and slowly repeat six times, 'My abdomen is warm.' Then, 'I am completely calm.'
9. Quietly and slowly repeat six times, 'My forehead is pleasantly cool.' Then, 'I am completely calm.'
10. Enjoy the feeling of relaxation, warmth and heaviness.

---

81 Hanh (1989).
82 Stetter and Kupper (2002).
83 Manzoni *et al.* (2008).

11. When you are ready, quietly say to yourself, 'Arms firm, breathe deeply, eyes open.'

Verbal guides to release

These affirmations can be used in a similar way, repeated to drop down from adrenal states and hypervigilance associated with constant busy-ness.

Dropping away from 'doing' and constant action

1. 'My whole body is still; I am occupying my whole body.'
2. 'My hands are still; there is nothing to do.'
3. 'My feet are still; there is nowhere to go.'
4. 'My jaw is relaxing; there is nothing to tense against.'
5. 'My face is softening; there is nothing to express.'

Softening to allow stillness

1. 'My throat is soft; there is nothing to say.'
2. 'My spine is moving with my breath; I am fluid.'
3. 'My brain is still; there is no reaction needed.'
4. 'My breath is softening; I feel peace.'
5. 'My whole body is still; I am able to let go.'

Embodied awareness via the breath

1. As I inhale, I know I am inhaling.
2. As I exhale, I know I am exhaling.
3. As I inhale, I allow the inhale to deepen.
4. As I exhale, I allow the exhale to slow down.
5. As I inhale, I allow my mind to calm.
6. As I exhale, I allow myself to feel ease.
7. As I inhale, I draw in what I need to nourish myself.
8. As I exhale, I release what no longer serves me.
9. As I inhale, I am here.
10. As I exhale, I know there is nowhere else to be.

Metta bhavana (loving-kindness practice)

May I be safe.
May I be happy.
May I be healthy.
May I be free.

This *mantra*, or affirmation, can be used in each stage of a *metta bhavana* practice (changing the preposition appropriately, for example 'May they be safe') in each section, offering compassion, friendliness, kindness and gentleness to yourself, someone close, a neutral person and someone with whom you have difficulty, then back to self or bringing all four people together. You may wish to set a timer to indicate movement between sections.

This practice is a safe way to start to explore interbeing, the diffusion of boundaries between all beings, but starting and ending with yourself, reaffirming your own safe boundaries. Self-compassion resources you to be able to offer out to others without depletion or fatigue.

A traditional Buddhist meditation, the practice fosters kindness and non-judgemental awareness, which can be healing where a sense of 'otherness' has evolved from trauma. We can recognise that we, and all others, are deserving of loving-kindness.

1. Sitting comfortably, bring attention to the breath, imagining it travelling through the body and experiencing being in the body, fully present, as an act of compassion. Slowly repeat the above phrase three times, contemplating, without judgement, how this feels. If there is distraction or discomfort – physical or emotional – come back to the breath, being in the body.
2. Bring into awareness someone who you feel natural warmth towards and repeat the phrase ('May they...'), again noticing how the breath and body respond when cultivating benevolence to this person.
3. Repeat, visualising someone you have no emotional attachment to at all, a neutral person such as someone you see in a shop or have passed in the street.
4. Now bring to mind someone more difficult. (Tip: start with someone relatively innocuous, working up to more challenging people over time, with practice.) How does it feel to offer this person the same

generosity and kindness? Do you notice any shift in the breath or physical sensations?

5. Visualise yourself and all the other people – recognise that all of you are deserving of the same compassion.

6. Finally, expand your awareness to include all sentient beings, recognising the interconnectedness of all beings.

7. Come back to yourself, your body, your breath.

Self-enquiry questions

1. How do the concepts of physical and emotional boundaries relate to each other for you?

2. When body functions and structures such as fascia, the digestive tract, epithelium and interstitial fluid are so unseen – and most beyond the realm of our conscious feeling – which qualities of attention or tuning inwards (interoception) help you relate to them?

3. How do you feel your own times of self-protection or being triggered ripple through your body tissues?

4. Can you listen and respond to the inner voice of 'enough' when it comes in, both during practice and off the mat?

5. Are you able to say 'no' – and 'yes' – appropriately within your whole being as well as in language in your life? How might embodiment in practice help us notice and express healthy boundaries in life beyond the mat?

Further resources

Tara Brach (2020) *True Refuge, Radical Compassion, Radical Acceptance*. London: Hay House UK [a collection of three books that can be bought singly].

Thich Nhat Hanh (1989) *The Miracle of Mindfulness: A Manual on Meditation: An Introduction to the Practice of Meditation*. Boston, MA: Beacon Press.

Stanley Keleman (1989) *Emotional Anatomy: The Structure of Experience*. Berkeley, CA: Center Press.

Bessel van der Kolk (2015) *The Body Keeps the Score: Brain, Mind and Body in the Healing of Trauma*. London: Penguin.

Charlotte Watts (2018) *Yoga Therapy for Digestive Health*. London and Philadelphia, PA: Singing Dragon.

Ed Yong (2017) *I Contain Multitudes: The Microbes Within Us and a Grander View of Life*. London: Vintage.

References

Acharya, V. (ed.) (no date). *Microbiome and Movement*. Physiopedia. Accessed 31/05/2022 at: www.physio-pedia.com/Microbiome_and_Movement

Albert Einstein College of Medicine (2020). *Researchers Detour to Confront the COVID-19 Crisis*. Albert Einstein College of Medicine. Accessed 31/05/2022 at: https://einsteinmed.edu/features/2356/researchers-detour-to-confront-the-covid-19-crisis

Ayoade, S. (2017) 'The differences between the germ theory, the terrain theory and the germ terrain duality theory.' *JOJ Nursing & Health Care 2*(4). Available at: https://juniperpublishers.com/jojnhc/pdf/JOJNHC.MS.ID.555631.pdf

Barnard, E. and Li, H. (2017) 'Shaping of cutaneous function by encounters with commensals.' *The Journal of Physiology 595*(2), 437–450. Available at: https://pubmed.ncbi.nlm.nih.gov/26988937

Bartlett, J.A., Fischer, A.J. and McCray, P.B. Jr (2008) 'Innate immune functions of the airway epithelium.' *Contributions to Microbiology 15*, 147–163. Available at: https://pubmed.ncbi.nlm.nih.gov/18511860

Becattini, S., Taur, Y. and Pamer, E.G. (2016) 'Antibiotic-induced changes in the intestinal microbiota and disease.' *Trends in Molecular Medicine 22*(6), 458–478. Available at: https://pubmed.ncbi.nlm.nih.gov/27178527

Bower, J.E. and Irwin, M.R. (2016) 'Mind-body therapies and control of inflammatory biology: A descriptive review.' *Brain, Behavior, and Immunity 51*, 1–11. Available at: www.ncbi.nlm.nih.gov/pmc/articles/PMC4679419

Braniste, V., Al-Asmakh, M., Kowal, C., Anuar, F., *et al.* (2014) 'The gut microbiota influences blood–brain barrier permeability in mice.' *Science Translational Medicine 6*(263), 263ra158. Available at: https://pubmed.ncbi.nlm.nih.gov/25411471

Brown, B. (2015) *Daring Greatly: How the Courage to Be Vulnerable Transforms the Way We Live, Love, Parent, and Lead*. London: Penguin Life.

Bryant, E.F. (2009) *Yoga Sutras of Patanjali*. New York: North Point Press.

Bush, Z. and Cummings, P. (2021) 'The innate immune system.' Available at: https://zachbushmd.com/innate-immune-system

Chen, Y.E. and Tsao, H. (2013) 'The skin microbiome: Current perspectives and future challenges.' *Journal of the American Academy of Dermatology 69*(1), 143–155. Available at: https://pubmed.ncbi.nlm.nih.gov/23489584

Clarke, S.F., Murphy, E.F., O'Sullivan, O., Lucey, A.J., *et al.* (2014) 'Exercise and associated dietary extremes impact on gut microbial diversity.' *Gut 63*(12), 1913–1920. Available at: https://pubmed.ncbi.nlm.nih.gov/25021423

Clayton, T.A., Baker, D., Lindon, J.C., Everett, J.R. and Nicholson, J.K. (2009) 'Pharmacometabonomic identification of a significant host–microbiome metabolic interaction affecting human drug metabolism.' *Proceedings of the National Academy of Sciences of the United States of America 106*(34), 14728–14733. Available at: https://pubmed.ncbi.nlm.nih.gov/19667173

Colbey, C., Cox, A.J., Pyne, D.B., Zhang, P., Cripps, A.W. and West, N.P. (2018) 'Upper respiratory symptoms, gut health and mucosal immunity in athletes.' *Sports Medicine 48*(1), 65–77. Available at: https://pubmed.ncbi.nlm.nih.gov/29363055

Damasio, A. (2000) *The Feeling of What Happens: Body, Emotion and the Making of Consciousness*, Reprint edn. London: Vintage.

de Punder, K. and Pruimboom, L. (2015) 'Stress induces endotoxemia and low-grade inflammation by increasing barrier permeability.' *Frontiers in Immunology 6*, 223. Available at: https://pubmed.ncbi.nlm.nih.gov/26029209

Eisenstein, C. (Host). (2020, July 28). Dr. Zach Bush: Life is a Community (No. 49) [Audio podcast episode]. In *A New and Ancient Story*. https://charleseisenstein.org/podcasts/new-ancient-story-podcast/dr-zach-bush-life-is-a-community-e49

Engen, P.A., Green, S.J., Voigt, R.M., Forsyth, C.B. and Keshavarzian, A. (2015) 'The gastrointestinal microbiome: Alcohol effects on the composition of intestinal microbiota.' *Alcohol Research 37*(2), 223–236. Available at: https://pubmed.ncbi.nlm.nih.gov/26695747

Fakhoury, H.M.A., Kvietys, P.R., Al Kattan, W., Al Anouti, F., *et al.* (2020) 'Vitamin D and intestinal homeostasis: Barrier, microbiota, and immune modulation.' *The Journal of Steroid Biochemistry and Molecular Biology 200*, 105663. Available at: https://pubmed.ncbi.nlm.nih.gov/32194242

Felitti, V.J., Anda, R.F., Nordenberg, D., Spitz. A.M., *et al.* (1998) 'Relationship of childhood abuse and household dysfunction to many of the leading causes of death in adults. The Adverse Childhood Experiences (ACE) Study' *American journal of preventative medicine 14*(4), 223–236. Available at: https://pubmed.ncbi.nlm.nih.gov/9635069

Foster, J.A., Rinaman, L. and Cryan, J.F. (2017) 'Stress & the gut–brain axis: Regulation by the microbiome.' *Neurobiology of Stress 7*, 124–136. Available at: https://pubmed.ncbi.nlm.nih.gov/29276734

Frati, F., Salvatori, C., Incorvaia, C., Bellucci, A., *et al.* (2019) 'The role of the microbiome in asthma: The gut–lung axis.' *International Journal of Molecular Sciences 20*(1), 123. Available at: www.ncbi.nlm.nih.gov/pmc/articles/PMC6337651

Galley, H.F. and Webster, N.R. (1996) 'The immuno-inflammatory cascade.' *British Journal of Anaesthesia 77*(1), 11–16. Available at: https://pubmed.ncbi.nlm.nih.gov/8703619

Gautam, S., Tolahunase, M., Kumar, U. and Dada, R. (2019) 'Impact of yoga based mind-body intervention on systemic inflammatory markers and co-morbid depression in active rheumatoid arthritis patients: A randomized controlled trial.' *Restorative Neurology and Neuroscience 37*(1), 41–59. Available at: https://pubmed.ncbi.nlm.nih.gov/30714983

Grice, E.A. and Segre, J.A. (2011) 'The skin microbiome.' *Nature Reviews. Microbiology 9*(8), 626. Available at: https://pubmed.ncbi.nlm.nih.gov/21407241

Guzman, J.R., Conlin, V.S. and Jobin, C. (2013) 'Diet, microbiome, and the intestinal epithelium: An essential triumvirate?' *BioMed Research International 2013*, 425146. Available at: https://pubmed.ncbi.nlm.nih.gov/23586037

Hanh, T.H. (1989) *The Miracle of Mindfulness: A Manual on Meditation: An Introduction to the Practice of Meditation.* Boston, MA: Beacon Press.

Hansen, E.S.H., Pitzner-Fabricius, A., Toennesen, L.L., Rasmusen, H.K., *et al.* (2020) 'Effect of aerobic exercise training on asthma in adults: A systematic review and meta-analysis.' *The European Respiratory Journal 56*(1), 2000146. Available at: https://pubmed.ncbi.nlm.nih.gov/32350100

Hanski, I., von Hertzen, L., Fyhrquist, N., Koskinen, K., *et al.* (2012) 'Environmental biodiversity, human microbiota, and allergy are interrelated.' *Proceedings of the National Academy of Sciences of the USA 109*(21), 8334–8339. Available at: https://pubmed.ncbi.nlm.nih.gov/22566627

Hedberg, N. (2020) 'Inflammation masterclass.' *Integrative Healthcare & Applied Nutrition* magazine, December.

Heller, L. and Lapierre, A. (2012) *Healing Developmental Trauma: How Early Trauma Affects Self-Regulation, Self-Image, and the Capacity for Relationship.* Berkeley, CA: North Atlantic Books.

Hyman, M. (Host). (2022, Jan 26). The Power Of Epigenetics To Transform Your Healthspan And Lifespan with Dr. Jeffrey Bland (No. 485) [Audio podcast episode]. In *The Doctor's Farmacy.* https://drhyman.com/blog/2022/01/26/podcast-ep485

Invernizzi, R., Lloyd, C.M. and Molyneaux, P.L. (2020) 'Respiratory microbiome and epithelial interactions shape immunity in the lungs.' *Immunology 160*(2), 171–182. Available at: https://pubmed.ncbi.nlm.nih.gov/32196653

Kayama, H. and Takeda, K. (2016) 'Functions of innate immune cells and commensal bacteria in gut homeostasis.' *Journal of Biochemistry 159*(2), 141–149. Available at: https://pubmed.ncbi.nlm.nih.gov/26615026

Keleman, S. (1985) *Emotional Anatomy: The Structure of Experience.* Berkeley, CA: Center Press.

Kennedy, P.J., Cryan, J.F., Dinan, T.G. and Clarke, G. (2014) 'Irritable bowel syndrome: A microbiome–gut–brain axis disorder?' *World Journal of Gastroenterology 20*(39), 14105–14125. Available at: www.ncbi.nlm.nih.gov/pmc/articles/PMC4202342

Koch, L. (2019) *Stalking Wild Psoas: Embodying Your Core Intelligence.* Berkeley, CA: North Atlantic Books.

Komegae, E.N., Farmer, D.G.S., Brooks, V.L., McKinley, M.J., McAllen, R.M. and Martelli, D. (2018) 'Vagal afferent activation suppresses systemic inflammation via the splanchnic anti-inflammatory pathway.' *Brain, Behavior, and Immunity 73*, 441–449. Available at: https://pubmed.ncbi.nlm.nih.gov/29883598

Lange, K., Buerger, M., Stallmach, A. and Bruns, T. (2016) 'Effects of antibiotics on microbiota.' *Digestive Diseases 34*(3), 260–268. Available at: https://pubmed.ncbi.nlm.nih.gov/27028893

Leslie, J.I. and Annex, B.H. (2018) 'The microbiome and endothelial function: An investigative fountain or analytical morass.' *Circulation Research 123*, 1015–1016.

Mackos, A.R., Maltz, R. and Bailey, M.T. (2017) 'The role of the commensal microbiota in adaptive and maladaptive stressor-induced immunomodulation.' *Hormones and Behavior 88*, 70–78. Available at: https://pubmed.ncbi.nlm.nih.gov/27760302

Maeng, S.H. and Hong, H. (2019) 'Inflammation as the potential basis in depression.' *International Neurology Journal 23*(S2), S63–S71. Available at: www.ncbi.nlm.nih.gov/pmc/articles/PMC6905209

Manzoni, G.M., Pagnini, F., Castelnuovo, G. and Molinari, E. (2008) 'Relaxation training for anxiety: A ten-years systematic review with meta-analysis.' *BMC Psychiatry 8*, 41. Available at: https://pubmed.ncbi.nlm.nih.gov/18518981

Marizzoni, M., Cattaneo, A., Mirabelli, P., Festari, C., *et al.* (2020) 'Short-chain fatty acids and lipopolysaccharide as mediators between gut dysbiosis and amyloid pathology in Alzheimer's disease.' *Journal of Alzheimer's Disease 78*(2), 683–697. Available at: https://pubmed.ncbi.nlm.nih.gov/33074224

Maseda, D. and Ricciotti, E. (2020) 'NSAID–gut microbiota interactions.' *Frontiers in Pharmacology 11*, 1153. Available at: www.ncbi.nlm.nih.gov/pmc/articles/PMC7426480/#B19

Mason, H., Vandoni, M., deBarbieri, G., Codrons, E., Ugargol, V. and Bernardi, L. (2013) 'Cardiovascular and respiratory effect of yogic slow breathing in the yoga beginner: What is the best approach?' *Evidence-Based Complementary and Alternative Medicine 2013*, 743504. Available at: www.ncbi.nlm.nih.gov/pmc/articles/PMC3655580

Maté, G. (2021) *The Wisdom of Trauma* [film]. Available at: https://thewisdomoftrauma.com

Montiel-Castro, A.J., González-Cervantes, R.M., Bravo-Ruiesco, G. and Pacheco-López, G. (2013) 'The microbiota–gut–brain axis: Neurobehavioral correlates, health and sociality.' *Frontiers in Integrative Neuroscience 7*, 70. Available at: https://pubmed.ncbi.nlm.nih.gov/24109440

National Institute of Environmental Health Services (2022). *Microbiome*. NIH. Accessed 31/05/2022 at: www.niehs.nih.gov/health/topics/science/microbiome/index.cfm#footnote9

Nishihara, H. and Engelhardt, B. (2020) 'Brain barriers and multiple sclerosis: Novel treatment approaches from a brain barriers perspective.' *Handbook of Experimental Pharmacology* (Part of the Handbook of Experimental Pharmacology book series). Available at: https://pubmed.ncbi.nlm.nih.gov/33237504

Painold, A., Mörkl, S., Kashofer, K., Halwachs, B., *et al.* (2019) 'A step ahead: Exploring the gut microbiota in inpatients with bipolar disorder during a depressive episode.' *Bipolar Disorders 21*(1), 40–49. Available at: https://pubmed.ncbi.nlm.nih.gov/30051546

Park, J.H., Choi, D.Y., Park, H., Lee, K.W. and Cho, J.A. (2020) 'Oxytocin modulates immunostatus, metabolic state and gut microbiome.' *Journal of Biological Regulators and Homeostatic Agents 34*(3), 1117–1124. Available at: https://pubmed.ncbi.nlm.nih.gov/32668897

Payne, A.N., Chassard, C. and Lacroix, C. (2012) 'Gut microbial adaptation to dietary consumption of fructose, artificial sweeteners and sugar alcohols: Implications for host–microbe interactions contributing to obesity.' *Obesity Reviews 13*(9), 799–809. Available at: https://pubmed.ncbi.nlm.nih.gov/22686435

Pennisi, E. (2022). 'Meet the Psychobiome.' *Science*. Accessed 31/05/2022 at: www.sciencemag.org/news/2020/05/meet-psychobiome-gut-bacteria-may-alter-how-you-think-feel-and-act

Petruccelli, K., Davis, J. and Berman, T. (2019) 'Adverse childhood experiences and associated health outcomes: A systematic review and meta-analysis.' *Child Abuse & Neglect 97*, 104127. Available at: https://pubmed.ncbi.nlm.nih.gov/31454589

Poroyko, V.A., Carreras, A., Khalyfa, A., Khalyfa, A.A., *et al.* (2016) 'Chronic sleep disruption alters gut microbiota, induces systemic and adipose tissue inflammation and insulin resistance in mice.' *Scientific Reports 6*, 35405. Available at: https://pubmed.ncbi.nlm.nih.gov/27739530

Prata, J., Machado, A.S., von Doellinger, O., Almeida, M.I., *et al.* (2019) 'The contribution of inflammation to autism spectrum disorders: Recent clinical evidence.' *Methods in Molecular Biology 2011*, 493–510. Available at: https://pubmed.ncbi.nlm.nih.gov/31273718

Pruimboom, L. and Muskiet, F.A.J. (2018) 'Intermittent living; the use of ancient challenges as a vaccine against the deleterious effects of modern life – A hypothesis.' *Medical Hypotheses 120*, 28–42. Available at: https://pubmed.ncbi.nlm.nih.gov/30220336

Ramsheh, M.Y., Haldar, K., Esteve-Codina, A., Purser, L.F., *et al.* (2021) 'Lung microbiome composition and bronchial epithelial gene expression in patients with COPD versus healthy individuals: A bacterial 16S rRNA gene sequencing and host transcriptomic analysis.' *The Lancet 2*(7), E300–E310. Available at: www.thelancet.com/journals/lanmic/article/PIIS2666-5247(21)00035-5/fulltext

Schleip, R. with Bayer, J. (2021) *Fascial Fitness: Practical Exercises to Stay Flexible, Active and Pain Free in Just 20 Minutes a Week*, 2nd edn. Chichester: Lotus Publishing.

ScienceDaily (2021) 'Revealing the logic of the body's "second brain".' Michigan State University, 1 October. Available at: www.sciencedaily.com/releases/2021/10/211001130230.htm

Skabytska, Y., Kaesler, S., Volz, T. and Biedermann, T. (2016) 'How the innate immune system trains immunity: Lessons from studying atopic dermatitis and cutaneous bacteria.' *Journal der Deutschen Dermatologischen Gesellschaft 14*(2), 153–156. Available at: https://pubmed.ncbi.nlm.nih.gov/26788792

Solis, A.G., Klapholz, M., Zhao, J. and Levy, M. (2020) 'The bidirectional nature of microbiome–epithelial cell interactions.' *Current Opinion in Microbiology 56*, 45–51. Available at: https://pubmed.ncbi.nlm.nih.gov/32653776

Spector, Prof T. (2020). '15 tips to boost your gut microbiome.' *Science Focus*. Accessed 31/05/2022 at: www.sciencefocus.com/the-human-body/how-to-boost-your-microbiome

Spychala, M.S., Venna, V.R., Jandzinski, M., Doran, S.J., *et al.* (2018) 'Age-related changes in the gut microbiota influence systemic inflammation and stroke outcome.' *Annals of Neurology 83*, 23–36. Available at: https://pubmed.ncbi.nlm.nih.gov/29733457

Stetter, F. and Kupper, S. (2002) 'Autogenic training: A meta-analysis of clinical outcome studies.' *Applied Psychophysiology and Biofeedback 27*(1), 45–98. Available at: https://pubmed.ncbi.nlm.nih.gov/12001885

Subramanya, P. and Telles, S. (2009) 'A review of the scientific studies on cyclic meditation.' *International Journal of Yoga* 2(2), 46–48. Available at: www.ncbi.nlm.nih.gov/pmc/articles/PMC2934575

Taneja, V. (2017). 'Microbiome: Impact of Gender on Function & Characteristics of Gut Microbiome.' In M.J. Legato, *Principles of Gender-Specific Medicine: Gender in the Genomic Era*, 3rd edn (Chapter 39). Elsevier. Available at: www.sciencedirect.com/topics/immunology-and-microbiology/microbiome

van der Kolk, B.A. (2015) *The Body Keeps the Score: Brain, Mind, and Body in the Healing of Trauma*. London: Penguin.

Vila, A.V., Collij, V., Sanna, S., Sinha, T., *et al.* (2020) 'Impact of commonly used drugs on the composition and metabolic function of the gut microbiota.' *Nature Communications* 11(1), 362. Available at: https://pubmed.ncbi.nlm.nih.gov/31953381

Walsh, J., Griffin, B.T., Clarke, G. and Hyland, N.P. (2018) 'Drug–gut microbiota interactions: Implications for neuropharmacology.' *British Journal of Pharmacology* 175(24), 4415–4429. Available at: https://pubmed.ncbi.nlm.nih.gov/29782640

Yong, E. (2016) *I Contain Multitudes: The Microbes Within Us and Grander View of Life*. London: HarperCollins.

Zenaro, E., Piacentino, G. and Constantin, G. (2017) 'The blood-brain barrier in Alzheimer's disease.' *Neurobiology of Disease* 107, 41–56. Available at: www.ncbi.nlm.nih.gov/pmc/articles/PMC5600438

Zhang, N., Liao, X. Zhang, Y., Li, M., Wang, W. and Zhai, S. (2019) 'Probiotic supplements for relieving stress in healthy participants: A protocol for systematic review and meta-analysis of randomized controlled trials.' *Medicine (Baltimore)* 98(20), e15416. Available at: https://pubmed.ncbi.nlm.nih.gov/31096437

Zhao, L., Xiong, Q., Stary, C.M., Mahgoub, O.K., *et al.* (2018) 'Bidirectional gut-brain-microbiota axis as a potential link between inflammatory bowel disease and ischemic stroke.' *Journal of Neuroinflammation* 15(1), 339. Available at: https://pubmed.ncbi.nlm.nih.gov/30537997

PART 5

EMBODIED AWARENESS

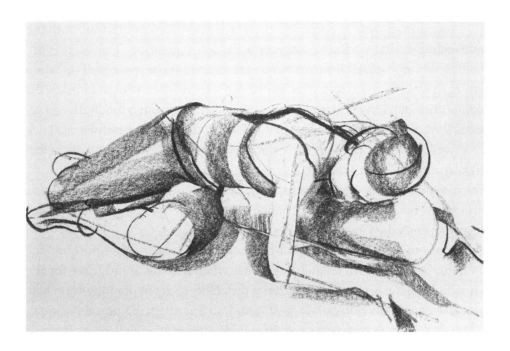

Exploring how we can support self-regulation and balance with interoception (sensing inwards), recognising that there is constant interplay between tuning in and kind attention, where we're shifting, where we're coming back to and insight via the movement of prana and the vayus.

We have been recognising how regulation in the autonomic system offers the potential for equilibrium with the immune and respiratory systems. This balance is often referred to as homeostasis – meaning coming back to the same – and referring to our baseline states, for example fluid balance, pH and glucose levels. A more accurate term is perhaps allostasis, which acknowledges that staying in balance doesn't mean always coming back to the same point, that changes according to internal and external variables are constantly occurring, relayed in via the nervous system.

This constant flux is also inherent in our embodied awareness, noticing and feeling so that we foster adaptation and self-regulation. The latter is the ability to calm yourself down when you're upset and cheer yourself up when you're down. That is, to find your way back to centre when you get knocked off course, the equanimity (page 298) we can cultivate through meditative practices. Without grounding we lose that sense of tether and an easeful route back to a steady central core. With this resource in place, we can self-regulate with a flexible range of emotional and behavioural responses that are well matched to the demands of their environment.[1] This can get knocked off course by trauma and stress, but our capacity for change (neuroplasticity) is great when we are fostering embodied awareness.[2]

Emotional self-regulation is healthy influence over our emotions, for example calming down an angry response when it is not appropriate for the situation. Behavioural self-regulation is the ability to act in our long-term best interest, consistent with our deepest values, so this might include choosing to come to a resting yoga practice or *pranayama* rather than collapsing in front of a screen.

Interoception

Interoception is our ability to 'read' our internal landscape, the route into embodied awareness – consciousness of our physical and breath bodies (*koshas*, page 150), which changes moment to moment: 'Interoception refers to the representation of the internal states of an organism, and includes the processes by which it senses, interprets, integrates, and regulates signals from within itself.'[3] This awareness isn't about identifying, labelling or analysing, but recognising the constantly changing nature of our interior space. This involves a relearning

---

1   Inzlicht *et al.* (2021).
2   Cook and Cook (2009).
3   Chen *et al.* (2021).

of our natural states, away from the conditionings and education of moving through childhood into adulthood as a modern human being.

Where interoception used to be understood as feeling something 'viscerally',[4] it is now more broadly related back to the homeostatic needs of the body or coming back to physiological equilibrium. If we are overly panicked, for example, our regulatory systems will seek what soothes, brings us down. The less resources we have, the more we might turn to quick-fix numbing soothers like sugar, alcohol, TV, screens – whatever we have learned quickly brings us down from agitated neurochemistry.

The neuroscientist Antonio Damasio talks about each individual's 'resources', defined as what supports health, where our ability to heal is directly linked to our resources and our ability to embody and bring awareness to these. The link between our experience of the world and our ability to process what comes in through the body is key:

> Pain and suffering act like a magnet that grabs our awareness. The journey to embody our experience is a big step in developing resources. The body gives a whole new theatre in which our experience and emotions can be played out. We can move towards and away from sensations, slow things down and control what is centre stage in our bodies in a way that is not possible with mental functioning alone. Learning that we have emotions and sensations and that we do not need to become them is very important. Pain is unlikely to be the only sensation possible. Stepping back and finding a wider context and other sensations is often a transformational shift.[5]

That tuning in, our barometer, is affective and motivational, changing how we react in relation to body maintenance and integrity, including safety and avoiding pain, physical or emotional. So, if we are overheating, we might take off some clothes or open a window. Similarly, we might move away from someone who feels unsafe, and if our system is upregulated to perceive danger at all corners (in chronic stress or trauma), those who feel cold might react to get that window shut as if it were more threatening than in reality, but it seems that imperative. These heightened reactions can be either conscious or unconscious, but the more we can bring them to consciousness, the less we are at their whim and can change our habitual responses (*samskaras*; page 279).

---

4   Schleip and Jäger (2012).
5   Quoted in Sumner and Haines (2010).

Trauma and chronic stress speed everything up, from the survival imperative that it is not safe to slow down, to stop and simply be, and most importantly, to feel. This *samskara*, that is tightly wound into our social and cultural behaviour – 'there's not enough time' – can also feed into attitudes to meditation and yoga practices, where we can struggle to be with the space of slowing down. The feeling is the journey back to ourselves as whole (healthful), to our true nature, unravelling woven-in patterns of armouring and self-labelling, and the compassionate holding of mindfulness (page 71).

The philosophy of interoception

Scientific interest in interoception has fluctuated during the years since Charles Sherrington's first usage of the concept in 1906. Its 'intrinsic' relevance dates back to important scientific milestones like Darwin's 'expression of emotion' (1872), Claude Bernard's 'milieu interior' (1878) or William James's 'principles of psychology' (1890). The recent years have witnessed a surge of interest in the topic of interoception, which is due to the 'embodiment paradigm shift' in psychology and neurosciences, recognising that intelligent or adaptive behaviour needs a body behaving within contexts, and which is promoted by findings highlighting the integral role of interoception in self-regulation, emotional experience, decision-making and consciousness.[6] Interoception, as the visceral dimension of embodiment,[7] has gained rapidly expanding interest in the study of the human mind.[8]

In 20th-century continental European philosophy, there was a profound reckoning with 'identity' and the 'self'. Thinkers like Foucault, Deleuze, Levinas and Derrida destabilised our notions of an autonomous self and in different ways showed how these notions are pervaded by difference and informed by the existence of the 'other'.[9]

According to Damasio's somatic marker hypothesis,[10] changes in heart rate, breathing, hormones, facial expression, muscle tone, etc. are like emotional fingerprints that signal to the brain, 'somatic markers', which can affect reaction or response. Emotional feelings can be the conscious experience of bodily sensations and vice versa: 'The ability to cognitively regulate emotional responses to aversive events is essential for mental and physical health. One prerequisite of

---

6   Khalsa and Lapidus (2016).
7   Herbert, Pollatos and Klusmann (2021).
8   Quadt, Critchley and Garfinkel (2018).
9   Kyle (2021).
10   Damasio (1996).

successful emotion regulation is the awareness of emotional states, which in turn is associated with the awareness of bodily signals [interoceptive awareness].[11]

Fascia, an interoceptive and proprioceptive organ

As well as shaping and giving our bodies structure, and enabling movement and transport of fluids, fascia is a communicative, sensory organ, an inextricable part of our sensing of our internal and external world. Around the organs and under the skin, fascial tissue contains immune cells, lymph and blood vessels, and nerves. Water and nutrient exchange occur within and through fascia:

> Physiologists nowadays consider the general metabolic function of the connective tissue as its central role within the body. And since the loose connective tissue under the skin runs like a network throughout our body, researchers have come to see it as a communication phenomenon: if the supply network is disturbed or damaged at any point, the reactions and stress responses within the connective tissue will span the entire body.[12]

The various receptors of fascia throughout the body communicate with the central nervous system to register motion, stretching, muscle positions, pressure changes – our proprioceptive sense (feeling where our body is in time and space). Interstitial receptors also connect to the autonomic nervous system, signalling pain and temperature. Pain and motion arise primarily in the fascia rather than in muscles. The musculoskeletal system's fascia, a sensory organ in its own right, provides essential information for brain function, crucial to embodiment:

> The number of interoceptors in fascia far exceeds the number of proprioceptors and mechanoreceptors (for movement, position, pressure, etc.). This highlights the great importance of these signals for the state and activity of the organs in the body. Our "gut feeling", as in our internal awareness of our bodily functions and organ activities, seems to depend largely on the fascia – the connective tissue around the intestines.[13]

Consciousness, our sense of self and emotional states could, therefore, depend on fascial signalling, with mental illnesses seen as interoceptive disorders. Schleip and Bayer explain that:

---

11 Füstös *et al.* (2013).
12 Schleip with Bayer (2021).
13 Schleip with Bayer (2021).

Yoga is based on the stretching of fascial tissue. Slow, methodical stretches held for a long duration have significant physiological effects. When fascial tissue is stretched, signals are transmitted to the autonomic nervous system. This reduces activity levels in the system responsible for stress – the sympathetic nervous system – which indirectly causes the body to relax.[14]

This leads back to immune regulation via the autonomic nervous system, namely through the recognition that stretching also impacts inflammation resolution in connective tissue,[15] meaning that it also has the possibility of reducing cytokine-induced depression (pages 154 and 213). When we are in inflammatory mode, energy may be sapped by the immune system being stuck in overdrive. This can cause 'cytokine sickness', where the constant signalling of the body's immune messengers in response to inflammation can lead to a feeling of being generally unwell, in the form of low-level flu symptoms, low mood and skin conditions that won't shift.[16]

Interoception in spiritual tradition

How does this compare to more contemplative traditions that arose in a time before the advent of the mirror and fully seeing 'our selves' in the 15th century? While life may have been very different, the inner human experience and responses may not have been. In the cultures from which the yoga lineage arises, it has been observed that Samkhya yoga, the basis of the *Yoga Sutra*, the distillation of the *Vedas* emanating from the Indus Valley circa 1500 BCE and Buddhism explore very similar themes to the 20th-century continental critiques on page 260. The Buddhist *anatman* ('non-self') and Samkhya yoga's *purusha* (consciousness) cultivate an experience of non-identity that is, according to their teachings, the source of liberation. This ties into the crisis of the over-actualised 'self' in the modern world, and the capitalist focus on individualism over community.

In Buddhist philosophy, *vedana* (feeling or sensation) refers to sensations arising from internal sense organs contacting external sense objects in consciousness. In psychology, this is identified as 'valence', the categorisation of emotions, events, objects or situations into binary good or bad, pleasant or unpleasant, or neutral, features of brain states that include interoception. Pleasant *vedana* sets up craving, clinging and attachment; unpleasant *vedana*

---

14 Schleip with Bayer (2021).
15 Berrueta *et al.* (2016).
16 Dantzer (2009).

EMBODIED AWARENESS

leads to aversion – both of which are states of suffering to be alleviated by concentrated awareness and clear comprehension.

> Withdrawal (*Pratyahara*) is the pivotal phase in the turn from outer to inner practises. Insofar as its aim is to disengage the senses from their objects, withdrawal is central to, and in some instances coextensive with, yoga itself.[17]

Internal rhythms

Interoception is attunement to the natural tides, rhythms and expressions of the autonomic nervous system that let us know where we are, often unconsciously, as well as overarching rhythms such as circadian, monthly, menstrual, seasonal, etc. The rhythm that we are most obviously able to sense is our breath, the inhale and the exhale. Movements like spine undulations (page 112 and Part 2 Practices) can help us tune into what may not be accessible. Where there is dissociation from the breath, this can cause anxiety in and of itself, so somatic guidance, in a held context, is vital for awakening this connection. Placing a hand on the heart can be similarly useful to help tune into the changing rhythm of the heartbeat, increasing a sense of agency over our own homeostasis.

Leah Barnett,[18] who co-teaches (with Charlotte) on the 'Yoga for Stress, Burnout and Fatigue' course run by Yogacampus, says:

> The whole being is animated by *prana* which is pulsed in and out of the body by the diaphragm. The movement of the diaphragm is replicated throughout the body and indeed all of life. This pulsing, expanding and contracting motion is called *spanda* – the movement of life. Via this incredible process of breathing the alchemical process of turning air (formless) into life force for each cell (form) is unfolding, breath by breath.

We may feel vasomotor activity – the constriction or dilation of blood vessels – in our pulse, sensing how the blood is flowing at particular points such as the temples or wrists, or deep in the belly – known as 'The Mother Pulse' in Thai Medicine. Digestive and bladder are larger motions, but we can tune into these visceral feelings changing through movement, the changes in intra-abdominal pressure, for instance, when we twist, forward fold or invert the body.

Rhythms like the breath or the pulse are objective, solid: we can feel them

---

17 Mallinson and Singleton (2017).
18 www.yogacampus.com/teachers/leah-barnett

263

at a point in time as an invitation to presence. Coming to these sensations in terms of tone or physical sensation without placing any projection of story or emotion onto them helps us to come back to the moment phenomenologically, how it is felt in its truest sense in that moment, without idea, projection or association.

Subjective experience

Our experiences are relative and subjective, to a degree. The more we can tune into when and how they are in the body, in time and space, associations that we bring relationally to others, our emotional landscape and our relationship to our own sensations, the more we can notice how these are linked into our past traumas, our unconscious memories. The more we can subsequently sift through and drop beneath what is and is not right here, right now.

Interoception can be dependent on:

- Emotional states.
- Decision-making (cognitive in terms of decision-making and more reactive, based on triggers of 'not safe').
- Perception of the physical world and how we move through it based on our *samskaras* – somatic markers laid down through experience that affects our decision-making (page 197 and 279).
- Peri-personal space, our sense of boundaries beyond the physical body: what we sense inwardly is massively affected by what we sense outwardly (see qi gong moving meditation, page 246).
- Sense of wholeness or fragmentation: stress, trauma or the modern medical perspective that reduces us to separate, disconnected body systems. The more we can bring a sense of wholeness through our somatic practices, the more cohesion we can feel. Coming back to the midline in the pause between different movement practices can be felt as a palpable relief from holding ourselves as fragmented parts. Fostering a sense of wholeness can allow fractured systems to heal.

Immunity and interoception

A large part of interoception is peripheral communication about the immune system to the brain:

> Immune communication from periphery to brain represents a major component of interoception. The signalling of systemic inflammation is communicated

to the brain via neural (predominantly vagus nerve) pathways, humorally via cytokines and directly via immune cells. Both acute and chronic states of inflammation influence emotion through a coordinated set of motivational changes conceptualised as "sickness behaviours". These include fatigue, anhedonia, social withdrawal and irritability, that is symptoms shared with depression.[19]

When immune responses occur, there is a whole cascade through the nervous system that dampens us down to inhibit us from doing more, so that we have energy available for healing mechanisms. Sickness behaviours are seen as a specific set of responses to reroute energy into the immune system. Interoceptive signals of 'I feel unwell' create the response of an ill person to shut down activity. Locking into this and overidentification with unwellness is where confused signalling may lie; this can also come from messages from childhood that we were 'sickly children' or 'not strong', for instance.[20]

A 2021 study showed that breath awareness helped to regulate neural oscillations in the brain, and activated areas of the brain that relate to emotions, autonomic endocrine responses and pain perception.[21] When pacing the breath, regions of the brain that related to empathy, love, trust, state of union, interoception and embodied recognition were activated, with emotional, cognitive and physiological regulation observed. Much current research into interoception is also exploring links with yoga,[22] meditation,[23] massage[24] and acupuncture,[25] to name a few.

Understanding of the link between the nervous and immune systems is growing. Recent years have seen the field of neuroimmunology continue to expand;[26,27,28] we are now also starting to appreciate the role of the immune system in healthy brain development and homeostasis,[29] and equally the importance of the nervous system in regulating the immune system.[30,31]

19   Critchley and Garfinkel (2017).
20   Lipton (2016).
21   Boyadzhieva and Kayhan (2021).
22   Rivest-Gadbois and Boudrias (2019).
23   Kang, Sponheim and Lim (2021).
24   Eggart, Queri and Müller-Oerlinghausen (2019).
25   Bai et al. (2009).
26   Nutma et al. (2019).
27   Gruol (2017).
28   Bechter, Brown and Najjar (2019).
29   Morimoto and Nakajima (2019).
30   Ben-Shaanan et al. (2018).
31   Caldwell et al. (2020).

Vestibular system – balance and body regulation

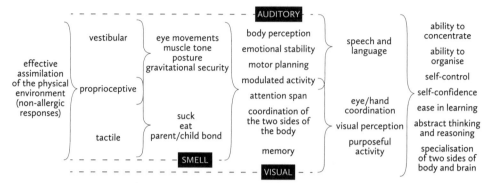

FIGURE 5A. SENSING THE WORLD AROUND US
Different ways of making sense of our experience, relating to the world around
us and to others, bringing information in, processing, sending it out to see
how it relates to the external world, bringing in responses, etc.

We sense the world around us through proprioception and balance through our vestibular system (Figure 5b), sensing where we are in relation to the ground at any given time. Registering safety through the autonomic nervous system therefore relies on immediately relaying this constantly shifting and adapting orientation, that can get knocked or thrown off balance (literally) by chronic stress and trauma:

> According to the *Gita*, one may say that reason alone is insufficient to lead us from the experience of the phenomenological world (*saṃsara*) to that of the sacred realm (*nirvaṇa*). While the more inorganic level of reality can be known through the senses and reasoning, the organic and sentient world seems to contain secrets only accessible through intuition, mostly in a state of contemplation, or deep meditation, when one is endowed with the highest levels of pure (*sattvic*) *sraddha*. How it is that the brain reflects this sense of soul-force named *sraddha* is something still beyond the reach of natural science. It is something which remains in the realm of spirituality – a category whose main concrete feature is the universal *sraddha*, which is at the core of all philosophical and religious insights.[32]

The vestibular system is another way we can link breathing, movement and posture:

---

32   Turci (2020).

Recent evidence has shown that the vestibular system participates in adjusting the activity of both upper airway muscles and respiratory pump muscles during movement and changes in body position... It is practical for the vestibular system to participate in the control of respiration, to provide for rapid adjustments in ventilation such that the oxygen demands of the body are continually matched during movement and exercise.[33]

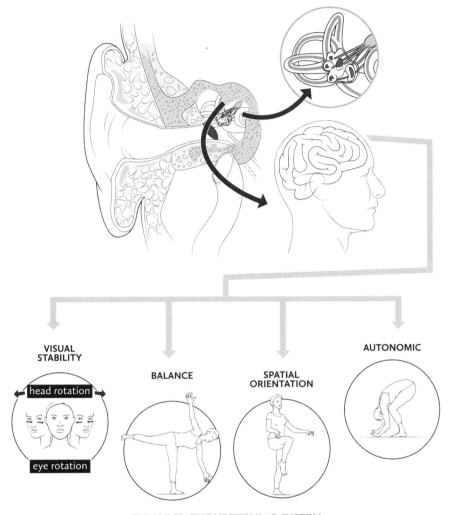

FIGURE 5B. THE VESTIBULAR SYSTEM

Trauma can keep us caught up in reactive states, sensing the outside and our inner worlds as essentially unsafe, or shutting off sensations – sensory motor amnesia, where we feel an absence or lack of interoception:

33   Yates *et al.* (2002).

Trauma can create...an "interoceptive moron", who may be unable to differentiate whether the visceral sensations at a given moment are signs of an empty
stomach, of stage fright-induced "butterflies", of empathy-driven "gut feelings"
about another person's dilemma, or may simply be an acute gastritis.[34]

Here there is an inability to discern appropriate cognition of a visceral feeling
that can then bring about its own cascade of inflammation and subsequent
trauma. Mindful movement practices and manual therapies that foster a sense
of internal listening skills, where attention to subtle sensations follow larger
motor movements, have been shown to have positive health-enhancing effects
with many modern, stress-related conditions, from irritable bowel syndrome
(IBS) to post-traumatic stress disorder (PTSD), where there is dissociation and
interrupted interoception.[35,36]

Balancing in practice

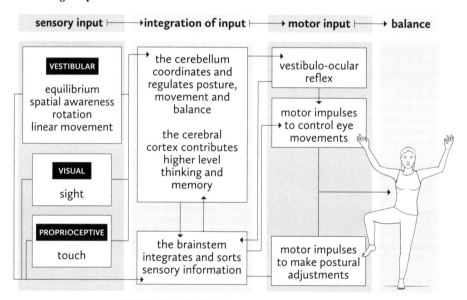

FIGURE 5C. THE HUMAN BALANCE SYSTEM
The physiological and neural mechanics of balancing the body: a blueprint for finding allostasis
in life off the mat – the changing point of equilibrium relative to need in that moment.

We explored standing practices in Part 4 coming from a place of support,
moving up from the ground. Tuning inwards, staying present to our inner

---

34   Schleip (2014).
35   Taylor *et al.* (2020).
36   Rosenow and Munk (2021).

sensations and 'riding the waves' of the less/more difficult without grasping at one or pushing away (or hiding from) the other, allows us to come physically and emotionally to allostasis, that ever-shifting equilibrium (page 141).

Literally, finding balance within our physical practice can allow us to explore calibrating to external changes. Tuning into transitions, adaptation and non-reaction are palpable tools we can learn in practice that support autonomic nervous system regulation and soothe inflammatory tendencies, as well as offering us a psycho-social framework for unpredictability and uncertainty in life. Subtleties such as the orientation we feel on turning the head or feeling balance across the foot are also opportunities to consciously mimic vigilance and foster safety.

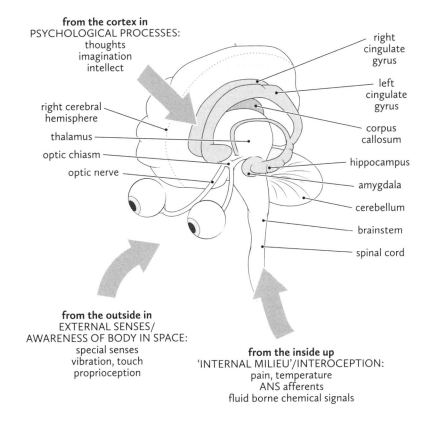

The brainstem, limbic system (emotional centre), thalamus and hypothalamus assess incoming information for danger and can trigger overwhelm responses that hijack the functioning of the whole body.

FIGURE 5D. WHAT THE BRAIN RECEIVES TO BE PROCESSED

Our sensory systems, how we experience the world, internally and externally, are key to how we develop and learn.

Source: Adapted from Sumner and Haines (2010), with thanks

The *pancha vayu* model – yoga and Ayurveda

The yoga and Ayurvedic models (page 276) are systemic, holistic perspectives, as are psycho-neuro-immunology, naturopathy and functional medicine approaches (to name a few). They always treat the body and mind as a whole, rather than separating us out into constituent parts, for example an eye specialist separate to an immunologist, separate to a psychologist.

This is different to a view of the (separate) body based on the function (or dysfunction) of organs – body and mind are viewed holistically, as intertwined and part of the symphony of the whole. Stephen Porges,[37] author of *Polyvagal Theory*, states that while the medical system excludes neural implications of illness with organ dysfunction (including emotional and psychological states), there is a failure to connect how the nervous system needs social engagement and touch for regulation and health. This is where reactions to COVID-19, for example, could be including issues of social isolation as damaging to the nervous, immune and respiratory systems, as we regulate within social engagement (ventral vagus mode; page 162).

The yoga tradition focuses on the movement of nourishment throughout the system. How is everything coming back into balance? If there is dis-ease, *dukkha*, the question to ask is not which organ system is affected (circulatory, digestive, immune, respiratory, etc.), but what is the underlying cause? Where do we go in to support the whole system to dissolve the stagnation or blockage to optimal function? Which direction of movement is causing trouble: taking stuff in, processing it, distributing it, eliminating it or growing from it? Which aspects of the movement of energy and health are being affected, and how do we support these?

In the *Prashnopanishad* of the *Atharva Veda* (1st millennium BCE), *pancha prana*, or *pancha vayu*, the five elements, are considered five supreme 'Gods' that reside in the body – Earth, Water, Air, Fire and Space. *Prana* (Air) is the most important: if it leaves the body, the other elements cannot function. *Prana* is converted into the other elements, the source of all living energy in the universe.

Prana constitutes energetic movement throughout the body, which can be seen through the following lenses:

- *Gunas* (page 274): the energies arising from *prakriti* (primal creative force). *Sattva*, coming to homeostasis, the more fiery energy of *rajas* or the heavy, listless quality of *tamas*.

---

37   Porges (2007).

- *Doshas* (page 276): in Ayurveda, depending on your constitution and the environment, *vata* is wind, 'that which moves' – *vata* dominance is common in modern society, more agitative and ungrounded; *pitta*, 'that which heats', is fiery, more inflammatory, angry and reactive to stress, also prevalent in our society; *kapha* is 'that which sticks', more grounded, but it can be more dull and heavy, where we move into burnout territory. Balance between the *doshas* is key.
- *Vital essences*: *prana* is vital life force, *tejas* is the spark of life and *ojas* is the fluid (page 277).
- *Chakras*: the organisation of the body and quality of energies throughout.

Throughout all these, we have the sense of too little or too much, excess or deficiency – out of balance – so with physical and subtle practices we can respond with appropriate warming or cooling. *Brahmana* practices are warm, and bring *agni* (fire), but where there is excess, this can slip over into inflammatory tones (stuck in *rajasic*). *Langhana*, cooling practices, can calm, but where there is lack of fire, this can lead to fatigue, stagnation (*tamas*).

Samkhya

Samkhya (translated as 'counting') philosophy classifies matter, listed in the *Bhagavad Gita* and a founding model for yoga: 'By focussing attention on the physical level, awareness is progressively trained to identify subtler forms of matter. If it is clear what purusha is not, one can transcend the mind… "Samkhya and yoga are one," Krishna says.'[38]

Yoga essentially adds practical methods to *samkhya* theory:

Samkhya has terms of its own, distinguishing consciousness (*purusha*) from matter (*prakriti*). All material things are part of *prakriti*, including the workings of the mind. This causes confusion – *purusha* is misidentified with thinking as well as the body, producing suffering. The aim of yoga is to end this mistake, disentangling *purusha* from everything else.[39]

Samkhya provides a metaphysical map that can be used to retrace manifestation to its source and presents a world of "direct experience" based on what we

---

38 Simpson (2021).
39 Simpson (2021).

experience during meditation. It classifies "inward" and "outward" states of perception experienced through yogic practices and the mystical experience of the Rishis, or sages. Yoga is the method to put these ideas into practice.[40]

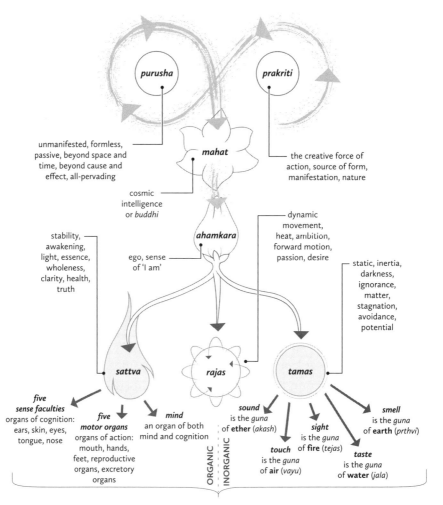

FIGURE 5E. THE *SAMKHYA* SYSTEM OF PSYCHO-PHYSICAL CATEGORIES

Samkhya

To count, enumerate, classify or organise; a psychological and philosophical system – yoga is the method to put these ideas into practice (guided by *sattva-rajas-tamas* in equilibrium).

A tool to make sense of our perception and interaction with the material world, illuminating the experience of 'close observation'.

Provides a metaphysical map to relate our direct experience back to the source of manifestation, based on what we experience during meditation.

Classifies 'inward' and 'outward' states of perception experienced through yogic practices and the mystical experience of the Rishis, or sages.

Source: With thanks to Heather Elton for this synopsis

---

40 Elton (2022).

In *samkhya*, 25 major principles (*tattvas*) explain all manifest reality. Twenty-four are *prakriti*:

- *Mula prakriti* (unmanifest state).
- *Buddhi/mahat* (intelligence), the decision-making part of the mind, discernment.
- *Ahamkara* (I-maker/ego): 'The faculty of self-referencing, for instance when you think something has to do with you, whether or not it actually does (hint: it usually doesn't)'.[41]
- *Manas* (mind), the part of the mind that senses, including the instruments of cognition (seeing, hearing, smelling, tasting and touching); of action (speech, hands, feet, anus and genitals); and the gross elements (space, air, fire, water and earth) that both manifest and unmanifest.
- *Gunas* (page 274): the above are animated by the interplay of the *gunas* (*sattva, rajas, tamas*), which brings impermanence and change.
- *Purusha*, the 25th *tattva* (consciousness).[42]

These spiritual traditions have aims to move towards pure consciousness, away from the body. In the modern world, where we can be caught up in the whirring of the mind, embodiment practices serve to bring us into the real, felt senses, which can tend to get lost. Amin *et al.* explain that: 'All information from the senses is conveyed to the *manas*. To make sense of this information, the *buddhi* scans the *citta* which is the memory storage. Information in this memory storage is organized into five categories, corresponding to the five senses.'[43] Just as in Patanjali's eight limbs of yoga, where *asana* (physical practice) precedes meditation and withdrawal of the senses on the journey to *samadhi* (liberation), embodiment – presence in the physical – must come before we can attain more expansive conscious states.

41 The Sutra Project (no date).
42 Sedlmeier and Srinivas (2016).
43 Amin *et al.* (2014).

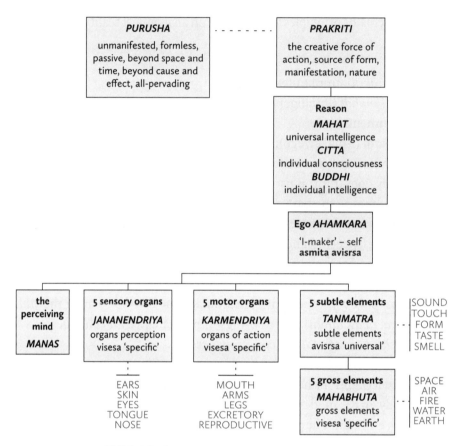

FIGURE 5F. *SAMKHYA* PHILOSOPHY OF CREATION

The *gunas* – three interconnected energies or qualities that animate our world including our thoughts, feelings and all mental activity.

As described in the *Bhagavad Gita*: *rajas* and *tamas* obscure the true self (*atman*) whereas *sattva* illuminates it.

Chapter 14, verse 5: 'Purity, passion and inertia, these are the *gunas*, qualities born of *prakriti*, bind fast the indestructible *atman* – self, to the body.'

Chapter 14, verse 10: 'They are in a constant state of flux resulting in our reality being governed by change – *parinama*.'

The gunas

In yogic practices, awareness and conscious manipulation of these energetic states can affect both physical and psychological outcomes:

- *Tamas*: darkness, chaos, inertia, inactivity, laziness, staleness, obstruction, materiality, heaviness, insentience, ambivalence
- *Rajas*: energy, activity, change, passion, dynamism, egotism, agitation, excitement, movement, attachment, motion, friction

- *Sattva*: lightness, balance, harmony, kindness, openness, clarity, intelligence, awareness, inspiration.

If we view dysfunction through the lens of the *gunas*, we can gain insight into what is needed to restore balance. Interoceptively, moment-to-moment observance of sensation and energy in relation to the *gunas* can guide an appropriate response. Cultivating this deep listening and responding on the mat lays a blueprint for more intuitive, holistic health beyond: 'Knowledge arises from *sattva* and greed arises from *rajas*. Negligence and delusion arise from *tamas*, and ignorance as well.'[44]

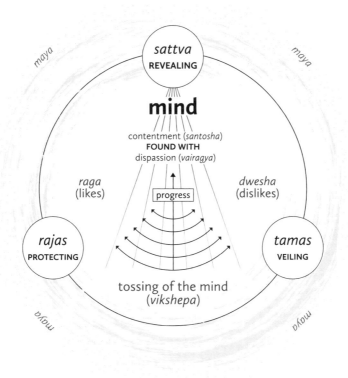

FIGURE 5G. THE *GUNAS* AND THE MIND

---

44   Easwaran (2007, verse 14:17).

Ayurveda

Note: This section is to stimulate enquiry. Ayurveda is a huge and complex system, and for the purpose of this book, this is just a taste in relation to immune and respiratory health.

The doshas

The *doshas* are three different constitutional types within Ayurveda: *vata*, *pitta* and *kapha*. They are biological energies derived from the five elements that lay down our tendencies, physical, emotional and beyond, through the *koshas* (the five 'sheaths' or 'veils' of awareness). These particularly pertain to the movements and quality of *agni* (digestive fire) and so can offer insight into digestive issues and immunity.

Balanced *doshas* manifest as good health, where physiological functions flow with ease and body systems orchestrate with ease. Where one or more *dosha* becomes imbalanced, bodily functions cannot operate smoothly and we are physically and emotionally affected, as effects ripple out through the whole system organisation. If this disturbance in balance becomes critical or is not redressed over time, the result is chronic disease.[45]

Dosha qualities

	Biological or physiological	Sleep	Temperament and endurance	When in balance	When out of balance
Vata	Related to the lower body; causes: elimination, inspiration and expiration. Sensitive to stress or lifestyle changes.	Interrupted, light	Nervous types with poor endurance; easily exhausted, need plenty of recovery	Inspirational, emotional balance, clear mind, enthusiasm, expression	Worry, insomnia, poor memory, anxiety, fear. Loss of energy, poorly healing wounds, depletion of body tissue. Loss of awareness. Poor circulation.
Pitta	Provides proper digestion, maintains body heat, suppleness, vision, hunger, thirst and appetite, skin health and formation of *ojas*.	Sound sleep, medium length	Motivated types with moderate but focused endurance	Strong heart, lucidity, intellect, courage, drive	Hypersensitivity and allergies. Inflammatory conditions. Anger, aggression, addictions, indecision. Excess hunger and thirst. Weakened digestion. Loss of lustre.

---

45 Rhyner (2017).

Kapha	Provides lubrication, fluidity, firmness of joints and immunity. Resistance to disease. Promotes healing and tissue building.	Sound, long, heavy sleep	Contented temperament with high endurance	Strength, love, patience, forgiveness	Irritability, lethargy, heaviness, reduced digestion, food sensitivities, loose joints. Inflammatory conditions, fatigue, frequent respiratory issues.

Within modern society, the two Ayurvedic *doshas* of *pitta* and *vata* tend to dominate. *Pitta*, which translates as 'that which cooks', is associated with heat and therefore inflammation, but also the tendencies in stress for anger and irritability. *Vata* translates as 'that which moves', and is responsible for the fluctuations and ruminations of the mind, that which can keep us in mental agitation, hypervigilance, worry and fear when we get 'stuck in the head' or overwhelmed.

Appropriately soothing practices, quality of awareness and full exhalations help soothe and help balance these energies. *Kapha* (that which sticks) tends to be duller, more listless, but we need it to ground, to bring the other two down.

We all have aspects of these three *doshas* within us, but will have a con-stitutional type – often a mixture, with one dominant. It is worth visiting an Ayurvedic practitioner to find your individual needs, and then understand these in the context of societal conditionings and expectations.

Ojas

In Ayurveda, *ojas* can be compared to immunity, and is all-pervasive, our resist-ance to decay. We can relate this to fluidity in the body, our ability to move things through: 'It is the *ojas* that keeps living beings refreshed. There can be no life without it. *Ojas* marks the beginning of the formation of the embryo and is the nourishing fluid.'[46]

Ojas is the subtle essence of all vital fluids, in yoga and Ayurveda. It is responsible for health, harmony and spiritual growth, said to give tissues health, strength and endurance. It is composed primarily of water and earth, the stuff things grow from.

Daily practice of deep diaphragmatic breathing increases *ojas* by supplying abundant life energy as *prana*. *Ojas* is depleted by things that get in the way of our life force, the quality of information coming in, for example, sitting at a

---

46   Rhyner (2017).

screen all day, gossiping or social media. Our true sense of vitality comes from being fully in the present moment.

Balam

In Ayurveda, *balam* means strength and, in the context of health, signifies strength of the mind and body, and often refers to the immune system in its most functional states. According to the medicinal and surgical text *Susrutha Samhita*[47] (one of the foundational texts of Ayurveda), *balam* is the quality that enables us to have stability and nourishment of *mamsa dhatu* (muscle tissue), and the ability to carry out different tasks efficiently; it is also the factor behind good complexion, clarity and pleasantness of voice, as well as the clear, efficient working of the sense organs, motor functions, mind and intellect.

Balam can be broken down into three types:

- *Sahajam*: innate immunity present since birth, where there is an equilibrium of the three *doshas* (*vata*, *pitta* and *kapha*).
- *Kalajam*: dependent on seasonal variations and age (*balam* is at its peak during middle age). The depleting strength during *aadanakalam* (summer season) and progressive gaining of strength during *visargakalam* (winter season) is interesting in relation to the eustress of meeting the elements (pages 101 and 156).
- *Yukthikritham*: immunity that we can engage with; diet, rest, exercise and *rasayana* (rejuvenation therapies).

Causes of disease

The following are factors that interrupt the flow of *prana* and deplete *ojas* and *balam*, affecting our ability to return to balance:

- *Parimana* (change): although change is constant, it is our adaptation to rerouting that determines our ability to come back to balance, our ability to maintain healthy boundaries, while allowing inevitable flux to go on its natural way – riding the waves, rather than sinking.
- *Tapa* (desire or expectation): desire is motivational, but when wants drive us in repetitive patterns that become interruptive to our interoception, we can struggle to feel contentment (*santosha*) in the present. Ideals of 'If I just had that I'd be happy' or constant striving based on

---

47   Susruta and Bhishagratna (2020).

how we 'should' be wear us down. Any value that comes from expectation rather than what is present (or a sense of deeper, true need)
interrupts our flow, creating doubt or *granthis*, knots.

- *Samskaras* (habit patterns): somatic markers, our tags where we feel
  safe or unsafe (page 197), which keep us going round in unconscious
  behavioural, relational loops. Bringing these into awareness through
  embodied practices gives us the opportunity to come down to a sense
  of *sukha*, ease.

- *Sanga* (attachment): not just as addiction, but repeating patterns of
  reacting and behaving that lead us into *samskaras*. Not the thoughts
  or desires or the labels, but the attachment to them, creating stories,
  becoming overly analytical. Loosening our grip and becoming more
  open to response in the moment is a key part of our practice.

- *Viyoga* (disconnection from reality): lack of clarity, that which yoga
  seeks to unveil. Trauma can hugely interfere with this, as there is a
  repetition in the mind of past events as if real and present, being stuck
  in what we think we are feeling, rather than true connection with
  visceral voices. Tuning into our felt, present sensations in a safe way is
  the path to freedom.

- *Vegadharana* (controlled or suppressed urges): rather than knee-jerk
  wants and desires, recognising our true needs, what keeps us safe, our
  boundaries (Part 4).

- *Guna vritti virodha* (disturbed natural cycle): poor sleep patterns, travel
  – all the stuff that modern life knocks out of whack. Coming back to
  our circadian rhythms, menstrual awareness, not being on screens
  late at night, etc., can all help us reconnect with natural rhythms.
  Overnight we need adequate rest and sleep to produce melatonin, a
  huge part of our immune system.

- *Ayuk taahara* (inappropriate diet): balancing diet using the model of
  the *gunas*, what is *sattvic*, or using the Ayurvedic model, eating to
  balance our *doshas*.

- *Ayuk tavihari* (inappropriate lifestyle): tuning into the autonomic
  nervous system; how we rest, respecting how we drop out of heightened states.

- *Kleshas* (hindrances or obstacles): of ignorance, ego, desire,
  aversions, fear.

The kleshas – obstacles to clarity

We can consider the *kleshas* in relation to any meeting of another, and, most importantly, to ourselves. According to Nicolai Bachman: 'The *kleshas* are arguably the most challenging aspects of ourselves to confront, yet the most liberating after they are weakened and eventually removed.'[48] Meeting and relating to our own shadows and needs allows us to turn up in an honest way in our lives and our teaching, where we will, of course, bring our story and mind habits to the table. Professor of Hindu religion and philosophy Edwin Bryant translates *Yoga Sutra* 2.12: 'Obstacles (*kleshas*) are the breeding ground for tendencies (*samskaras*) that give rise to actions and the consequences (*karma*) thereof. Such obstacles are experienced as visible or invisible obstacles.'[49]

Consciousness of our patterns and how we bring them into relation with others and teaching isn't about annihilating 'who we are', but rather, cultivating the aspects of ourselves that support both us and others. This means recognising when we have wandered into our shadow-selves, knowing where we can step out to, and how to navigate the territory – without shame, guilt or self-criticism. Neuroscientist Antonio Damasio explains that:

> The part of the mind we call self was, biologically speaking, grounded on a collection of nonconscious neural patterns standing for the part of the organism we call the body proper... The brain reconstructs the sense of self moment by moment... Our sense of self is a state of the organism.[50]

THE *KLESHAS*

- *Avidya*: ignorance, misconceptions, misunderstandings, incorrect knowledge. The misconception of our true reality, believing that the temporary is eternal, the impure is pure, and pleasure to be painful. This false representation of reality is the root *klesha* and produces the four others.
- *Asmita*: over-identifying with the ego, false identification, mistaking mind, body or senses for the true Self. We create a self-image of ourselves that we believe is us, but is not. This view of self can contain both external ('I am poor') and internal

48 Bachman (2011).
49 Bryant (2009, *Yoga Sutra* 2.12).
50 Damasio (2000).

('I am a bad person') judgemental narratives. We become trapped within the projections of our lives that we have created.

- *Raga*: desire, attachment to pleasure and the attraction for things that bring satisfaction. Our desire for pleasurable experiences creates mindless actions and blind-sighted vision; when we cannot obtain what we desire, we suffer. When we do obtain what we desire, our feelings of pleasure soon fade and we start pleasure seeking again, becoming trapped in an endless cycle. These are the traps of addictive behaviours.
- *Dvesha*: avoidance, aversion to pain, the opposite of *raga*, aversion towards things that produce unpleasant experiences. If we cannot avoid the things we dislike, we suffer – even thinking about unpleasant experiences produces suffering.
- *Abhinivesha*: attachment to fear, fear of death, clinging to life, will to live, the deepest and most universal *klesha*, remaining with us until our deaths. We know that one day we will die, yet our fear of death is deeply buried in our unconsciousness.

Sources of *prana*

Sources of *prana*, or life force, abundant within and about us, can be seen as coming from and through different aspects of our being and the world we are interbeing with:

- Land: this is the more material aspect of grounding, our muscles and bones, the *annamaya kosha*, physical body – matter. In many traditions, bones are seen as the spiritual essence of us, our ancestors.
- Water: the fluid body, the blood and other bodily fluids – *pranamaya kosha*.
- Fire: constant body temperature generated by metabolism, *agni*, our digestive fire, and *ojas*, our life essence. This is the stuff of the third *chakra* at the solar plexus (diaphragm area), our sense of self.
- Air: coming up into the heart, air coming in at the interface between the lungs and the heart. Primarily oxygen and carbon dioxide, but also other gases in the body.
- *Akash*: subtle currents, the higher realms or *chakras*. What flows throughout the body, including the *vayus* (page 283). This is our

animation, in terms of our ability to become more connected with what is outside of ourselves.

According to the *Hatha Yoga Pradipika*: As long as the breath is restrained in the body, the mind is calm. As long as the gaze is between the eyebrows there is no danger of death. When all the channels have been purified by correctly performing restraints of the breath, the wind easily pierces and enters the aperture of the *sushumna*. At the end of the breath-retention in *kumbhaka*, make the mind free of support. Through practising yoga thus one attains the *rajayoga* state.[51]

Modification of the breath

The breath is used as a means of connecting internal and external senses, referenced in Patanjali's *Yoga Sutras*: 'The modifications of the life-breath are either external, internal or stationary. They are to be regulated by space, time and number and are either long or short.'[52]

Prana, life force, is drawn from the external to the internal world, from *purusha* (formless) into *prakriti* (form), with the *Yoga Sutras* stating that this is obtained through breath that is both *dirgha* (long and steady) and *sukshma* (fine and subtle). This correlates with the modern suggestion that the most healthy and efficient breath is (as referred to in the Oxygen Advantage® programme[53]) that which emphasises deep, slow and light breathing to engage the diaphragm and create intra-abdominal pressure. There is also an emphasis on 'nose, low and slow', which does not differ from yogic recommendations (see also page 312):

- *Dirgha* (long and steady): nasal breathing slows down the rate at which breath comes in. This has been studied for the inhalation on runners, where they might gasp at the air through the mouth when their breathing is less efficient at oxygenating ('air hunger'); breathing in through the nose has shown to slow the breath down by an average of 22 per cent, resulting in 'easier, less effortful respiration.'[54]
- *Sukshma* (fine and subtle): that which is felt when putting a finger below the nostrils, but not down to chin level; if it reaches that far, it is being moved with too much force.

51 Swami Muktibodhananda (1998).
52 Sri Swami Satchidananda (2012, *Sutra* 2.50).
53 McKeown (2015).
54 Dallam *et al.* (2018).

As the only autonomic function we can consciously affect, the *Sutras* say 'Calm is restored by controlling the exhalation or retention of the breath.'[55] In changing breathing patterns, 'we are communicating to the brain using the language of the body, a language the brain understands and to which it responds'.[56]

Yoga teacher Donna Farhi references the journey of the breath as beginning in the womb, an interior movement that pulses through us. At birth, we become threaded into the universal rhythm through the breath. Robin Rothenberg, C-IAYT yoga therapist, describes *pranayama* (page 307) practices this way:

> Reinforcing breath retention throughout the day is the most effective way of changing respiratory chemistry and reducing a strong ventilatory response (urge to breathe)… Focus on the breath synchs your mind with all of your physiological functions… Framed by the monitoring of the breath, the pranayama leaps to the forefront of the mind and every choice becomes a choice either to move towards homeostasis or stay stuck in the rut of duhkha.[57]

A 2018 study explored that neural oscillations in the brain could be regulated by breath awareness alone, and that parts of the brain responsible for emotions – empathy, compassion, interoception and feelings of cohesion – as well as autonomic endocrine responses and pain perception, could be activated.[58]

The vayus (subtle winds)

In the yogic tradition (distinct from the *vayus* in Ayurveda) the ten *vayus* are the subtle winds that pervade the body and all interface with each other. The five *prana vayus* are the major winds of the inner body (within the *pranamaya kosha*; page 151), while the *upaprana vayus* are minor ones:

- *Naga* removes excess air, for example burping.
- *Kurma* controls contracting movements, for example blinking, which is slow and steady, like the tortoise it is named after.
- *Krikala* governs sneezing.
- *Devdatta* controls yawning, which can be satisfaction or tiredness

---

55   Bryant (2009, *Yoga Sutra* 1.34).
56   Brown and Gerbarg (2012).
57   Rothenberg (2019).
58   Herrero *et al.* (2018).

(see how we can move towards satisfaction within pandiculation on pages 56 and 290).

- *Dhananjaya* controls the functioning of heart valves, the fire that remains in the body ready for composition.

THE *PRANA VAYUS* (MAJOR INNER WINDS)[59]

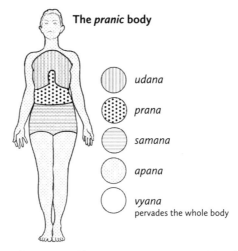

FIGURE 5H. THE *VAYUS* (FIVE WINDS) IN THE *PRANAMAYA KOSHA* (*PRANIC* BODY)

Awareness of these major *vayus* can offer us awareness and focus to support immune-respiratory health, as we tune into the direction of movement (or any lack of) within our physical movement and expression. See more on page 310.

---

59 Sen-Gupta (2012).

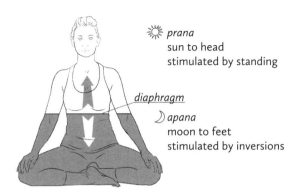

FIGURE 51. THE POLARITY OF *PRANA* AND *APANA VAYUS*
We can see the relationship between *prana* and *apana* when we are standing, rising
up away from ground force and gravity. Where we find the balance between the
polarities of lifting out of compression and dropping back down the earth to ground,
the homeostasis between the front and back body, lightness and heaviness.
Source: This illustration first appeared in Yoga Therapy for Digestive Health *by Charlotte Watts*

Prana vayu (up-breathing)
(This is different to *Prana* as life force.)

An inward and upward motion. Seated in the heart (*anahata chakra*) between
the diaphragm and throat, it governs and affects:

- Hunger, thirst and swallowing.
- Chest motions, including circulation and respiration.
- When *prana vayu* is weak, the mind cannot focus, and experiences
  excess worry.
- Disturbed *prana vayu* can lead to shortness of breath, anxiety, low
  energy or poor immune defences.
- Upwards-moving *prana* in the eyes and ears, heart and lungs, and in
  and out of the nose.
- Rises from the diaphragm up to the head, stimulated upon standing.

Practices that support *prana vayu*:

- *Nadi shodhana* (page 318) and *ujjayi* breathing (page 248).
- Third eye meditations (the *nadi shodhana* seal can be performed with
  fingers on the third eye for focus).
- Heart-opening poses, such as back arches.

- Inversions for flow back upwards, allowing us to have the heart pumping slower with help from gravity.
- Arms above shoulders (for example, *virabhadrasana* (warrior pose), *utkatasana* (chair pose)).
- Awareness of *prana vayu* in any pose creates a focus to lift, lengthen and open the upper body.

Apana vayu (down-breathing)
A downward and outward motion. Seated in the anus (*muladhara chakra*), it reaches down below the diaphragm and navel, and is associated with:

- Outpourings from the lower body: defectation, flatulence, urination, menstruation, ejaculation, conception and childbirth. It is important to see that all of these are things leaving the body, equally part of the cycle of health, none more or less desirable or acceptable.
- Full digestive function for immunity.
- Physical stability and steadiness, associated with the root and down to the feet; *sthira.*
- Earth element and the root (*muladhara chakra*).
- Weak or dysfunctional *apana vayu* creates feelings of ungroundedness and weakness in the legs. The exhale back down to the ground is really important for re-establishing this.

Practices that support *apana vayu*:

- The stomach-churning practice of *nauli* (or rotating tailbone; page 128) and *mula bandha*, sensitively, tuning into interoception.
- Calming and tension-releasing poses such as forward bends and seated twists.
- Poses with strength through the legs.
- Focus on grounding.

Udana vayu (out-breathing)
An upward and outward motion, circulating around the head. Seated in the throat above the larynx (*vishudda chakra*) and above, it:

- Holds the body upright; associated with *kundalini* rising up the spine, our being here in the world, related to expression, how we vocalise our boundaries.

- Governs speech, self-expression and growth, music and humming.
- Controls all automatic functions in the head and maintains body heat and falling asleep.
- Is the Air element, blue-green in colour.
- Can manifest as speech difficulties, if weak or dysfunctional – not being able to state our needs, shortness of breath and diseases of the throat. Also hindrances around the breath affecting the microbiome through stress responses (page 213).
- Relates to lack of self-expression, uncoordinated movement or loss of balance, if disturbed.

Practices that support *udana vayu*:

- *Ujjayi* (page 248), *brahmari* (page 319) and *jalandhara bandha* (page 336), where we draw energy around the throat, where the chest rises to meet the chin.
- Practising inversions and back-arching poses that bring awareness to the neck, shoulders and head. *Viparati karani* (page 304), where a natural back arch is supported, hips lifted and the chest is opened up to the chin. Part of a *langhana* (cooling, quietening) practice.

Samana vayu (on-breathing)

A horizontal motion, equalising. Seated in the navel (*manipura chakra*), maintains digestive fire (*agni*), processing all experience, not simply food, activating and regulating digestion in the belly, heart to the navel area, where it is responsible for:

- Movements of fluids and energy from the centre to the periphery.
- Digesting and assimilating our capacity of the human mind-body system; both food and life experiences; sustenance, toxicity or stress are all inputs into the body and we digest as we need. A full digestive process is breaking down whatever comes in and absorbing it or not, assimilating it or keeping outside of the body, recognising what is to be drawn in and what rejected. Also by-products of digestion: where these toxins build up it is called *ama* in Ayurveda; completing

transformation of these products, thoughts or experiences is vital to healthy immunity.
- Water element; light and cool (yin); white colour.
- A weak or dysfunctional *samana vayu* can manifest as poor judgement, low confidence and a lack of motivation and desire; also digestive issues, with an imbalance between fire and water.

Practices that support *samana vayu*:

- *Kapalabathi* ('breath of fire', 'skull shining breath' – *shatkarma* or purification, particularly of the sinuses) with *uddiyana bandha*. This should be done sensitively and with guidance (in one-to-one teaching with a regular student, rather than group classes). Where there is holding in the diaphragm, this could be triggering if trauma is present, and could also feed into already dysfunctional breathing patterns. The exhalation is active (short, forceful) while inhalation is passive, the opposite of normal breathing.
- Twisting and core focus poses, which bring awareness to the fascial and fluid movement around the belly area as much as honing strength and stability here.

Vyana vayu (outward-moving)

'Pervading one', a circular motion, out from the heart and lungs to flow throughout the entire body; a combination of *prana* and *apana* (and their polarities); moves through all the *nadis*, affecting:

- Activities on the periphery, such as senses and nerve impulses, how we move.
- Circulatory, lymphatic and nervous systems, the fluid body.
- Associated with the Ether element, sky-blue in colour/also water.
- Regulated by *samana*, so we can see the relationship between fire and water. These may seem in opposition but need to be in balance. Digestion is vital to these constant cycles.
- Its action is circulation; its expression is alignment.
- Weak or dysfunctional *vyana vayu* can create feelings of separation and alienation; disjointed, fluctuating and rambling thoughts – which can be a symptom of low serotonin and so depression and/or anxiety. Also poor circulation, skin disorders and nervous breakdowns.

Practices that support *vyana vayu*:

- Coherent breathing (page 131) or breath retention practices (*kumbhaka*, page 312).
- Moving *asana*; see page 181 for an alternative to the commonly practised *vinyasa* with *chaturanga dandasana* that can be compressive on the shoulders. This is especially important for those who may come from office work, for example, and could potentially bring the patterning of sedentary posture into their practice.
- Somatics to move circulation and lymphatics.
- Whole-body awareness in any pose or movement. This *vayu* really helps us to foster embodied awareness.

Autonomic release or shifts in Prana

We can interoceptively attune to shifts in *Prana* ('life force' rather than *prana vayu*) and consciously create what are usually subconscious responses to help autonomic release. Allowing these to happen helps us respond naturally as part of our sensory expressions. These might manifest as:

- Sighs and other involuntary noises
- Yawns
- Murmurs
- Tingles
- Shivers
- Shakes
- Sensations at the base of the skull
- Inner ear shifts
- Tears
- Fluids gurgling
- Burps and farts!

All these things allow us to bring to conscious and unconscious patterns laid down over time, and to drop down into parasympathetic dominance. We have the choice to welcome and rejoice at these natural expressions of release, where 'civilisation' has often restricted and limited them.

Moving this to a subtle body viewpoint, the Tantric text *Yoga Spandakarika* describes how *prana* manifests in our awareness like *spanda* – a pulse, vibration or tremor.[60] Within our phenomenological experience, if we close our eyes and sense subtle pulses, or see internal colour or light, within the yoga canon, this means we are beginning to access our *pranic* body.

Pandiculation

Pandiculation (page 56) is that combined yawn and stretch, which brings autonomic release throughout the nervous system. Naturally, we would do this about 17 times throughout the day, as it's a fundamental part of our neuromuscular functioning. Babies do this regularly to embed and grow their neuromuscular wiring. Without this resetting of the nervous system, muscles and fascia can lose responsiveness and movement, and pain and postural issues can follow. When people feel self-conscious to do this regularly, an important part of the nervous system release is lost. It prepares animals (including us!) for normal sensing and moving, readying the voluntary motor cortex for efficient functioning and movement.[61] Animals don't tend to have the psycho-social stress or self-judgement that humans might carry to interrupt our flow.

What we do in a pandiculation is threefold:[62]

1. Tighten a specific muscle or muscle group tighter than it already is.
2. Slowly lengthen and release that muscle or muscles to their full and comfortable length.
3. Completely relax the muscles. The more conscious this is, the greater the potential for neuromuscular resetting. In order for the brain to receive the feedback it needs to reset muscle length, the muscle needs about six seconds of moving into tension to fully release.

Pandiculation affects the sensory motor cortex or 'brain map'. It is 'our nervous system's natural way of waking up our sensory-motor system and preparing us for movement'.[63] The pandiculation isn't simply feeding back to the brain; it is keying in to how the brain moves us. We're not just moving the body and that's telling the brain something. The sensory part closer to the brainstem senses the input from the body. The motor part, closer to the forebrain, is affecting how we move the body. It is the brain that moves the body, but we are then sensing back in and moving out again, responding to sensory input.

---

60 Odier (2005).
61 Bertolucci (2011).
62 Peterson (2012).
63 Somatic Movement Center (2019).

Mind is the composer
Breath is the conductor
Body is the orchestra
Movement is the music.[64]

The sensory and motor cortexes

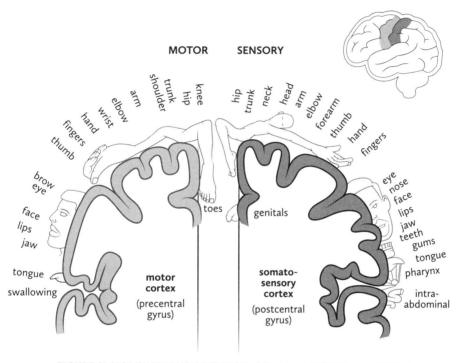

FIGURE 5J. HOMUNCULUS OF THE SENSORY AND MOTOR CORTEXES

Considering that we move from the brain to the peripheral body and somatic nervous system (page 81), it is an important guide within physical practice that there is the greatest neural connectivity to the hands and face (reaching out into these in pandiculation completes the circuit). The homunculus (Figure 5j) is a hypothesised map of the human cortex creating a 'little man', with all of these parts visited in the guided journey of *yoga nidra* (sleep yoga, in delta brainwaves; page 348). From this model, we can see that more neural circuitry is required at the sensorily concentrated sites of the face and hands. This offers insight into how hand gestures and facial awareness can connect us deeper

---

64   Laurie Booth, quote within a somatic movement session: www.lauriebooth.com

inwardly.[65] According to Tonja Bennett of the Homunculus Yoga Project:[66] 'If the cortical homunculus model is correct, I propose we could amplify our state of being with a smile and finger gesturing to accentuate neural plasticity.'

This is one of the ways we can see that practising *mudras* can be powerful beyond the esoteric (page 188) – hand therapies 'have been shown to improve cognition in diseases such as Alzheimer's'.[67] Smiling stimulates brain activity and chemical release (in ventral vagus mode; page 162), which induces pleasure and wellbeing, and can also have profound effects on our immunity and our body's ability to heal from a state of balance.

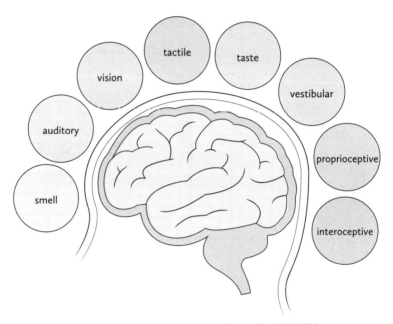

FIGURE 5K. WAYS WE PROCESS VIA THE SENSES

If we view this sensing through the lens of *samkhya* philosophy, *tanmatras* (protoelements; Figure 5f) – sound, touch, colour, taste and smell – and sense organs 'are products of self-awareness and do not form part of the gross elements... It is not because of the body alone that sense exists. The sense faculties and protoelements have an existence of their own and hail from finer particles of evolution, self-consciousness (*ahankara*).'[68]

The *karmendriyas* are the tactile motor organs or 'working senses' signalled

---

65   Koeppen and Stanton (2018).
66   "Sunflower" (2020).
67   Bahar-Fuchs, Clare and Woods (2013).
68   Freeman (2015).

by the brain – speech, handling, locomotion, evacuation and reproduction.[69] *Jnanendriya* are the cognitive organs of perception, ears, skin, eyes, tongue and nose.

Sighing

Another most-often subconscious response that we can bring into consciousness to affect the autonomic nervous system is sighing. Sighing is an involuntary inhalation (inspiration) that is 1.5–2 times greater than the usual tidal volume – some say it should be at least twice normal volume – to prompt the sigh out. It primarily involves the upper chest, dorsal muscles or upper sternum, but can be part of thoracic breathing, where people sigh in a more pathological way (see below).

During sleep, we sigh on average 1–25 sighs per night, often with pandiculation; both reset fascia: 'It has been noted that if we don't sigh every five minutes or so, the alveoli will slowly collapse causing lung failure. This is why patients in early iron lungs had such problems, because they never sighed.'[70]

Sighing can be long, deep breaths expressing sadness, relief or exhaustion, but occur spontaneously every few minutes to reinflate alveoli. We might even allow a sigh to be a kind of *pranayama*, conscious sighing, either within a physical practice (an extension of release through tissues and *koshas*) or in a more contained way, for example a two-part *krama* breath on the inhalation (page 316) with a sigh on the exhalation.

Excessive sighing is, however, regarded as a symptom of abnormal or dysregulated breathing since normal breathing in healthy subjects is regular or periodic. Frequent uncontrolled sighing is considered a sign of panic disorder,[71] anxiety states[72] or low back pain.[73] Back in the 1920s and 1930s this was seen as part of a hysterical/psychiatric picture.

Frequency of sighing increases under hypoxia (low oxygen), stress and certain psychiatric conditions, highlighting the need for autonomic reset in these circumstances, where people cannot access self-soothing.

---

69 Rhyner (2017).
70 Li *et al.* (2016).
71 Abelson *et al.* (2001).
72 Aljadeff *et al.* (1993).
73 Keefe, Wilkins and Cook (1984).

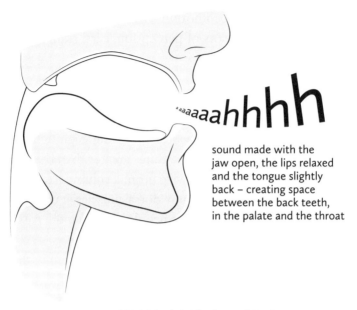

ᵃᵃaaaaahhhh

sound made with the
jaw open, the lips relaxed
and the tongue slightly
back – creating space
between the back teeth,
in the palate and the throat

FIGURE 5L. 'AHH' VOWEL SOUND
Consciously releasing an 'ahh' sound creates the opening of the palate and the
throat for autonomic reset, also bringing release around the skull and jaw.

Touch

Touch is another important aspect of autonomic release. It releases oxytocin, the 'love molecule', creating ventral vagus tone (page 162): 'The subcutaneous connective tissue has a special sensory system for touch that indicates affection. This system is connected to the brain and so influences our emotional state, empathy and interpersonal skills.'[74] Oxytocin is released from the pituitary gland (third eye) in the brain after about 20 seconds of sustained touch (a too-quick hug doesn't quite work!) and can bring us down from anxious states. It is found to reduce levels of fear by reducing the activity of the amygdala, the (lower) mammalian centre of the brain responsible for detecting danger and reacting to perceived emergencies (including via the immune system). Touch also reduces stress hormones like cortisol, and elevates mood so that we can experience safety, creativity and joy.

When we lose our sense of self through stress or trauma, feeling a real sense of our edges and where our internal world meets the external creates a palpable sense of safety that ripples back through the enteric nervous system. This form of practice is crucial connection in a society dominated by visual and auditory input. Kinaesthetic (tactile) communication is often under-valued, and

---

74 Schleip with Bayer (2021).

many feel the loss of not living within a physically and emotionally supportive extended family or tribe. We can feel this as a lack of safety in the gut–brain axis. Touch brings us back into our bodies, our physicality. We are, after all, pack mammals – warm-blooded creatures that have evolved to respond with reward to actions that secure cohesion of the tribe.

There are obvious implications here when we experience any form of social isolation or distancing. When we cannot touch others, self-soothing touch can be just as effective however: rubbing, stroking, tapping, compression, even hands together at the heart or on the belly has a powerful effect, evoking self-connection and compassion: 'We should not think of touch working by changing local tissue dynamics. There is much more going on. Touch can help us reconnect to, and in some cases change, primal experiences of how we created our sense of self.'[75]

The Tantric ritual *nyasa* (placing), of touch, or focus, also helps us create a proprioceptive map of the body. The *rishi* (seer) chants specific *mantras* to 'place' at specific points on the body, uniting the individual with the divine. How we place the body in *asana*, *pranayama* or meditation, or where we direct *mantras* or visualise specific locations of the subtle body as an anchor, can help us bring focus to what is here and now, cutting through the noise of the mind.

---

75   Haines (2021).

PHYSICAL PRACTICE: REST AND RECOVERY

Moving towards embodied awareness, we now arrive into practices that allow deep rest within the tissues and nervous system, the fully parasympathetic activity our immune and respiratory systems need for full and balanced function. This offers us places with plenty of time and space to bring the considerations of mindfulness (pages 69–73) and occupy a non-judgemental, introspective realm.

As most modern humans' fluids and lymphatics tend towards stagnation (*tamasic*) and need some fluidity, somatic movements (as explored in previous parts) are useful before settling into restorative positions, to avoid simply dropping into mind-body inertia. They also serve to gather awareness (possibly in the face of sensory motor amnesia; page 53) into areas with pulsing, rocking, rolling, reaching, kneading, etc., to cultivate a sense of 'the whole' that we are returning to. This is not simply hanging about or dropping off, but retaining a curious and compassionate awareness of the movements of *prana*, interoceptive rhythm and other moment-to-moment shifts and nuances. It is easy to let the mind take over in these held positions, finding places where we do not have to work to stay there, so less intense bodily feelings to take up our attention. This means that these practices are a whole lot more challenging for many, and offer us great depth (including deeper brainwave states; page 347) when we develop the *samskaras* of staying (and coming back when we wander) in the here and now.

When teaching or guiding embodied awareness, we have the opportunity to hold this space in restorative positions through calming language, tone and presence. Studies have shown that slow, meditative *yoga asana*, *pranayama* and meditation practice raise levels of the calming neurotransmitter GABA (gamma-amino butyric acid), shown to be low in those with high anxiety levels in the body.[76] GABA inhibits persistent and worrying thoughts (literally, 'stilling the mind'), regulating brain activity, relaxation and sleep. Tailoring sessions to focus on or include GABA-inducing practices may be helpful for those who tend to the 'unsafe' mode that creates constant rumination. Restorative practices can communicate to a heightened nervous system that it is safe to come

---

76   Streeter *et al.* (2010).

down: 'Relaxation, breath regulation and meditation [were] very important or essential for people with anxiety.'[77]

One of the researchers of The Shamatha Project (a long-term, continuing control group study of the effects of meditation training on mind and body, supported by the Dalai Lama), Tonya Jacobs, said, 'The more a person reported directing their cognitive resources to immediate sensory experience and the task at hand, the lower their resting cortisol' and also that 'people who dwell on painful past memories, or who develop anxiety about their future, typically have higher stress levels'.[78] On a specific study within the project on immune markers, it was concluded: 'Our results suggest that practice of concentration meditation influences interference control by enhancing controlled attention to goal-relevant task elements, and that inflammatory activity relates to individual differences in controlled attention.'[79]

TEACHING CONSIDERATIONS

When guiding ourselves or others towards greater interoceptive awareness, we may sometimes navigate choppy waters. Attuning to kinaesthesia (interoception and proprioception combined, our sixth sense) can help us distinguish between what we feel physically and observing our responses to it – sensory integration. In this way we can feel and be with emotional reactivity and retain a sense of equilibrium and healthy distance – not being swept up with a sense that these feelings define us, but retaining a clear sense of self and therefore safety.

In meeting our *kleshas* and *samskaras* through mindful attention and embodied, conscious awareness in the space of a slower practice – where we slow down to feel, including our vulnerabilities – we can bring along the following supportive qualities:

Aparigraha (non-grasping/-attachment or -greed): open to all experience like a river; letting it all come and go; observing any arising sensation and watching it dissolve in time; not gripping on to create emotions (or interpretations) from the feelings (*bhava*) that then have a story and life of their own – something else to cling to:

---

77   de Manincor *et al.* (2015).
78   Quoted in Sahdra *et al.* (2011).
79   Shields *et al.* (2020).

- Keep bringing students back to the present moment.
- Guide how to watch sensations arise and pass.
- Assure that any preoccupation, revelation, insight, decision, etc. will be there after the practice.
- Teach the courage to 'loosen their grip'.

Loving kindness (*metta/maitri*): spirit of generosity leads to possibility and availability, not needing to protect oneself against oneself (also compassion; page 343):

- Continually emphasise self-kindness and listening in.
- Practise from a viewpoint of curiosity and exploration.
- Encourage making decisions from body and breath, not mind or ideals.

Energy (*virya*): courage, diligence, enthusiasm, effort – an attitude of gladly engaging in wholesome activities, energy to accomplish wholesome or virtuous actions – to keep going on the journey. Trusting the way through reluctance, despair, doubt – *sattva* rather than *rajas*, sustainability:

- Support the energy that the student is lacking; if they are *tamasic*, energising; helping those with *rajasic* tendencies to drop down.
- Equally create healthy boundaries to preserve one's own energy to avoid resentment or 'compassion fatigue'.
- Foster the value of self-care and that 'more' is never simply 'better'.

Calm, equanimity (*upeksa*): equanimity is the ability to trust in the midst of uncertainty, being able to live with a sense of 'not knowing':

Neither a thought nor an emotion, it is rather the steady conscious realization of reality's transience. It is the ground for wisdom and freedom and the protector of compassion and love. While some may think of equanimity as dry neutrality or cool aloofness, mature equanimity produces a radiance and warmth of being. The Buddha described a mind filled with equanimity as "abundant, exalted, immeasurable, without hostility and without ill-will."[80]

- Co-regulate a calm presence for the student.
- Hold space for others that neither depletes nor excites you.
- Remain non-reactive through your own grounding.
- Step back when you need, recognising when you need space.
- Acknowledge that students' reactions to a teacher are rarely personal, although they may feel so to both parties.
- Come back to kindness.

Trust (*vishvasa*): trusting the way (Dao, *dharma*), staying power in the face of the struggles, brambles, stockades that pop up during life – firm determination:

- Being truly yourself; from a resourced place; real, and therefore compassionate and trustworthy.
- Showing that you are human and face the same difficulties.
- Modelling that you have some tools to navigate your path.

Reconditioning to allow restoration

Many people in modern society are attracted to stronger, faster practices, either because of their personal *samskaras*, to a degree their physiological and psychological make-up – but largely because society conditions us to be better, more productive, and this can create much resistance (and fear) to slowing down. Spending time with these considerations in more quiet practices or meditation can lay supportive foundations to still be able to access them when a practice becomes more 'busy' or strong, or space beyond the mat becomes more demanding.

This practice is relatively 'simple' and quietening, with lots of time and space opening out, encouraging downregulation to the parasympathetic, and specifically occupying the space of ventral vagus mode. Tuning into the subtle energies of the *gunas*, the movement of the *vayus* and autonomic nervous system states via the breath, which (as we have seen) has profound effects on our respiratory and immune health.

---

80 Fronsdale (2016).

To penetrate the hardest armour, use the softest touch
Yielding melts resistance
Density is filled with light
Good work accomplished without effort
In silence the teachings are heard
In stillness the world is transformed.

(Tao Te Ching, verse 36, aka 'The soft and the weak overcomes the hard and the strong')

It should be noted that many students seem surprised how tired they feel after a more gentle, somatic, restorative practice, even though they don't feel that they have 'done much'. This can be for several reasons:

- We hold fatigue in our fascia that gets 'locked in' from freeze responses and releases when we ease it out with movement that doesn't add in yet more stress.
- Our bodies and minds receive the communication that we are allowing ourselves to stop; this doing less and dropping beneath striving gives the signal that we can recover after 'holding it all together'. This is a sign we need more rest and quality sleep in our lives, less doing and more simply being (and in nature), but also to go into states of acknowledging and being with fatigue or lower energy; not to judge these as 'bad' (we get scared we will be less productive or won't 'get it all done', and often feel our value in society comes from how much we are 'doing') but as necessary to regroup, have a relationship with ease (*sukha*) and to nourish. To be able to say 'I am tired' without judgement.
- The result of meeting inflammation and beginning a resolution response through parasympathetic action and presence – again, going into 'recovery mode', where energy is rerouted to repair and renewal. Growth can only occur when survival needs feel met via safety.

Fatigue can be one of many feelings of release, alongside discomfort, irritability, tears, laughter, sadness, joy, confusion, ambivalence...any of the full spectrum of human experience, recognising shifts and changes as we transition through states and adapt to the new with self-compassion and kind attention:

We amplify this process by creating a steady even breath while we are practicing *asanas*. As we come up against the discomfort of tight muscles or challenging positions, we learn to soften and breathe into our tightness or breathe through our difficulty. When an upsetting emotion arises during meditation, we learn to give this feeling room by allowing our breath to rise and fall. This teaches us that while we cannot control what is going to happen to us, we can control our response. We can choose to open up or to shut down, to soften or to harden.[81]

In this restorative practice we explore moving inwards, interoception. Because the *vayus* (page 283) can seem abstract as an intellectual exercise, we will bring their movement, energy and direction into practice. When considering the *vayus* as teachers, it may become apparent that we include them implicitly rather than explicitly, guiding directional energetics:

> Gliding, undulating, and pulsating, we move with little effort, sensing how movement emerges from within. As we penetrate layer by layer into our interior, we experience not only physical but psychic absorption. This soaking inward is profoundly healing for both body and mind. It is like being in the amniotic sea of embryological development. The experience of soaking inward is akin to states of Samadhi celebrated in the teachings of yoga.[82]

Sensing inwardly (focus on the *vayus*)

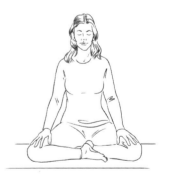

Sensing inwardly (interoception) is to move the focus of our eyes inwards – you may need to orient looking around the room or inwardly before you can settle your attention to the interior, introspection.

Access to sensing into the whole body can also involve moving into and releasing tension in the jaw. It is not uncommon for we, modern humans, to feel that we only exist as though caught up in the head, especially when we are often conditioned to think rather than feel our way through life. Much of our head architecture, gut–brain signalling and nervous system response is centred round the jaw, and we can habitually clench there. To allow access to our whole being can involve bringing awareness to the subtle, even slight, tightening that can accumulate in the temples, cheeks and base of the skull and show up as the forehead knot (*rudra granthi*).

---

81 Farhi (2005).
82 Little and Little (no date).

1. From a seated position, hips raised above the knees, settle onto the front edge of the sitting bones to invite uplift through the curve of the spine.

2. Palms down onto thighs – this is a more grounding *nyasa* (hand placement) than receptive palms up. Allow the weight of the arm bones to hang down, facilitating release in the shoulders (hands on the knees may create a forwards pull, depending on arm length).

3. To orientate first, look around, and get a sense of the external space in order to settle inwards.

4. Move the jaw to release as you close your eyes to draw attention inwards – bring your focus to internal spaces such as the nostrils and sinuses, the mouth, the temples and around the eyes and cheeks.

5. Notice the quality of the breath. No interpretation or analysis, more moment-to-moment awareness of tones, textures.

6. Observe the polarity of *apana* – the downwards movement of the exhale down the back body – and *prana* – the upwards motion through the front body on the inhale. Notice how this calibrates uplift in the body, the ventral and dorsal.

7. Notice any autonomic release (page 289) that expresses through sighs or spontaneous sounds.

Seated spinal undulation

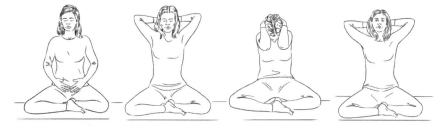

Undulating on any plane (sitting, lying, standing, z-legs, lunging, all-fours and more) before coming to resting or restorative positions brings an awakening and aliveness to all parts of us, radiating out from this centre. It also frees up tensions laid down as self-protecting bracing into the centre of the body – fascia, muscles, tendons and nerves – in towards the articulating chain of the spine. They can even feel warming as they release energy locked in; diffusing heat throughout the whole body out from the centre.

In this seated position, we are bringing awareness to the skull-sacrum channel and its relationship with our upright organisation. Raising our seat onto a lift (blocks, bolster, cushion, even a chair) that allows us to sit up from the front of our sitting bones and our spine, we can rise up out of the pelvis and feel the rib cage floating above, easily changing in volume with the breath. From there, we have the space to clasp the hands and play around with lifting the occiput (the base of the skull), feeling where the ears lift, the sinuses open and the temples release – room to allow movement of the breath and *vayus*, and to sense these subtleties.

1. Place the hands on the belly, feeling a meeting of hands and body. Notice the invitation of the breath to meet the presence of the hands and *samana vayu* – the quality of the breath at the navel.
2. Notice any sighs, autonomic releases. Allowing dropping towards the ground, the easy movement of the diaphragm.
3. Interlink the hands behind the skull, feeling the breath responding to the arms above the shoulders, the shift in circulation. Settle the shoulders, soften the eyes. *Udana vayu* – breath circulating in the head.
4. Come back to *apana/prana*, undulating the spine to lift, inhaling to rise, then exhaling to curl back in. Feel the relationship to holding the head.
5. Back in neutral, arms released, take three 'hums' (page 319), noticing the vibration in the skull, feeling the assimilation of that resonance. Feel the breath body occupying the physical body, a sense of *vyana vayu*, pervading all parts, regulated by *samana* at the belly.

Supported *balasana* (child's pose)

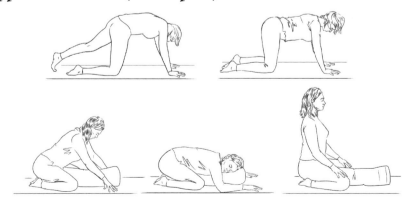

Here is space to explore and recognise that a pose or position isn't simply the endpoint of a shape; it is the whole story – preparing, arriving, entering, staying, anticipating moving in.

1. From all-fours, lengthen out each leg, feeling out any motion that facilitates the breath.
2. Pad through the hands, through the knees, to settle through all points connecting to the ground. Rotate the tailbone (page 128), limiting the motion in the shoulders. This is an alternative to the deeper practice of *nauli* (stomach churning), bringing attention to the centre.
3. Drop back into *balasana* (child's pose) with the support of a bolster. Lay the front body down onto the lift to draw attention to the diaphragm and the breath as it meets that surface.
4. Find where is most comfortable for the arms and shoulders so the fleshier parts drop, the bones release, shoulder blades moving away from each other.
5. Develop a curious inwards focus, interest in nuances, tones and shifts.
6. Draw the head back to centre, drawing the chin in towards the throat to gather up into the spine and roll up, using very little push with the arms. Rise up to let *prana* lift through the front spine.

Supported *viparati karani* (upside-down practice)

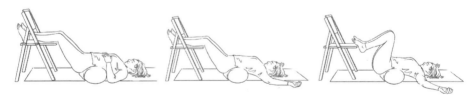

This supported inversion practice cools; the heart gets to rest, which down-regulates hypervigilance, fluids dropping towards the heart and head, relieving the work of the circulation. With the legs supported in this way, softness at the backs of the knees allows ease through the whole back body, which may not be as accessible with legs up the wall if the hamstrings are tight.

Bring attention to softness around the eyes, the physicality of the head, softness in the scalp. As the bones settle in relation to the flesh there may be micro-adjustments, allowing that settling 'ahh' of autonomic release.

1. *Viparati karani* (upside-down practice) raises the hips above the heart; this fully supported version supports *jalandhara bandha* (page 336). Place the bolster a fair way from the chair (depending on the length of your legs), so that the calves are fully supported when you lie down. Find the position where the bolster or lift is underneath the whole of the lower back and waist, so the tailbone and pubic bone can drop. Feel the change in relationship with gravity.

2. Find where the arms naturally release to allow weight and dropping down through the shoulders. If there is any discomfort in the breath or diaphragm, the hands can rest on the lower ribs to sense movement, the quality of breath in the belly, *samana vayu*.

3. Bring the soles of the feet onto the front edges of the chair, like an inverted squat, arms out to the side, open across the spine, allowing the arch into the back, naturally deepening *jalandhara bandha*.

Supported *apanasana* (wind-relieving pose)/ *ananda balasana* (happy baby pose)

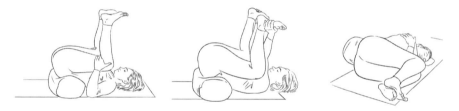

Take long, open time for each stage, including preparation for coming up from the side with eyes and front brain soft; focus on smoothly transitioning. Opening the pelvic floor with a supported inversion can ripple release up the whole of the spine and into the channel of the throat and jaw; breathe space between the back teeth, into the palate and around the eyes.

1. From *viparita karani* (or a supported bridge pose over a bolster), bring the knees into the chest, supported by the hands on the thighs. Essentially this is an inverted, raised foetal position, feeling *apana*, releasing energy, that which no longer serves us.

2. Bring the elbow to the inner legs and either hold the thighs or the outside of the feet, without creating compression. Feel the opening of the pelvic floor and the rippling through the dorsal fascia.

3. Roll the legs into the chest, draw into the centre line and roll slowly onto the side, off the lift, resting in a side foetal position to calibrate.

Supported z-legs twist

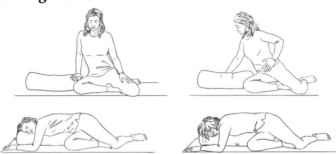

In the final resting position before *savasana* (page 67), the head may turn away from the legs, but only if this is a fully easeful place to feel the polarities of the spine. In restorative positions, we are not bringing in effort to stay or looking to feel anything in particular, so only turn the head if that comes with ease (and no pull in any part of the neck), retaining awareness down the spine as a whole passage of the breath and supporting your arms as needed.

Sthira is the quality of steadiness within practice, kindly bringing the attention back to the present, feeling the sensory feedback of the bolster and the ground, providing support and navigating back to the tides of the breath whenever we need a guide back into the here and now.

1. From a z-legs position with the bolster close in towards the front thigh, press down into the hand to lift the spine, creating space between the vertebrae. Lift and turn towards the bolster.
2. Slide the front hand across the side of the pelvis and the front of the belly to encourage a twisting movement and visceral connection. Use soothing touch to bring awareness through the abdomen.
3. Roll down to the bolster, head turned in the same direction as the knees so that there is full support, ease and release, shoulders dropping away from each other. Close the eyes to find that inner space for *udana vayu*, to move with ease in the head.

SUBTLE PRACTICES:
TRADITIONAL *PRANAYAMA*

Pranayama is the subtle or vital dimension of *prakriti* in the *panchamaya*.[83] The scholar, yoga teacher and author of *The Truth of Yoga*, Daniel Simpson, traces the history of pranayama from the *Vedas* through to modern-day practices: forms of *pranayama* have been explored and developed throughout yoga's evolution, intrinsically linked to the stilling of the mind and the journey to greater subtle awareness.[84] This differs to other systems; the same techniques are recommended in *dharma* texts as ways to restore chaste purity after misbehaving, and the earliest mentions in Vedic texts were more to do with effective performance of ritual. Studies have shown that *pranayama*, as part of a regular yoga practice, can improve psychological states, our ability to self-regulate:[85] 'By voluntarily changing the rate, depth and pattern of breathing, we can change the message being sent from the body's respiratory system to the brain. In this way, breathing techniques provide a portal to the autonomic communication network.'[86]

In a modern context, we can choose to control or bring consciousness to breath. Where our nervous systems are already pushed into overdrive, a less regimented, more spacious approach than some of the more stimulating ascetic practices may be more beneficial.

83 Rothenberg (2019).
84 Simpson (2018).
85 Kumar and Singh (2021).
86 Brown and Gerbarg (2012).

Pranayama: The basics

Prana: breath, respiration, life force, vitality, energy, strength – constancy, a force in constant motion.

Prana mainly flows through the body in the *nadi*, or nerve channels of the astral body, of which there are said to be between 2000 and 72,000, depending on sources.

Poor health can result from blocked *nadis*; *pranayama* (and later *asana*) were developed to clear these channels.

Ayama: stretch, extension, expansion, length, breadth, regulation, prolongation, restraint, control.

Pranayama:
conscious control of the breath to extend and expand vital life force energy

Pranayama (*prana*, energy + *ayama*, expansion) follows the *satkarma* (*shatkarmas*, purifications) in Hatha yoga – preparation is through *asana* and dietary moderations. *Asana* helps performance in *pranayama* by bringing elasticity to the lung fibres.

'The controlled intake and outflow of breath in a firmly established posture.' (*Yoga Sutras, Pantanjali*)

Process by which the internal *pranic* store is increased or expanded > quantity of *prana* is activated to a higher frequency.

The breath allows us to develop a nuanced awareness of *prana* (energy) as it moves through our inner landscape. This more subtle focusing of the mind is the beginning of yoga; quality of presence.

Pranayama prepares us for meditation by allowing us the freedom and creativity to follow the breath – there is no goal to establish a particular breath or create a certain relationship between the out-breath and in-breath; these are merely techniques along the way.

'In contrast to the modern fixation on bodily postures, the defining practice in traditional texts is *pranayama*.' (Simpson 2018)

The regulation of the breath through *pranayama* expands to stilling the patterning of consciousness and we are drawn less by thoughts, desires and actions.

Pranayama: Puraka, rechaka and *kumbhaka* – with *ujjayi*

Puraka (inhalation) corresponds to the sun, fire, the heart and the life force; it is heating.

(Rechaka) (exhalation) corresponds to the moon; it is a cooling breath associated with the lungs and death.

Kumbhaka (pause, retention) is a complete cessation of movement of air and muscles but also of all awareness of such movement and tendencies > exhibits control over the urge to inhale or exhale and is the ultimate goal of *pranayama*.

Ujjayi (victorious breath) is a form of *pranayama* and is sometimes called 'snake breath', the 'sounding breath' or 'ocean sounding breath'. It involves narrowing the back of the throat while breathing to create a series of 'hhh' sounds while breathing in and a series of 'sss' when breathing out. As well as the benefits, it helps us to hear and identify our breath.

Generates internal heat

Increases parasympathetic tone

Focuses the mind

Lengthens respiration, improves oxygen saturation, air volume in lungs

Rechaka and *puraka* need to be developed first to plant the seeds for *ujjayi* – these three form the basis for other practices, for example *kumbhaka ujjiya* and *viloma* (pauses without a breath).

Four stages of breathing (Tantric terminology)

1. *Puraka* (inhalation)
The process of drawing in air, with an aim for this to be smooth and continuous. Any pausing within a single inhalation is described as a broken *puraka* rather than as a series of *purakas*. The process of controlling the urge to exhale.

2. *Abhyantara kumbhaka* (pause after inhaling)
Full pause: conscious cessation of the flow of air, leading to retention of the air in the lungs. Any movement of lungs or body is suspended.

3. *Rechaka* (exhalation)
Like inhalation, looking to be smooth and continuous. Exhaling differs, however, as simply a relaxing of tensed muscles, while inhaling involves muscular action. Reducing the tendency to add force to the exhale is beneficial. The process of controlling the urge to inhale.

4. *Bahya kumbhaka* (pause after exhaling)
Empty pause: completes the cycle that terminates as the pause ends and a new inhalation begins. The stoppage is deliberate or prolonged.

Kevala kumbhaka (perfectly peaceful pause; spontaneous retention) is a state of complete rest. Urgency, interest, motive, will, desire, hatred, fear, ambition, love, anxiety, hunger and thirst are all gone for that specific moment.

By developing the practice of *kumbhaka* (breath retention) for longer periods, we can manipulate and direct currents of prana (energy) through the *pranamaya kosha*.

Pranayama: The *vayus*

Five types of *pranic* energy or *vayu*: meaning air or breath (primary nerve force) with the attributes of *ruksa* (dry), *laghu* (light), *sita* (cold), *khara* (rough), *sukshma* (minute) and *cala* (mobile).

of these, *prana* and *apana*:

In the *Upanisad* (Upanishads), *prana* is equated with *atman*, the innermost non-physical self.

Pranayama that includes elimination and provides the energy for this.

Prana – that which enters the body IN-BREATH

Apana – that which leaves the body OUT-BREATH

Prana is not just in-breath, but the power behind out-breath too; it is in all forms of life and living.

Refers to the lower abdomen and the stagnation we can collect there.

Breath transports *prana* from the external world to the internal world, from the formless (*purusa*) into the form (*prakriti*).

When practising *pranayama* and observing change of mind, *prana* has already entered the body. *Prana* enters the body in the moment when there is a positive change in the mind.

Too much *apana* is seen as heavy and slow (*tamasic*), so the out-breath clears the way for energy as *prana*.

As with all *pranic* forces, we need *apana* as energy, but when it is left as debris it can stop *prana* from entering the body; an efficient minimum is best.

The out-breath unblocks the mind.

Prana exists as a negative energy as well as a positive energy; too much can cause harm.

Prana is physical, mental, intellectual, sexual, spiritual and cosmic energy.

GREATER CLARITY

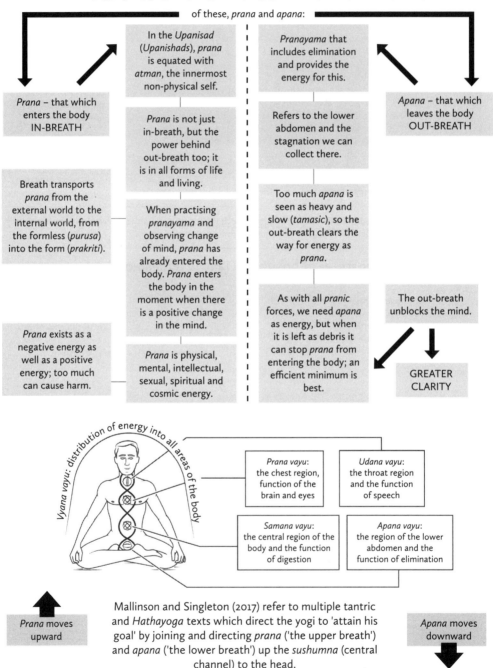

Vyana vayu: distribution of energy into all areas of the body

Prana vayu: the chest region, function of the brain and eyes

Udana vayu: the throat region and the function of speech

Samana vayu: the central region of the body and the function of digestion

Apana vayu: the region of the lower abdomen and the function of elimination

Prana moves upward

Mallinson and Singleton (2017) refer to multiple tantric and *Hathayoga* texts which direct the yogi to 'attain his goal' by joining and directing *prana* ('the upper breath') and *apana* ('the lower breath') up the *sushumna* (central channel) to the head.

Apana moves downward

Pranayama: The subtleties of *prana*

The symbiotic relationship between *prana* (vitality) and *citta* (mind) is a consistent theme in all of the Vedic teachings.

In yoga, when the breath is still, *prana* and *citta* are both still.

All the vibrations and fluctuations to which we are exposed come to a standstill when *prana* and *citta* are steady and silent.

Pranayama is the key practice in yoga, the root of spiritual knowledge or that of the true self (*atma jnana*).

With the breath reminding us we are alive, this links to the *kleshas* (hindrances or afflictions) – ignorance or lack of insight, aversion, desire, ego attachment, clinging to life – that awareness can move beyond for liberation.

'Everything that moves, breathes, opens and closes lives in the self.'
(*Mundaka Upanisad* 2.1)

- - - - - - - - - - - - - - -

Donna Farhi (2013) makes a philosophical connection between the words *prana* (energy) and *atman* (self/ pure consciousness), which stems etymologically from 'to breathe'. This points to a connection between expanding the breath and consciousness.

Pranayama is one of five *pancakosas* (*pancha kosha*, aka *koshas* in some lineages) and involves the manipulation of vital energy.

Maya is often translated as 'illusory', referring to the impermanent, changeable nature of *prakriti*.

- -

If all the *prana* is within the body, we are free of physical and mental symptoms.

If we feel unwell, the quality of *prana* and its density within the body is reduced.

The more peaceful and well balanced we are, the less our *prana* is dispersed outside the body.

Too little *prana* in the body can leave us feeling stuck or restricted, no drive, listless or depressed.

Pranayama helps to move blockages and rubbish out of the body so that *prana* can flow in.

Physical ailments can occur when there is not enough *prana* in the body, or its flow is interrupted.

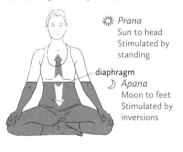

☀ *Prana*
Sun to head
Stimulated by standing

diaphragm
☽ *Apana*
Moon to feet
Stimulated by inversions

'Still others offer as sacrifice the outgoing breath in the incoming breath, while some offer the incoming breath into the outgoing breath. Some arduously practice *pranayam* and restrain the incoming and outgoing breaths, purely absorbed in the regulation of the life-energy. Yet others curtail their food intake and offer the breath into the life-energy as sacrifice. All these knowers of sacrifice are cleansed of their impurities as a result of such performances.' (*Bhagavad Gita*, 4.29–30)

The more content a person is and the better they feel, the more *prana* is inside.

Yogic and Ayurvedic models: because we can influence the flow of *prana* through the flow of our breath, our quality of breath influences our state of mind.

The more disturbed a person is, the more *prana* is dissipated and lost.

'The quality of *prana* in the people we commune with evokes responses in us, leaves impressions, and shapes our inner motivations. Likewise, our unconscious and conscious thoughts, emotions, and actions move our *prana* out into the world. This reciprocity is a constant reflective of the intake and output of every breath.' (Rothenberg 2019)

Pranayama: The practices

'*Pranayama* is the means to cultivate a healthy *pranic* reservoir for the vessel we call the body. Therefore, to restore our *prana*, practice must be adapted or titrated appropriately, according to the practitioner's starting point.' (Rothenberg 2019)

> According to *Yoga Sutra* 2.50 (Patanjali), the quality of the breath should be both:
>
> *Dirgha* – long and steady   *Sukshma* – fine and subtle

Starting practices (*Hathayogapradipika*) are simple observations of:

Puraka – sipping the inhalation
Rechaka – controlled exhalation

Then moving to easeful extension of the exhalation/then of the inhalation after practice of ease with the more calming out-breath. Then can add in *ujjayi*...

Others mentioned include:

Nadi shodhana (*nadi* purification):

alternate nostril breathing to balance the channels of *ida* and *pingala*; *mudra* to close the nostril not receiving or releasing breath supports the *kumbhaka* (pause)

Suryabheda (piercing the sun):

breathing into the right nostril and out of the left (moon/*chandra* cooling version is reverse)

Brahmari (black bee):

a 'buzzing' hum while exhaling – suitable in most positions and for most levels

Retentions:

after out-breath *sahita bahya kumbhaka* (deliberate external retention) can be practised with sensitive *uddiyana bandha*

after in-breath *sahita antara kumbhaka* (deliberate internal retention) can be practised with sensitive *mula bandha*

'*Jalandharabandha* is to be done at the end of inhalation. *Uddiyanabandha* is to be done at the end of [internal] *kumbhaka* and the beginning of exhalation.' (*Hathayogapradipika* 2:45)

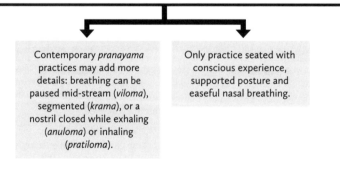

Contemporary *pranayama* practices may add more details: breathing can be paused mid-stream (*viloma*), segmented (*krama*), or a nostril closed while exhaling (*anuloma*) or inhaling (*pratiloma*).

Only practice seated with conscious experience, supported posture and easeful nasal breathing.

Pranayama: Practice guide

Lying down *pranayama* is suitable for all because it:

Removes worry about the posture.
Keeps body and mind tension-free.
Supports the chest for full and easy breathing.

When practice is too long, *prana* backs up and forces itself wherever it can flow; this may cause an overflow there. This is most common in the head and/or the solar plexus and can lead to headaches or being over-'fired up' (*rajasic*).

Under no circumstance should we be forceful (practice *satya*). If the *nadis* are not open and one forces it's like pushing against a coiled-up spring; eventually it pushes back.

Check for these factors if headaches, tension or irritability are occurring during or after practice:
• Forceful? • Posture? • Too long? • Running before walking; too advanced too soon?
• Eyes open or tense? • Jaw clenched? • Diaphragm 'stuck'?

During lying down practice, the diaphragm needs to keep releasing. The abdomen does not over-inflate, but we use its movement to feed the chest and so provide room for the diaphragm. Observe the experience above all else; keep the abdomen soft and notice any force creeping in.

The intercostal muscles elevate the ribs and need to be opened and loosened through *asana* practice. Preparing the pelvic and thoracic diaphragms is also necessary.

Ideally keep the eyes closed during *pranayama*. Breathe through the nose when possible.

Although in *pranayama* we are breathing into the chest we must keep the abdominal area free. This is not a case of 'either/or', but a subtle balance between the abdomen and the chest. This is particularly important towards the end of an in-breath so that the spleen, liver and stomach can release, allowing more downward-feeling in the diaphragm, feeding more upward-feeling in the chest.

Keep the brain passive, imagining energy flowing in (sun) and tension flowing out (moon).

'These are practices of *pratyahara*, requiring a fine attunement to the inner senses with *dharana* (focus, concentration). If the mind becomes distracted, the subtlety and rhythm will be lost.' (Rothenberg 2019)

Cultivate a sense of lengthening the abdomen to feed the chest. If the chest is taking time to release and inflate, then the abdomen acts as an 'overflow'.

B.K.S. Iyengar recommended (2013) practising before the sunrise, freshly awake and alert, or post-sunset as the heat of the day subsides. Where this relates to traditional practice in India, we can adapt to suit Western climate and lifestyle.

Before beginning a *pranayama* cycle, 'tidal air' should be expelled. This empties the lungs of any build-up of the air taken in from the breathing of the day to begin anew.

This is done by taking a slightly deeper breath and fully expelling the tidal air.

Like with *asana*, meditation, mantra and *bhakti* (devotion), if there is a feeling of force then we are stepping outside the advice of the *yamas*.

Build up practice honestly, analyse and mould the breath with thorough understanding, clarity and wisdom.

When extending the length of the in-breath imagine the marathon runner and consider pace.

If a breathing cycle is interrupted for any reason, for example airways become blocked, swallowing mid-cycle, losing concentration or drifting off, first try to finish that cycle without force. If any tidal air is breathed in during rectification of the problem, then this must be expelled again before returning to the *pranayama*.

'The practice of attuning our breath requires the attention of the mind, and attendance to the subtle movement of *prana* within us, as well as around us.' (Rothenberg 2019)

Pranayama: Health and the modern lens

BENEFITS OF BREATH PRACTICES – FULL, CONSCIOUS

- Increased oxygenation in the lungs, leading to the elimination of toxins, better sleep, recovery, immune function and the link between mind, body and spirit. As we age, lung cells contract and take in less oxygen, so *pranayama* keeps them open and has an anti-ageing effect, aiding red corpuscles to circulate.

- Increased digestion and assimilation of food. Oxygenation of both the digestive organs and the food lead to more efficient digestion (and microbiome health), as well as eating in a calmer state, when the body is ready to receive food.

- Improvement in the health of the nervous system. This is due to the calm that encourages the parasympathetic state of the autonomic nervous system, which increases oxygenation, spares vital nutrients, reduces heart rate, relaxes muscles and reduces anxious states. This increases all-over communication throughout the body, including the brain, spinal cord and nerves, and so the mind quietens, and inflammatory tendencies are reduced.

- Calm, longer breaths are equated with longer life; *pranayama* helps to lessen our usual 15 breaths per minute.

- The brain needs three times more oxygen than the rest of the body. The glands in the brain that affect mood are rejuvenated, including the pituitary and pineal glands.

- The movements of the diaphragm during deep breathing massage the abdominal organs. The upper movement of the diaphragm also massages the heart, stimulating visceral blood and lymphatic circulation.

- The lungs become healthy and powerful, a good insurance against respiratory problems. Increased elasticity in the lungs and rib cage promotes habitual full breathing.

- Deep, slow yoga breathing reduces the workload for the heart, especially during lying-down practices when the chest is supported. The result is a more efficient and stronger heart; more oxygen is brought into contact with blood sent to the lungs by the heart and so it doesn't have to work as hard to deliver oxygen to the tissues. Full breathing creates greater lung pressure differential, increasing circulation, allowing the heart to rest.

- Expansive, fluid breathing can support efficient metabolic function (related to COVID-19 risk). Extra oxygen burns up any excess fat more efficiently in those who are holding on to weight. For those who are underweight, the extra oxygen feeds the starving tissues and glands.

BENEFITS OF NASAL BREATHING

Cold air coming into the nose cools down the frontal lobe of the brain, which calms its activity.

Warms up air entering the lungs and body.

Nasal hairs prevent impurities entering the body; glands in the inner nose destroy bacteria.

The body produces nitric oxide when we breathe in through the nose; this opens up the cells in the lungs to receive oxygen. It is also important to immune function.

Why is *pranayama* so relevant for us today?

- Many of us are in constant states of excitation, anger, irritation or anxiety from the constant stimuli of the modern world; this leads to fast and shallow breathing. We tend to be in this 'fight or flight' sympathetic state of the autonomic nervous system, constantly reacting, which causes shallow breathing and an emphasis on the in-breath. This leaves us deficient in oxygen and in metabolic acidosis from the build-up of carbon dioxide, associated with inflammation and other immune imbalances.

- We are in too much of a hurry and our movements and breathing follow this pattern, keeping us stuck in survival mode.

- A sedentary lifestyle tends to use only one-tenth of our total lung capacity, leaving us poorly oxygenated; this is linked to heart disease, cancers and inflammatory conditions. Poorly exercised lungs lose some of their function.

- As life becomes more automated we lose the need to breathe deeply for exertion. Low oxygen levels leave us unable to produce full, vital energy and affect all body systems.

- With increasing pollution and less fresh air, the body instinctively takes more shallow breaths to protect itself from potentially harmful pollutants and pathogens. The body takes in just enough air to tick over.

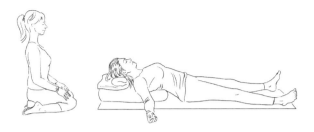

Pranayama can be practised seated in supported *vajrasana* (hero pose), with a bolster, blocks or meditation pillow, or in a comfortable cross-legged position such as *siddhasana* (accomplished pose) or *sukhasana* (comfort/easy pose), again with support to lift the hips and provide space. Seated *pranayama* can be conducive to alertness, but can be a strain on the postural muscles, and therefore the nervous system, to stay upright. Supported supine (lying) *pranayama* can be more restful, although the challenge here can be staying alert and awake!

Support for supine *pranayama*

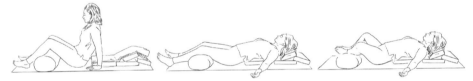

A traditional *savasana* (corpse pose) or *pranayama* lift (such as in the Iyengar yoga tradition) may use a bolster for chest support and opening the chest and throat. Alternatively, four yoga blocks can be used with a folded blanket over for comfort – this lower height than a bolster may be more suitable for many lower backs. A bolster under the knees can ease the back of the legs and therefore soften the lower back.

This lift can be used for other supine restorative positions, such as *supta baddha konasana* (supine bound angle pose).

1. To create a *pranayama* lift, you may use a soft bolster with a blanket for your head or with four blocks, which sets the relationship with the chest and the skull. Two blocks end to end, portrait, then one or two (angled) landscape, for the head, with a folded blanket over the blocks. Whatever lift is used, assure that the chest is lifted, there is no jamming into the lower back and the chin is drawn in towards the chest.

Any pinching in the lower back can be soothed by manually taking the buttock flesh down away from the back to elongate and create space. Arms out to the side – some people may need blocks under the arms to support tight shoulders (or shorter arms) so that there isn't excessive pulling across the upper chest.

2. Bring spacious attention to the release of the body right to the periphery, fluidity of the breath, perhaps sighing out some deeper exhalations. Introduce a little *antara kumbhaka* – internal retention after the inhalation, holding the 'full pot' natural pause before the exhale naturally falls out, without any sense of grasping (page 50). Feel the energy of *prana* at the top of the inhalation. Return to the natural flow of the breath, observing how it flows, regulates in response to the needs of the body, moment to moment, checking into soft eyes, soft jaw periodically.

3. Wake up the toes and the feet, sliding the legs towards the pelvis, soles of the feet onto the bolster (knees pointing up) to settle into the lower back, noticing sensations around the pelvis. Roll to the side to come up slowly.

Krama pranayama (stepped breath extension) with *nyasa* (hand placement)

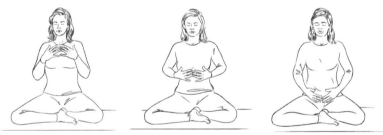

In *krama pranayama*, the focus is on long inhalations and exhalations that move continuously through the body. Adding pauses to both the inhales and exhales, the breath and lung capacity are expanded. With relaxed attention, this can lead the practitioner's mind and body towards steadiness and calm.

1. Sitting in a comfortable seat, such as *siddhasana* (accomplished pose) or *sukhasana* (comfort/easy pose), on a bolster (or on a chair), bring

awareness to height in the spine, the atlas of the skull supported over the pelvis.

2. Begin with the hands on the chest, then, with an inhalation, feel the hands move down to the belly and then to the diaphragm. On the exhalation, move the hands back up from the belly, to the diaphragm, to the chest. Tune into *apana* and *prana*, moving respectively down and up with the natural flow of the breath, connected to its physicality.

There are three ways to practise *krama* breathing where there is more of a specific breath pause:

- Three pauses within the exhale: this form is more pacifying and best practised for those with sympathetic dominance or trauma. Begin with a full cycle of breath (inhale and exhale), then take a long inhale, hold it at the top as long as comfortable, then exhale one-third of the way (pause), another third (pause) and, for the last third, empty out the breath completely, pausing at the bottom of the breath. Notice that moment after the exhale where the pause of *bahya kumbhaka* sits as a still moment, the potential of the bliss body, *anandamaya kosha*. Follow with a full deep breath (recovery breath), then begin another round of *krama* breath. Complete 5–10 rounds.
- Three pauses within the inhale: this is more activating and uplifting, and often recommended to ease symptoms of depression when practised with sensitivity. Its active tone means it is more suitable in the morning or before dynamic practice.
- Three pauses within both the inhales and exhales: after much experience with the first two, here we balance out their energies, when we can practise retaining ease (*sukha*). Then it can be supportive preparation for the steadiness of meditation and autonomic nervous system regulation.

Nadi shodhana (alternate nostril breathing) with *mrigi mudra* (deer seal)

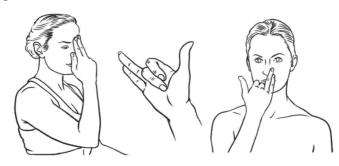

With variations of placement (*nyasa*) of the *mudra*, play with positioning to find where the shoulder of the raised arm can be most comfortable and without tension. If you cannot find that place, you can visualise this hold instead, so no strain is brought into the practice.

Either way of focusing the alternating breath regulates *prana* and the *nadis*, links the third eye and root to ground, and calms the mind in preparation for meditation. Physiologically, this supports respiratory function, rejuvenates the nervous system and balances left and right brain hemispheres. Research has demonstrated that right-nostril breathing is indeed involved with relatively higher sympathetic activity, and left-nostril breathing with relatively more parasympathetic activity. See also moon piercing breath on page 131.[87,88]

1. Sit comfortably with a sense of length in the spine, chest open.
2. Bring the right hand to the face and rest the index and middle finger at the centre of the brows. Close the eyes and draw the attention inwards to the breath.
3. Inhale and exhale smoothly and completely to clear the lungs.
4. Close the right nostril with the thumb, ensuring that the septum is not pushed off centre, and breathe in through the left nostril.
5. Close the left nostril with the ring finger noticing the natural pause, *kumbhaka*, at the top of the inhale, then open the right nostril and breathe out slowly.
6. Inhale through the right, then close this nostril for a brief, comfortable pause before opening and breathing out through the left side.

87 Niazi *et al.* (2022).
88 Sinha, Deepak and Gusain (2013).

7. Repeat for 5–10 cycles, ensuring that the breath is smooth and easeful.

Brahmari (black bee breath) with *shanmukhi mudra* (six gates seal, aka 'Closing the seven gates of perception')

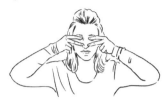

Sealing the tragus (ear), nose and eyes is conducive to *pratyahara*, the drawing in of the senses. This can help to relieve the incessant pull of mental chatter and can help in shifting unhelpful emotional patterns, or anxiety. The elongation of the exhale increases vagal tone and the resonance of the humming vibrates tissues in the lungs to loosen any mucus there.

1. In a supported, comfortable seated position such as *siddhasana* (accomplished pose) or *sukhasana* (comfort/easy pose) (or sitting in a chair), use the thumbs to close the ear apertures with the tragus. The index fingers gently seal the eyelids shut and the middle fingers partially close the nostrils.
2. *Pranayama* should always start with a cleansing breath – a deep, fluid inhale and exhale to clear the lungs, and soften shoulders, jaws, eyes.
3. Following this cleansing breath, inhale through the nose with the mouth closed.
4. Exhale slowly through the nose while making a humming sound in the back of the throat – practice 4–10 rounds.

THE POWER OF THE HUM

The oscillating airflow produced by humming on the exhalation increases nasal nitric oxide levels,[89] which could help reduce viruses entering the respiratory system and improve immune responses to COVID-19.[90] Increased nitric oxide levels have also been linked to reduction in sinus inflammation, improving respiratory issues such as rhinitis.[91] Humming extends the exhalation, creating vibration in the upper torso and throat. The 'mmm' sound created vibrates into the cerebral cortex, said to nourish the pituitary gland for endocrine and autonomic nervous

---

89 Weitzberg and Lundberg (2002).
90 Kobayashi (2021).
91 Eby (2006).

system/vagus regulation (see Part 6 for further vibrational practices), as well as deactivating the limbic fight-or-flight response,[92] stimulating serotonin production.

Humming can be brought in any time within a physical or meditative practice as a focus on inner vibration (*spanda*), particularly in the silence that follows.

Self-enquiry questions

1. Which circumstances, positions or practices most enable you to tune inwards, to sense interoception?
2. Are you able to sense breathing patterns easily from the beginning of a practice, or do you need bodily movement to help you tune in?
3. Can you tune into the different movements of the *vayus* to feel a sense of whole?
4. Can you notice any movement positions or practices that naturally incorporate pandiculation?
5. In positions held for longer times – for example, restorative, yin, static *asana*, meditation, *pranayama* – can you notice the different nature of autonomic release as you drop into deeper layers, with their differing energies of support/effort?

Further resources

Steve Haines and Sophie Standing (2021) *Touch is Really Strange*. London and Philadelphia, PA: Singing Dragon.

Tias Little (2020) *The Practice Is the Path: Lessons and Reflections on the Transformative Power of Yoga*. Boulder, CO: Shambhala Publications.

James Mallinson and Mark Singleton (2017) *The Roots of Yoga*. London: Penguin.

Hans H. Rhyner (2017) *The Complete Book of Ayurveda*. Woodbury, MN: Llewellyn.

Robin L. Rothenberg (2019) *Restoring Prana: A Therapeutic Guide to Pranayama and Healing through the Breath for Yoga Therapists, Yoga Teachers and Healthcare Practitioners*. London and Philadelphia, PA: Singing Dragon.

Daniel Simpson (2021) *The Truth of Yoga: A Comprehensive Guide to Yoga's History, Texts, Philosophy, and Practices*. New York: North Point Press.

John Stirk (2021) *Deeper Still: Authentic Embodiment for Yoga Teachers*. Pencaitland: Handspring Publishing Ltd.

---

92 Kalyani *et al.* (2011).

References

Abelson, J.L., Weg, J.G., Nesse, R.M. and Curtis, G.C. (2001) 'Persistent respiratory irregularity in patients with panic disorder.' *Biological Psychiatry 49*(7), 588–595. Available at: https://pubmed.ncbi.nlm.nih.gov/11297716

Aljadeff, G., Molho, M., Katz, I., Benzaray, S., Yemini, Z. and Shiner, R.J. (1993) 'Pattern of lung volumes in patients with sighing breathing.' *Thorax 48*(8), 809–811. Available at: https://pubmed.ncbi.nlm.nih.gov/8211870

Amin, H.D., Sharma, R., Vyas, H.A. and Vyas, M.K. (2014) 'Importance of *Manas Tattva*: A searchlight in Yoga Darshana.' *Ayu 35*(3), 221–226. Available at: www.ncbi.nlm.nih.gov/pmc/articles/PMC4649565

Bachman, N. (2011) *The Path of the Yoga Sutras: A Practical Guide to the Core of Yoga.* Boulder, CO: Sounds True.

Bahar-Fuchs, A., Clare, L. and Woods, B. (2013) 'Cognitive training and cognitive rehabilitation for mild to moderate Alzheimer's disease and vascular dementia.' *The Cochrane Database of Systematic Reviews 2013*(6), CD003260. Available at: https://pubmed.ncbi.nlm.nih.gov/23740535

Bai, L., Qin, W., Tian, J., Dong, M., *et al.* (2009) 'Acupuncture modulates spontaneous activities in the anticorrelated resting brain networks.' *Brain Research 1279*, 37–49. Available at: https://pubmed.ncbi.nlm.nih.gov/19427842

Bechter, K., Brown, D. and Najjar, S. (2019) 'Editorial: Recent advances in psychiatry from psycho-neuro-immunology research: Autoimmune encephalitis, autoimmune encephalopathy, and mild encephalitis.' *Frontiers in Psychiatry 10*, 169. Available at: https://pubmed.ncbi.nlm.nih.gov/31001151

Ben-Shaanan, T.L., Schiller, M., Azulay-Debby, H., Korin, B., *et al.* (2018) 'Modulation of anti-tumor immunity by the brain's reward system.' *Nature Communications 9*(1), 2723. Available at: https://pubmed.ncbi.nlm.nih.gov/30006573

Berrueta, L., Muskaj, I., Olenich, S., Butler, T., *et al.* (2016) 'Stretching impacts inflammation resolution in connective tissue.' *Journal of Cellular Physiology 231*(7), 1621–1627. Available at: https://pubmed.ncbi.nlm.nih.gov/26588184

Bertolucci, L.F. (2011) 'Pandiculation: Nature's way of maintaining the functional integrity of the myofascial system?' *Journal of Bodywork and Movement Therapies 15*(3), 268–280. Available at: https://pubmed.ncbi.nlm.nih.gov/21665102

Boyadzhieva, A. and Kayhan, E. (2021) 'Keeping the breath in mind: Respiration, neural oscillations, and the free energy principle.' *Frontiers in Neuroscience 15*, 647579. Available at: https://pubmed.ncbi.nlm.nih.gov/34267621

Brown, R.P. and Gerbarg, P.L. (2012) *The Healing Power of the Breath: Simple Techniques to Reduce Stress and Anxiety, Enhance Concentration, and Balance Your Emotions.* Boulder, CO: Shambhala Publications.

Bryant, E.F. (2009) *Yoga Sutras of Patanjali.* New York: North Point Press.

Caldwell, L.J., Subramaniam, S., MacKenzie, G. and Shah, D.K. (2020) 'Maximising the potential of neuroimmunology.' *Brain, Behavior, and Immunity 87*, 189–192. Available at: https://pubmed.ncbi.nlm.nih.gov/32201255

Chen, W.G., Schloesser, D., Arensdorf, A.M., Simmons, J.M., *et al.* (2021) 'The emerging science of interoception: Sensing, integrating, interpreting, and regulating signals within the self.' *Trends in Neuroscience 44*(1), 3–16. Available at: https://pubmed.ncbi.nlm.nih.gov/33378655

Cook, J.L. and Cook, G. (2009) *Child Development Principles and Perspectives.* London: Pearson.

Critchley, H.D. and Garfinkel, S.N. (2017) 'Interoception and emotion.' *Current Opinion in Psychology 17*, 7–14. Available at: https://pubmed.ncbi.nlm.nih.gov/28950976

Dallam, G., McClaran, S.R., Foust, C.P. and Cox, D.G. (2018) 'Effect of nasal versus oral breathing on Vo2max and physiological economy in recreational runners following an extended period spent using nasally restricted breathing.' *International Journal of Kinesiology and Sports Science 6*(2), 22–29. Available at: www.researchgate.net/publication/325521734_Effect_of_Nasal_Versus_Oral_Breathing_on_Vo2max_and_Physiological_Economy_in_Recreational_Runners_Following_an_Extended_Period_Spent_Using_Nasally_Restricted_Breathing

Damasio, A. (1996) 'The somatic marker hypothesis and the possible functions of the prefrontal cortex.' *Philosophical Transactions of the Royal Society of London. Series B, Biological Sciences 351*(1346), 1413–1420. Available at: https://pubmed.ncbi.nlm.nih.gov/8941953

Damasio, A. (2000) *The Feeling of What Happens: Body, Emotion and the Making of Consciousness*, Reprint edn. London: Vintage.

Dantzer, R. (2009) 'Cytokine, sickness behavior, and depression.' *Immunology and Allergy Clinics of North America 29*(2), 247–264. Available at: https://pubmed.ncbi.nlm.nih.gov/19389580

de Manincor, M., Bensoussan, A., Smith, C., Fahey, P. and Bourchier, S. (2015) 'Establishing key components of yoga interventions for reducing depression and anxiety, and improving well-being: A Delphi
method study.' *BMC Complementary and Alternative Medicine 15*, 85. Available at: https://pubmed.
ncbi.nlm.nih.gov/25888411

Easwaran, E. (2007) *The Bhagavad Gita*, 2nd edn. Totnes: Nilgiri Press.

Eby, G.A. (2006) 'Strong humming for one hour daily to terminate chronic rhinosinusitis in four days: A
case report and hypothesis for action by stimulation of endogenous nasal nitric oxide production.'
Medical Hypotheses 66(4), 851–854. Available at: https://pubmed.ncbi.nlm.nih.gov/16406689

Eggart, M., Queri, S. and Müller-Oerlinghausen, B. (2019) 'Are the antidepressive effects of massage therapy
mediated by restoration of impaired interoceptive functioning? A novel hypothetical mechanism.'
Medical Hypotheses 128, 28–32. Available at: https://pubmed.ncbi.nlm.nih.gov/31203905

Elton, H. (2022) 'Yoga philosophy and practice: Part 5 – Sāṃkhya.' Available at: www.eltonyoga.com/blog/
yoga-history-and-philosophy-samkhya

Farhi, D. (2005) *Bringing Yoga to Life: The Everyday Practice of Enlightened Living*, Reprint edn. London:
Harper One.

Freeman, R. (2015) *The Yoga Matrix: The Body as a Gateway to Freedom* [audiobook]. Boulder, CO: Sounds
True.

Fronsdale, G. (2016) *The Buddha before Buddhism: Wisdom from the Early Teachings*. Boulder, CO: Shambhala Publications.

Füstös, J., Gramann, K., Herbert, B.M. and Pollatos, O. (2013) 'On the embodiment of emotion regulation:
Interoceptive awareness facilitates reappraisal.' *Social Cognitive and Affective Neuroscience 8*(8), 911–917.
Available at: https://pubmed.ncbi.nlm.nih.gov/22933520

Gardiner, M. (2013) 'The window in: Following the breath – by Donna Farhi.' Manaia Yoga &
Wellbeing, 22 September. Available at: https://manaiawellbeing.co.nz/the-window-in-following-
the-breath-by-donna-farhi

Gruol, D. (2017) 'Advances in neuroimmunology.' *Brain Sciences 7*(10), 124. Available at: https://pubmed.
ncbi.nlm.nih.gov/28953216

Haines, S. (2021) *Touch Is Really Strange*. London and Philadelphia, PA: Singing Dragon.

Herbert, B.M., Pollatos, O. and Klusmann, V. (2021) 'Interoception and health, psychological and physiological mechanisms.' *European Journal of Health Psychology 27*, 4. Available at: https://econtent.
hogrefe.com/doi/full/10.1027/2512-8442/a000064

Herrero, J., Khuvis, S., Yeagle, E., Cerf, M. and Mehta, A.D. (2018) 'Higher neural functions and behavior.'
Journal of Neurophysiology 119, 145–159. Available at: https://journals.physiology.org/doi/pdf/10.1152/
jn.00551.2017

Inzlicht, M., Werner, K.M., Briskin, J.L. and Roberts, B.W. (2021) 'Integrating models of self-regulation.'
Annual Review of Psychology 72, 319–345. Available at: https://pubmed.ncbi.nlm.nih.gov/33017559

Iyengar, B.K.S. (2013) *Light on Pranayama*. London: HarperCollins.

Kalyani, B.G., Venkatasubramanian, G., Arasappa, R., Rao, N.P., *et al.* (2011) 'Neurohemodynamic correlates
of "OM" chanting: A pilot functional magnetic resonance imaging study.' *International Journal of Yoga
4*(1), 3–6. Available at: https://pubmed.ncbi.nlm.nih.gov/21654968

Kang, S.S., Sponheim, S.R. and Lim, K.O. (2021) 'Interoception underlies therapeutic effects of mindfulness meditation for posttraumatic stress disorder: A randomized clinical trial.' *Biological Psychiatry.
Cognitive Neuroscience and Neuroimaging S2451-9022*(21), 00280-9. Available at: https://pubmed.ncbi.
nlm.nih.gov/34688923

Keefe, F.J., Wilkins, R.H. and Cook, W.A. (1984) 'Direct observation of pain behavior in low back pain
patients during physical examination.' *Pain 20*(1), 59–68. Available at: https://pubmed.ncbi.nlm.nih.
gov/6238269

Khalsa, S.S. and Lapidus, R.C. (2016) 'Can interoception improve the pragmatic search for biomarkers in
psychiatry?' *Frontiers in Psychiatry 7*, 121. Available at: https://pubmed.ncbi.nlm.nih.gov/27504098

Kobayashi, J. (2021) 'Lifestyle-mediated nitric oxide boost to prevent SARS-CoV-2 infection: A perspective.'
Nitric Oxide 115, 55–61. Available at: https://pubmed.ncbi.nlm.nih.gov/34364972

Koeppen, B.M. and Stanton, B.A. (2018) 'Organization of Motor Function.' In B.M. Koeppen and B.A.
Stanton, *Berne & Levy Physiology*, 7th edn (Chapter 9). Elsevier. Available at: www.sciencedirect.com/
topics/neuroscience/primary-motor-cortex

Kumar, N. and Singh, U. (2021) 'Yoga for improving mood and cognitive functions – A brief review.'
Yoga Mīmāṃsā 53(1), 39–45. Available at: www.researchgate.net/publication/353411228_
Yoga_for_improving_mood_and_cognitive_functions_-A_brief_review

Kyle, J. (2021) Notions of the Self [online course]. Embodied Philosophy.

Li, P., Janczewski, W.A., Yackle, K., Kam, K., *et al.* (2016) 'The peptidergic control circuit for sighing.' *Nature* 530(7590), 293–297. Available at: https://pubmed.ncbi.nlm.nih.gov/26855425

Lipton, B. (2016) *The Biology of Belief: Unleashing the Power of Consciousness, Matter and Miracles*, 10th Anniversary edn. London: Hay House UK.

Little, T. and Little, S. (no date) SATYA (Sensory Awareness Training for Yoga Attunement). [course training manual]. Accessed 2019.

Mallinson, J. and Singleton, M. (2017) *The Roots of Yoga*. London: Penguin.

McKeown, P. (2015) *The Oxygen Advantage: Simple, Scientifically Proven Breathing Techniques to Help You Become Healthier, Slimmer, Faster, and Fitter*. New York: William Morrow & Company.

Mohan, A. (2010) *Krishnamacharya: His Life and Teachings*. Boulder, CO: Shambhala Publications.

Morimoto, K. and Nakajima, K. (2019) 'Role of the immune system in the development of the central nervous system.' *Frontiers in Neuroscience 13*, 916. Available at: https://pubmed.ncbi.nlm.nih.gov/31551681

Niazi, I.K., Navid, M.S., Bartley, J., Shepherd, D., *et al.* (2022) 'EEG signatures change during unilateral Yogi nasal breathing.' *Scientific reports 12*(1), 520. Available at: https://pubmed.ncbi.nlm.nih.gov/35017606

Nutma, E., Willison, H., Martino, G. and Amor, S. (2019) 'Neuroimmunology – The past, present and future.' *Clinical and Experimental Immunology 197*(3), 278–293. Available at: https://pubmed.ncbi.nlm.nih.gov/30768789

Odier, D. (2005) *Yoga Spandakarika: The Sacred Texts at the Origins of Tantra*. Rochester, VT: Inner Traditions.

Peterson, M. (2012) *Move Without Pain*. New York: Sterling.

Porges, S.W. (2007) 'The polyvagal perspective.' *Biological Psychology 74*(2), 116–143. Available at: https://pubmed.ncbi.nlm.nih.gov/17049418

Quadt, L., Critchley, H.D. and Garfinkel, S.N. (2018) 'The neurobiology of interoception in health and disease.' *Annals of the New York Academy of Sciences 1428*(1), 112–128. Available at: https://pubmed.ncbi.nlm.nih.gov/29974959

Rhyner, H.H. (2017) *Llewellyn's Complete Book of Ayurveda: A Comprehensive Resource for the Understanding and Practice of Traditional Indian Medicine*. Woodbury, MN: Llewellyn.

Rivest-Gadbois, E. and Boudrias, M.-H. (2019) 'What are the known effects of yoga on the brain in relation to motor performances, body awareness and pain? A narrative review.' *Complementary Therapies in Medicine 44*, 129–142. Available at: https://pubmed.ncbi.nlm.nih.gov/31126545

Rosenow, M. and Munk, N. (2021) 'Massage for combat injuries in veteran with undisclosed PTSD: A retrospective case report.' *International Journal of Therapeutic Massage & Bodywork 14*(1), 4–11. Available at: https://pubmed.ncbi.nlm.nih.gov/33654501

Rothenberg, R. (2019) *Restoring Prana: A Therapeutic Guide to Pranayama and Healing Through the Breath for Yoga Therapists, Yoga Teachers and Healthcare Practitioners*. London and Philadelphia, PA: Singing Dragon.

Sahdra, B.K., MacLean, K.A., Ferrer, E., Shaver, P.R., *et al.* (2011) 'Enhanced response inhibition during intensive meditation training predicts improvements in self-reported adaptive socioemotional functioning.' *Emotion 11*(2), 299–312. Available at: https://pubmed.ncbi.nlm.nih.gov/21500899

Schleip, R. (2014) 'Interoception: Some suggestions for manual and movement therapies.' *Terra Rosa E-magazine 15*. Available at: https://issuu.com/terrarosa/docs/terra_rosa_e-mag_issue_15

Schleip, R. with Bayer, J. (2021) *Fascial Fitness: Practical Exercises to Stay Flexible, Active and Pain Free in Just 20 Minutes a Week*, 2nd edn. Chichester: Lotus Publishing.

Schleip, R. and Jäger, H. (2012) 'Interoception: A New Correlate for Intricate Connections between Fascial Receptors, Emotion, and Self Recognition.' In R. Schleip, T.W. Findley, L. Chaitow and P.A. Huijing (eds) *Fascia: The Tensional Network of the Human Body* (Chapter 2.3). Edinburgh: Churchill Livingstone. Available at: www.sciencedirect.com/science/article/pii/B9780702034251000477

Sedlmeier, P. and Srinivas, K. (2016) 'How do theories of cognition and consciousness in ancient Indian thought systems relate to current western theorizing and research?' *Frontiers in Psychology 7*, 343. Available at: www.ncbi.nlm.nih.gov/pmc/articles/PMC4791389

Sen-Gupta, O. (2012) *Vayu's Gate – Yoga and the Ten Vital Winds*. Vijnana Books.

Shields, G.S., Skwara, A.C., King, B.G., Zanesco, A.P., Dhabhar, F.S. and Saron, C.D. (2020) 'Deconstructing the effects of concentration meditation practice on interference control: The roles of controlled attention and inflammatory activity.' *Brain, Behavior, and Immunity 89*, 256–267. Available at: https://pubmed.ncbi.nlm.nih.gov/32640286

Simpson, D. (2018) 'Yogic breathing: *Pranayama*.' Available at: www.danielsimpson.info/archive/yoga-breathing-pranayama-sahapedia

Simpson, D. (2021) *The Truth of Yoga: A Comprehensive Guide to Yoga's History, Texts, Philosophy, and Practices*. New York: North Point Press.

Sinha, A.N., Deepak, D. and Gusain, V.S. (2013) 'Assessment of the Effects of Pranayama/Alternate Nostril Breathing on the Parasympathetic Nervous System in Young Adults.' *Journal of Clinical & Diagnostic Research* 75(5), 821–823. Available at: https://www.ncbi.nlm.nih.gov/pmc/articles/PMC3681046

Somatic Movement Center (2019) 'What is pandiculation, and why doesn't stretching work?' Available at: https://somaticmovementcenter.com/wp-content/uploads/2018/10/Pandiculation-and-Stretching.pdf

Sri Swami Satchidananda (2012) *Yoga Sutras of Patanjali*, Revised edn. Integral Yoga Publications.

Streeter, C.C., Whitfield, T.H., Owen, L., Rein, T., *et al.* (2010) 'Effects of yoga versus walking on mood, anxiety, and brain GABA levels: A randomized controlled MRS study.' *Journal of Alternative and Complementary Medicine* 16(11), 1145–1152. Available at: www.ncbi.nlm.nih.gov/pmc/articles/PMC3111147

Sumner, G. and Haines, S. (2010) *Cranial Intelligence – A Practical Guide to Biodynamic Craniosacral Therapy*. London and Philadelphia, PA: Singing Dragon.

"Sunflower", T. (2020). 'The Homunculus Yoga Project.' *Embodied Philosophy*. Accessed 31/05/2022 at: http://embodied.bestdevserver.com/yoga/the-homunculus-yoga-project

Susruta, S. and Bhishagratna, K.L. (2020) *An English Translation of the Sushruta Samhita, Based on Original Sanskrit Text, Vol. 1 of 3: Sutrasthanam*. London: Forgotten Books.

Swami Muktibodhananda (1998) *Hatha Yoga Pradipika*, 4th reprinted edn. India: Bihar School of Yoga.

Swami Niranjanananda Saraswati (2009) *Prana and Pranayama*. India: Yoga Publications Trust.

Taylor, J., McLean, L., Korner, A., Stratton, E. and Glozier, N. (2020) 'Mindfulness and yoga for psychological trauma: Systematic review and meta-analysis.' *Journal of Trauma & Dissociation* 21(5), 536–573. Available at: https://pubmed.ncbi.nlm.nih.gov/32453668

The Sutra Project (no date). *What is The Sutra Project?* The Sutra Project. Accessed 31/05/2022 at: https://www.thesutraproject.com

Turci, R. (2020) 'The Yoga of the *Bhagavad Gita*: Spirituality, Meditation, and the Rise of a New Scientific Paradigm.' In S. Telles and R.K. Gupta (eds) *Handbook of Research on Evidence-Based Perspectives on the Psychophysiology of Yoga and Its Applications*. Medical Information Science Reference.

Weitzberg, E. and Lundberg, J.O.N. (2002) 'Humming greatly increases nasal nitric oxide.' *American Journal of Respiratory and Critical Care Medicine* 166(2), 144–145. Available at: https://pubmed.ncbi.nlm.nih.gov/12119224

Yates, B.J., Billig, I., Cotter, L.A., Mori, R.L. and Card, J.P. (2002) 'Role of the vestibular system in regulating respiratory muscle activity during movement.' *Clinical and Experimental Pharmacology and Physiology* 29(1–2), 112–117.

PART 6

GOOD VIBRATIONS

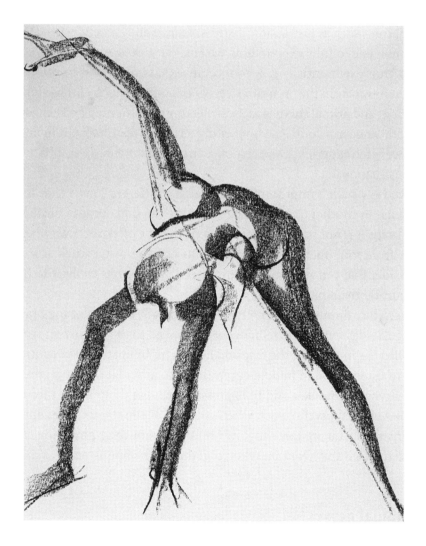

A dive into the mouth and throat as entry points for our health, both in terms of the breath and our immunity; also how sound and mantra can support health through vibration and support of tissues in the throat and mouth territory – as our first defence and gateway to the vitality of the breath.

We both take in (food, drink, air, even smoke) and expel (air, speech, spit, vomit) through the mouth and throat, and as such busy junctions, they need continual maintenance. Beyond these more perfunctory parts, there is the resonance of words, language, song and chant – all enabled through our breath; this is a truly expressive part of our whole system and: 'Calm is restored by the controlled exhale or retention of the breath.'[1]

This refers to the feedback loop between mental states and disturbed breathing patterns, linked by signs of unease in the autonomic nervous system via symptoms such as distraction, distress, despair and anxiety, especially when we are not able to fully express how we feel, our needs, our boundaries, fears or pain.[2] It is experientially easy to recognise that breath and emotions are in constant interplay in the orchestration of our system. Much of these responses are ancient and primal survival tactics, meeting conditioning and expectations born of the modern world – an interesting recipe for dissonance at many times, which we often experience as a response that might not be appropriate for the current situation.

If we view such 'symptomology' through a different lens – that it would make sense in another circumstance – then we can find our way through with more clarity. It is not particularly surprising that we often feel overwhelm and anxiety from too much electronic stimulus or from being stuck at a desk, if we consider that our psycho-emoto-physiological beings evolved to live and move constantly in nature.

When the calming vagus emerged in mammals, the area of the brainstem that regulated the newer myelinated vagus linked to the brainstem areas that controlled the muscles of the face and head. This brainstem area controls our ability to listen through middle ear muscles, to articulate through the laryngeal-pharyngeal muscles, and to express emotion and intention through the face: 'As a clinical psychologist, when you look at the clients' faces and listen to their voices, you are inferring information about their physiological state because the face and heart are wired together in the brainstem.'[3]

The cranial nerves

This all occurs with constant orchestration with the cranial nerves, including the 10th, the vagus (page 158), relaying sensory information around the face and head to the whole body and vice versa, up from the organ body (Figure 2a).

---

1   Bryant (2009, *Yoga Sutra* 1.34).
2   Yang *et al.* (2020).
3   Porges (2017).

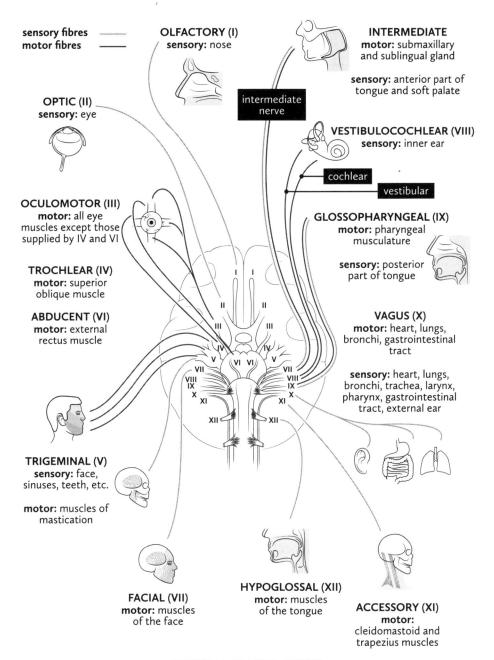

sensory fibres ———
motor fibres ———

OLFACTORY (I)
sensory: nose

INTERMEDIATE
motor: submaxillary
and sublingual gland

sensory: anterior part of
tongue and soft palate

intermediate
nerve

OPTIC (II)
sensory: eye

VESTIBULOCOCHLEAR (VIII)
sensory: inner ear

cochlear
vestibular

OCULOMOTOR (III)
motor: all eye
muscles except those
supplied by IV and VI

GLOSSOPHARYNGEAL (IX)
motor: pharyngeal
musculature

sensory: posterior
part of tongue

TROCHLEAR (IV)
motor: superior
oblique muscle

ABDUCENT (VI)
motor: external
rectus muscle

VAGUS (X)
motor: heart, lungs,
bronchi, gastrointestinal
tract

sensory: heart, lungs,
bronchi, trachea, larynx,
pharynx, gastrointestinal
tract, external ear

TRIGEMINAL (V)
sensory: face,
sinuses, teeth, etc.

motor: muscles of
mastication

FACIAL (VII)
motor: muscles
of the face

HYPOGLOSSAL (XII)
motor: muscles
of the tongue

ACCESSORY (XI)
motor:
cleidomastoid and
trapezius muscles

FIGURE 6A. CRANIAL NERVES

Cranial nerves – showing how we sense and relate; social engagement, for example through
the facial muscles and expression, and gut feelings up from the vagus nerve, gut to brain.

There are 12 cranial nerves (Figure 6a):

I. Olfactory, sensory: nose
II. Optic, sensory: eye
III. Oculomotor, motor: eye muscles
IV. Trochlear, motor: superior oblique muscle
V. Trigeminal, sensory: face, sinuses, teeth, etc.; motor: masticulating muscles
VI. Abducent, motor: external rectus muscle
VII. Facial, motor: muscles of the face
VIII. Vestibulocochlear, sensory: inner ear
IX. Glossopharyngeal, motor: pharyngeal musculature; sensory: posterior part of tongue, tonsil, pharynx
X. Vagus, motor: heart, lungs, bronchi, gastrointestinal tract; sensory: heart, lungs, bronchi, trachea, larynx, pharynx, gastrointestinal tract, external ear
XI. Accessory, motor: sternocleidomastoid and trapezius muscles
XII. Hypoglossal, motor: tongue muscles

Many of these cranial nerves affect how we move our face and sense in through the nose, ears and mouth. This shows the whole orchestration of how our head receives sensory input and relates out in terms of our response and our expression. The breath completely interplays these effects down into the brainstem, the respiratory pacemaker, and other neuronal complexes in the brain.

The respiratory pacemaker

The regulatory processes of the breath are governed in that same area, the brainstem. It is only fairly recently that the respiratory pacemaker – which keeps the regulation – was recognised as a region of neurons within the older part of the brain: 'The respiratory pacemaker has, in some respects, a tougher job than its counterpart in the heart. Unlike the heart's one-dimensional, slow-to-fast continuum, there are many distinct types of breaths: regular, excited, sighing, yawning, gasping, sleeping, laughing, sobbing.'[4]

This highlights the multifactorial and expressive part of us that responds to input from unconscious or conscious associations in our world or our sensory experience.

---

4 Mark Krasnow, quoted in Goldman (2017).

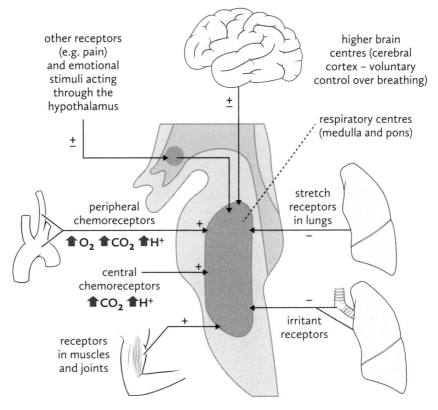

other receptors
(e.g. pain)
and emotional
stimuli acting
through the
hypothalamus

higher brain
centres (cerebral
cortex – voluntary
control over breathing)

respiratory centres
(medulla and pons)

peripheral
chemoreceptors

$\uparrow O_2$ $\uparrow CO_2$ $\uparrow H^+$

stretch
receptors
in lungs

central
chemoreceptors

$\uparrow CO_2$ $\uparrow H^+$

irritant
receptors

receptors
in muscles
and joints

FIGURE 6B. RESPIRATORY PACEMAKER

Breath, emotion and cognition

There is a distinct connection between breath, emotion and cognition – where we make sense of the world in our front brain – in relation to the emotional and more instinctive reactions of the older part of the brain. The preBötC (the pre-Bötzinger complex) is a region of the more primal (reptilian) brain that is the breathing control centre.

The preBötC coordinates all phases of the breathing cycle, breathing with orofacial (face in relation to the mouth) behaviours, and strongly influences, and is influenced by, emotion and cognition.[5] This draws attention to how our breath and facial communication, our expressions, are in constant interplay with our social engagement, how we relate to the world. Coming back to central vagal tone, where we are able to fully socially engage and our breath can

5   Del Negro, Funk and Feldman (2018).

drop down into these more easy, regular and more coherent patterns – we feel safety and connection with others.

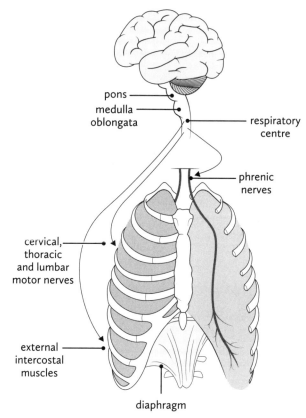

pons
medulla oblongata
respiratory centre
phrenic nerves
cervical, thoracic and lumbar motor nerves
external intercostal muscles
diaphragm

FIGURE 6C. RESPIRATORY CENTRE

The mouth

This brings us down into the territory of much of our expression, the mouth. This gateway area is full of lymphatic tissue and lymphoid organs – adenoid tonsil, two tubal tonsils, two palatine tonsils, lingual tonsils – anything that takes away what enters the body that is potentially harmful. This boundary is protected and lubricated by nasal breathing, where mouth breathing and postural habits – dropping the head forwards of the shoulders – dries out the tissues and brings in more potentially damaging particulates. Within the lymphoid organs, M cells (microfold cells, epithelial cells that act as antigen delivery in the intestine, lung and nasopharynx) then alert the underlying B cells and T cells (see Part 1); tonsils also make T cells directly, while others come from the lymphatic system. We also have here sIgA cells and the potential for acquired immunity. This whole protective area is our gateway to the lungs and gut, protecting the mucosa, the epithelial tissues of the interior of the lungs.

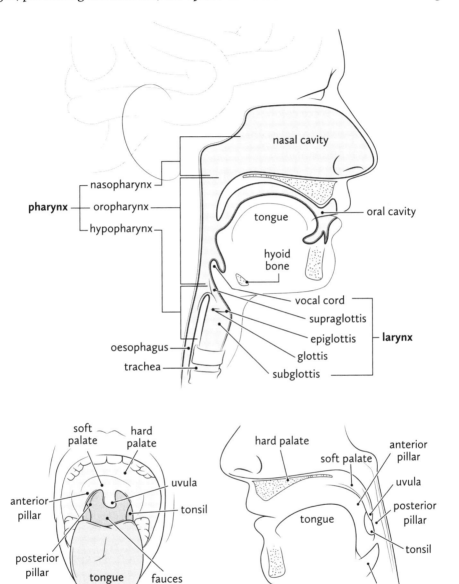

FIGURE 6D. MOUTH AND THROAT ANATOMY

The larynx (voice box)

The larynx is situated behind the mouth, nasal cavity and the trachea, and above where the tubes to the stomach and lungs branch off. The larynx is the voice box: it is involved in breathing, producing sound and protecting the trachea against food aspiration into the lungs. Human beings evolved to have a larger voice box for language, but we have become less efficient at stopping food going down the wrong way – we are the only animals that can choke to death![6]

The larynx is innervated by branches of the vagus nerve on each side, so pitch and tone of voice, our ability to express ourselves clearly, relies on the tones we can come to in the vagus nerve – as soon as we go into sympathetic tone, the pitch of the voice can be affected by the breath being higher and faster (or very low if we need to be stealthy). The larynx houses the vocal folds and manipulates pitch and volume.

Situated level with the C3–C6 vertebrae, the larynx can also be affected by tension in the neck and spine.

The respiratory muscles move the vocal cords apart for breathing and the phonatory muscles move the vocal cords together for the voice: this is another polarity interplaying within the body.

The pharynx

Sitting above and held by the larynx is the pharynx. This makes up a large part of the structure of the back of the neck, the part that we can feel lengthening when we consciously make space up into the back of the skull. Behind the mouth and the nasal cavity and above the oesophagus, the pharynx is part of the digestive system and the conducting zone – which regulates communication – of the respiratory system. It encompasses:

- The hyoid muscles, which open the oesophagus for swallowing.
- The temporal muscles connected to the jaw for chewing. Any tension coming up from the diaphragm or even below can be held in this area, playing into tension pulling down into the base of the skull.

The pharynx is the seat of *jalandhara bandha*, so when we come into that lifting of the breastbone to draw the chin in, we are opening up the pharynx as a protective space to hold the softness and the energy of growth within.

---

6   Lieberman (2014).

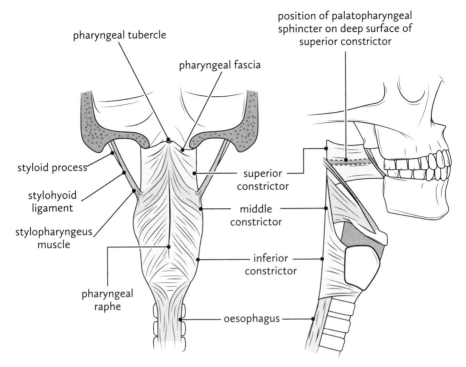

FIGURE 6E. PHARYNGEAL RAPHE

THE RIB CAGE

The rib cage is perhaps the least regarded body structure. Its function is most frequently described as that of being a protective shield of the lungs and heart. Beyond that, very little attention is paid to it. Its importance as a generator of kinetic patterning is underrated or ignored in most movement training. We must focus on this unique form and reevaluate our relationship with it.

First, consider how a dog or a horse pull and lead from their chest. The power of the animal is expressed in a strength which finds its focus in a mid-point between the two front limbs. When you see an animal run, you can often fail to see how the rib cage conducts and releases tension through the limbs. If we take a closer look, we can see that the ribs operate as a living Jack-in-the-box or even a "Slinky". They conduct pressure from the body centre to the periphery and mediate the relationship between the skull and the pelvis, allowing them to counterbalance each other.

In the evolutionary narrative of vertebrates, the ribs precede the development of the more specialised limbs. The lateral movement of the vertebral limb is THE primary movement pattern and in a sense all other kinetic patterns are variations of this one theme. The ribs support and initiate the tubular shape of the vertebral body and combine strength with suppleness. So our movement training must allow our ribs to be more articulate. When the ribs underachieve the consequences are multiple. The spine will have reduced motility in the thoracic region, the lungs and heart can be compressed, the lower back and neck may suffer from over use and the consequent uneven weight distribution will affect the limbs. And let's not forget the emotional cost – a pervading sense of alienation and disconnection is symptomatic of a kinetically compromised rib cage.

Laurie Booth[7]

The eight diaphragms

As well as the thoracic and pelvic diaphragms, we have in total eight diaphragms in the body, stacking up from the bottom, where we calibrate in our most easeful curves up from the ground. We can see how they lift above each other, and the quality of their 'bounciness', as opposed to rigidity, can really affect how we stand up from the ground, the quality of our breath, how we adapt with fluidity. This can affect our immune capacity, how we can come down from inflammation or being on constant alert.

- The plantar fascia, at the instep, is the starting point, how we lift up from the ground, our base of being.
- The tibiotalar diaphragm is much smaller, in the ankle, affecting how we move and articulate, stepping up and moving out from the feet.
- The popliteal diaphragm, at the knees, is a place of support and bearing weight. The faster we go, the more we need the space held there.
- The pelvic diaphragm supports the whole of the spine, viscera and upper body, responding emotionally in terms of how we can also bring a responsive *mula bandha*.
- The respiratory diaphragm (page 45) divides the thoracic and abdominal cavities.
- The vocal cord diaphragm – the quality of voice – how we express

---

7   Laurie Booth, choreographer, gyrotonic instructor and movement investigator, quote requested: www.lauriebooth.com

ourselves – can be dependent on how we stack ourselves up from the ground.

- The palatine diaphragm, at the palate, where we place the tip of our tongue in *kechari mudra*, meeting nerve endings to the brain.
- The tentorium cerebelli in the skull, holding the brain.

How we feel the ease of nasal breathing, softness up into the eyes and back down into our expression around the throat is dependent on the fluidity moving upwards between our diaphragms.

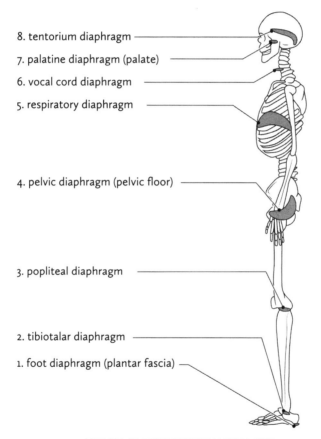

8. tentorium diaphragm

7. palatine diaphragm (palate)

6. vocal cord diaphragm

5. respiratory diaphragm

4. pelvic diaphragm (pelvic floor)

3. popliteal diaphragm

2. tibiotalar diaphragm

1. foot diaphragm (plantar fascia)

FIGURE 6F. THE EIGHT DIAPHRAGMS

Key horizontal sheaths at different levels from the ground – support from the base up, that is, need pliable insteps for ease further up.

Influence each other and meet other fascial sheaths and lines as a continuum – respond to stress, trauma, etc. by locking upwards ready for self-protecting movements and tightness as protection.

Affected by postural divergence from centre where compensation of force transmission creates stress from within.

Source: With thanks to Tias Little

The throat
Jalandhara bandha

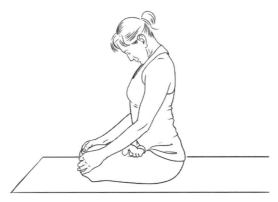

FIGURE 6G. *JALANDHARA BANDHA*

Breaking it down, *jal* means 'throat', *dharan*, 'stream', and *bandha* is 'lock'. We should think of *jalandhara bandha* as an energetic gathering rather than a lock, which could feel tight or hard. The more modern sensibility, a sensitive 'gathering' rather than 'locking' here, more readily embodies *ahimsa* (non-violence). It can also be translated as 'upwards-pulling net', referring to drawing *prana* into the torso, the net bringing in water analogy that is often used around the throat, also referring to *jala*, meaning 'water'. The throat is compared to a river, containing the flow of *prana* – breath and food – coming in through the throat. It is where the back of the throat draws into the safety of its cave and a nourishing compression in *jalandhara bandha*.

Tucking the jawbone down against the sternum lifts the heart. When we move into *jalandhara bandha* it is the sternocleidomastoid that lifts the breastbone towards the chin to facilitate the lifting of the heart, the softening of the head, not simply a dropping of the chin. We may do this in the fuller way, or we might find a lighter, more naturally occurring *jalandhara bandha* in *viparita karani* (upside-down pose; page 304) or supported *setu bandhasana* (bridge pose).

When we squeeze the area around the thyroid (which regulates energy and metabolism) and throat, parathyroid (which regulates calcium levels) and lymph ducts, this supports whole body and digestive, immunity and metabolic processes.

This is the area where many physical and subtle aspects converge – not just sensory channels to the mouth and ears, but also passageways for the respiratory, digestive, vocal and lymphatic systems. Particularly where the neck is open, there is an open channel, releasing a major *granthi* (knot) where the head gets locked into thinking. Bringing consciousness into this area can be incredibly important for reconnecting where there is dissociation from the body, from the gut, below: according to the *Hatha Yoga Pradipika* 'It stops the opening (hole) of the group of *Nadis*, through which the juice from the sky [from the *soma* or *chandra* in the brain] falls down. It is, therefore, called the *jalandhara bandha* – the destroyer of a host of diseases of the throat.'[8]

The territory of *jalandhara bandha* contains branches of the vagus nerve. It affects our ability to self-soothe, to be able to come into softening of the front brain in towards the heart, how we take in experience and move through, how we let go what doesn't serve us or our health.

Vishuddha, the fifth chakra

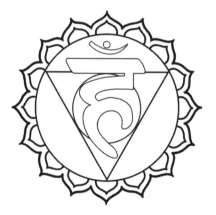

FIGURE 6H. *VISHUDDHA*, THE FIFTH *CHAKRA*

Vishuddha chakra, at the throat is at a pivotal point between skull and spine – connecting to both anterior and posterior aspects of the neck is important to explore when we consider the dynamics of skull-sacrum polarity.
If we consider the throat as gateway to the body for what comes in through both the mouth and nose, it becomes clear that purifying this area – whether through the *niyama* (internal discipline, first in Patanjali's eight-limbed yoga path) of *sauca* (cleanliness), meditation or movement through *vishuddha*, or *pranayama* – has profound effect on the whole body-mind.

Jalandhara bandha is also associated with the expression and purification of the fifth *chakra*, *vishuddha*, which takes in the neck and throat area, including the jaw, mouth, tongue and larynx. *Visha* means 'impurity' or 'poison', and *suddhi* 'to purify', so *vishuddha* (or *vishuddhi*) clears space around us, signified by its element, ether or space. Sound, expression and language are fostered here. Health can be supported by learning authentic expression from the heart below: if we're able to express ourselves fully, then good health can follow.

---

8   Swami Muktibodhananda (1998).

This viewpoint is bringing in the often super-imposed Jungian theory of the 1930s[9], which adds psychological inferences to the *chakras* (so, importantly, not part of yogic theory). More traditionally, *chakras* would have been associated much more with their elements, the focuses for meditation.

Deficiency around *vishuddha* can manifest, (again in modern *chakra* theory) as difficulty communicating or speaking one's mind, even anxiety around self-expression, a sense of feeling stuck here. Shame, the 'demon of the solar plexus *chakra*', can prevent expression of thoughts or beliefs, which can be felt physiologically as tightness and constriction in the diaphragm leading up to the throat area, collapse in the chest, meaning less movement of *prana* up into the throat, physically and somato-emotionally.

'Too much' at the fifth *chakra* can be experienced as overwhelm – this could come from overly fierce *uddiyana bandha*, excessive ego or an overflow upwards – and can result in excessive talking. This could be talking too fast as a defence mechanism, through anxiety, or always having to speak and fill silence with an inability to ground or earth; where there is overabundance of nervous energy.

Shatkarmas (*satkarmas* or *shatkriyas*)

The *shatkarmas* are the six (or more) purifications outlined in the *Hatha Yoga Pradipika* to prepare the body for *moksha* (liberation). An integral part of Hatha yoga, many of these are focused around the mouth and throat, the nasal passages, the sinuses, down into the gut, all of the places where toxins can come into the body. We can see from the wide spaces in the sinuses needed for full nasal breathing (Figure 6i) that there is a large surface area (epithelium, page 206) to keep healthy.

The *shatkarmas* can be seen as part of the *niyama* of *sauca*, cleanliness, as they help eliminate accumulated toxins (*ama*), which can also be the build-up of anything in the body that doesn't get fully processed or resolved, including experience. So these practices help to cleanse those places in contact with the outer world (air, food matter or waste). They support the flow of *prana* into the organs, build up resistance to diseases for immunity, and detoxify:

- *Jala neti* uses saline solution to cleanse the sinuses. This can be a useful practice to support the nasal biome. *Sutraneti*, using a cloth to

---

9   Jung (1999).

cleanse, is a less common, more advanced practice. Both should be done with instruction.

- *Kapalabathi* cleans the sinuses, using forced exhalation through the nose.
- *Trataka* cleans the eyes by focusing on one steady gaze until the eyes water.
- *Basti* (enema).
- *Dhauti* (swallowing cloth), a much less practised *kriya*.
- *Nauli* (stomach churning) to clear and tone, bringing lymphatic movement into the gastrointestinal (GI) tract. This can be done in a softer way, rotating the tailbone (page 128).

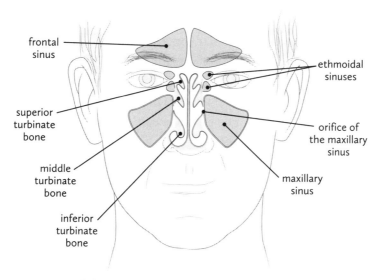

FIGURE 61. NASAL BREATHING PHYSIOLOGY

Health of the linings (epithelium, page 206) is an important barrier function against pathogens. Nasal inflammatory conditions such as allergic rhinitis have shown significant symptom reduction with supplementation of probiotics, where the Lactobacillus species *L. acidophilus*, *L. paracasei* and *L. rhamnosus* were supplemented, especially alongside vitamin D (crucial for immune function).[10,11,12]

Nasal passages have shown particularly high levels of ACE2 (page 107), which is a cellular entry receptor for SARS-CoV and SARS-CoV-2 to enter

---

10 Ishida *et al.* (2005).
11 Lin *et al.* (2014).
12 Jerzynska *et al.* (2016).

the bloodstream. The binding affinity of ACE2 (and the S protein produced alongside) was found to be a major determinant of SARS-CoV replication rate and disease severity.[13,14] Furthermore, 'nasal epithelial cells, including two previously described clusters of goblet cells and one cluster of ciliated cells, show the highest expression (of ACE2 expression) among all investigated cells in the respiratory tree'.[15]

Nasal health, including cleansing methods, nasal breathing and steam, can be an important part in the larger picture of immune and respiratory self-care.

Oral health

The oral microbiome, the beneficial bacteria in the oral cavity, cannot be minimised (page 168) – it is linked to heart disease, inflammatory conditions and neurological diseases such as Alzheimer's: 'The oral cavity has the second largest and diverse microbiota after the gut harboring over 700 species of bacteria...crucial to health as it can cause both oral and systemic diseases.'[16]

Many of the bacteria that come into the mouth will be pathogenic. When our oral microbiome is in balance, it will keep these toxins at bay, but if it is compromised, it can contribute to any of the above disease states and more.

Gargling

Gargling as a practice within Ayurveda and many other traditional cultures is an important cleansing remedy that can be effective as part of immune defence support: 'Simple water gargling was effective to prevent URTIs among healthy people. Even when a URTI (upper respiratory tract infection) occurred, water gargling tended to attenuate bronchial symptoms.'[17]

Gargling with ½ teaspoon of salt in a glass of warm or hot water, to enervate the mucosal linings:

- Causes the liquid in your mouth to bubble and creates a vibration in your throat. This helps the liquid cover various parts of your throat and all or most of the oral mucosa.
- Draws pathogens from the tissues of the mouth and throat. Gargling

---

13   Hoffmann *et al.* (2020).
14   Matsuyama *et al.* (2010).
15   Sungnak *et al.* (2020).
16   Deo and Deshmukh (2019).
17   Satomura *et al.* (2005).

with warm salt water three times a day may decrease the risk of developing an upper respiratory tract infection by 40 per cent.[18]
- Breaks up mucus in throat, respiratory tract and nasal cavity.
- Relieves inflammation caused by cold, flu, sinus infections and tonsillitis.[19]
- Promotes vagal tone through vibration, which activates the vagus nerve.

Gandusha (oil pulling)
In Ayurveda, the practice of *gandusha*, oil pulling, is also used to cleanse the oral cavity – balancing *kapha*, the *dosha* that tends towards more mucous stickiness, and *vata*, the windy element that can tend towards sympathetic dominance. This can also help those with more *pitta*, inflammatory, profiles.

A tablespoon of a warming oil such as sesame oil (or other plant oils, for example, coconut) is swirled around the mouth, filling it completely for 3–15 minutes, then released and pulled through the interdental spaces. This can combat bacteria in the mouth, so helping to improve oral hygiene, but can also affect the microbiome. *Gandusha* is believed to be beneficial for migraines, inflammation of the mouth and throat, fatigue, limb and joint pain and rheumatic diseases. In addition, 'Oil pulling therapy showed a reduction in the plaque index, modified gingival scores, and total colony count of aerobic microorganisms in the plaque of adolescents with plaque-induced gingivitis.'[20]

Kavala graha is where a more comfortable amount of fluid is retained with the mouth closed for about three minutes and then gargled.

Chewing
Chewing roots, for example liquorice root, promotes anticavity action, reduces plaque and has an antibacterial effect. Liquorice also supports the mucosal lining of the mouth and throat and can reduce ulceration in the oesophagus and stomach. The consumption of soft, processed food post industrialisation[21] has led to a general decrease in the size of human jaws and a subsequent narrowing of airways and associated respiratory and dental disorders. Chewing whole food can vastly improve oral health, respiration and therefore our immune defences around the mouth.

18 Sakai *et al.* (2009).
19 Emamian, Hassani and Fateh (2013).
20 Asokan, Emmadi and Chamundeswari (2009).
21 Lieberman (2014).

Heart–brain axis and compassion

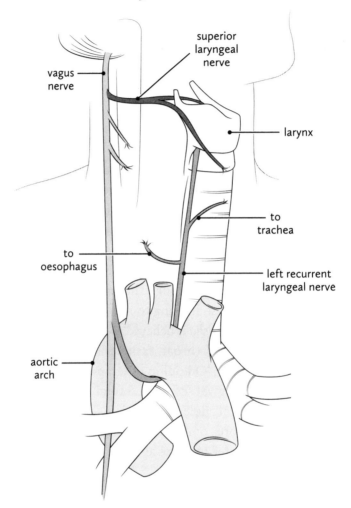

FIGURE 6J. VAGUS TO HEART

The face, mouth and inner ear have a direct link via the vagus to the heart, including the larynx – the heart–brain axis (also see page 217) – and can be put in the context of our ability to show compassion, to come into ventral vagus modes. When we can express from the fifth *chakra*, coming from a place of tolerance, openness, that's when we can express responsively rather than reactively, with space.

The work of the self-compassion researcher Kristin Neff has led to a body of work clearly supporting self-compassion and psychological health via the vagus nerve activity of self-soothing. A paper that cites her work says: 'CFT (compassion-focussed therapy) is grounded in a theoretical assumption that we have three affective systems (threat, drive and soothing) and that enhancing the soothing system helps us manage negative thoughts and emotions through promoting social bonding and positive self-repair behaviours.'[22]

Neff has drawn on traditional spiritual practice to present a psychometric measure of self-compassion, the Self Compassion Scale,[23] which comprises six separate subscales including three positive and three negative: the positive subscales include self-kindness, common humanity and mindfulness, while the negative subscales include self-judgement, isolation and over-identification. Viewing these in relation to the components of mindfulness (pages 69–73) and the hindrances (*kleshas*; page 280) guides us into practice that drops beneath our stories and ruminations, liberating us from the identification that our thoughts and projections are 'us'. Neff says:

> Drawing on the writings of Buddhist scholars, I have defined self-compassion as having 3 main components: (a) self-kindness versus self-judgment, (b) a sense of common humanity versus isolation, and (c) mindfulness versus overidentification [Neff 2003]. These components combine and mutually interact to create a self-compassionate frame of mind. Self-kindness refers to the tendency to be caring and understanding with oneself rather than being harshly critical or judgmental. Instead of taking a cold "stiff-upper-lip" approach in times of suffering, self-kindness offers soothing and comfort to the self. Common humanity involves recognizing that all humans are imperfect, fail and make mistakes. It connects one's own flawed condition to the shared human condition so that greater perspective is taken towards personal shortcomings and difficulties. Mindfulness, the third component of self-compassion, involves being aware of one's present moment experience in a clear and balanced manner so that one neither ignores nor ruminates on disliked aspects of oneself or one's life.[24]

Through kind and compassionate focus, we can positively impact the neural regulation of the heart, also including sounding and chanting (Part 6 Practices), smiling (sincerely!), humming, releasing the jaw, etc., all of which soften and support the architecture of this heart–brain axis region. Compassion has been shown to be whole body, with evidence that the immune modulating slgA antibodies on the gut wall (page 214) can be used as an 'indicator of

---

22 Wilson *et al.* (2019).
23 Neff (2003).
24 Neff (2009).

immunocompetence after a Mindfulness and Self-Compassion-Based Intervention', alongside the reduction in the stress hormone cortisol observed.[25]

In stress responses and compromised rib, diaphragm and lung movement, there may not be enough breath coming up from the heart *chakra* and the voice may struggle to have life. If we feel depleted, our voice may come out in a diminished way (see also the phrenic nerve, page 83). We can experiment with this, sounding before movement, then during and after, to listen in to the changing quality in tone, pitch and steadiness in the voice.

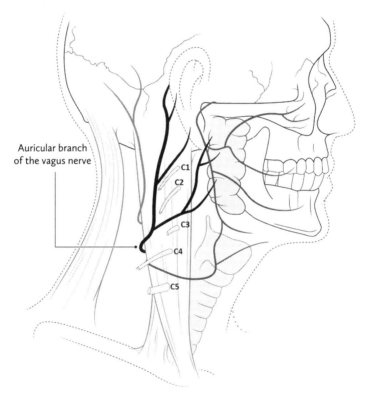

Auricular branch
of the vagus nerve

C1
C2
C3
C4
C5

FIGURE 6K. AURICULAR BRANCH OF THE VAGUS NERVE
Supplies sensory innervation to the skin of the ear canal, tragus and auricle, activated when
closing the tragus (ear flap) for *bhramari pranayama* – also part of the cough reflex.

The auricular nerve is also a part of this axis – it is the only part of the vagus nerve that is peripheral; reaches to the outer part of the body, rather than deeply internal as is the rest of the vagus. This means this is a useful part of the body to access with gentle touch and feel the resonance of sound here as it meets this entry into the interior.

25   Bellosta-Batalla *et al.* (2017).

Research has shown that auricular acupuncture and acupressure elicits vagal tone: 'It is described as a reflexive treatment of physical, emotional, and neurological dysfunctions via specific zones on the ear where these dysfunctions are reflected.'[26]

Listening can be powerfully affecting, depending on the source and quality of the sound. Our ability both to physically listen and to be able to listen in deeply to inner sensations and experience demand calm vagal tones, the space to be calm and still in body and mind. Sounding and *mantra* can provide these vehicles inwards, and voices that bring compassion with them have a deep resonance with soothing and healing (this joins up with the pharyngeal branch of the vagus nerve; see the pharynx, page 332).

So that sense we have, of 'speaking from the heart', is real, where we come from a place of emotional intelligence that can override logic. Neurocardiology research into the heart shows that the heart has its own nervous system that can act independently of the cranial brain: 'Communication between heart and brain actually is a dynamic, ongoing, two-way dialogue, with each organ continuously influencing the other's function.'[27]

Researchers for the HeartMath Institute state that the heart communicates with the brain and the rest of the body in four ways:[28,29,30]

- Neurological communication (nervous system)
- Biochemical communication (hormones)
- Biophysical communication (pulse wave)
- Energetic communication (electromagnetic fields).

When the heart is coherent, it generates a stable, oscillating wave-like pattern, which positively affects the body and brain. Benefits include deeper intuition, clarity and decision-making ability.[31] The heart also produces a hormone, atrial natriuretic factor (ANF), or atrial peptide, which helps regulate the blood vessels, the kidneys, adrenals and parts of the brain: 'Increased atrial peptide inhibits the release of stress hormones, reduces sympathetic outflow and appears to

---

26 Wei *et al.* (2012).
27 HeartMath Institute (2016).
28 Armour (2003).
29 Armour (2008).
30 Forssmann *et al.* (1989).
31 McCraty *et al.* (2009).

interact with the immune system. Even more intriguing, experiments suggest atrial peptide can influence motivation and behaviour.'[32]

Heart–brain communication is being studied in people who are critically ill with COVID-19, with emerging research reporting 'new insights into pathogenic role of the deregulation of the heart–brain axis (HBA)...in leading to severe multiorgan disease syndrome (MODS) in patients with confirmed infection with severe acute respiratory syndrome coronavirus 2 (SARS-CoV-2)'. The researchers concluded that heart–brain axis dysfunction might worsen the outcome of the COVID-19 patients.[33]

Anahata, the fourth chakra

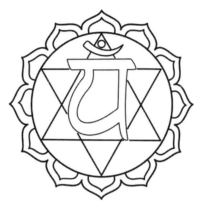

FIGURE 6L. *ANAHATA*, THE FOURTH *CHAKRA*
Both the physical heart and *anahata chakra* (at the heart) sit at the central point between head and body, at the midpoint in the seven *chakra* system. Tias Little[34] makes the connection that the heart intermediates between what is above and below, pointing to the heart's complete inclusivity, synthesising all impulses and energies, and reflected in the sacred geometry of its symbol; *anahata chakra yantra* – focus for meditation.

The heart *chakra* is the support underneath the throat. The translation is 'unstruck', 'unhurt' or 'unbeaten', rooted in the Sanskrit for 'sound produced without touching two parts', the sound of silence, referring to the Vedic 'unstruck sound' of the celestial realm. It can also mean 'pure', 'clean' or 'stainless', but all these nuances come back to the potential of openness, vastness and space, what we are looking to open out into. It is related to air, the wind element, circulation and moving around. When we practise yoga, we are often guided to expand this area, physiologically and emotionally, both drawing in

32   HeartMath Institute (2016).
33   Lionetti *et al.* (2021).
34   Little (2016).

with the intention to nourish and resource ourselves, and moving out to bring compassion in our interactions with others.

The human heart, in addition to its other functions, possesses a heart-brain composed of around 40,000 neurons – these can sense, feel, learn and remember, but, like the gut, this is not cognitive thinking as such. Not only does the heart-brain send messages to the head-brain about how the body feels, there is also research showing that the heart appears to receive and respond to intuitive information,[35] describing it as a 'psychoneuroendocrine and immunoregulatory organ'.[36] One study measured the effects of anger and frustration, showing a significant increase in total mood disturbance and heart rate, with inhibition of immunity as measured by sIgA levels (page 214) when these states were held for five minutes. These effects were reversed with five minutes' focus on care and compassion – both self-induced and prompted by watching a video.[37]

Brainwaves

Meditation has always been believed to have profound effects on the mind and body, but modern scientific tools such as the MRI and EEG have offered more measurable insights, so we can map the effects on brainwaves. Neurons pulsing in the brain produce synchronised electrical impulses, the frequency of which determine our physical and emotional states.

During meditation – with time, presence and attunement – the subject typically starts off with high beta (thinking), and then experiences more alpha, followed by more theta, and finally delta, the deepest level (where we may also go more quickly in *yoga nidra*). After some time, the reverse process takes place, bringing the person back to beta, feeling awake and refreshed, sometimes with new insights.

35 McCraty, Atkinson and Bradley (2004).
36 Lin, Tona and Osto (2018).
37 Rein, Atkinson and McCraty (1995).

Gamma (40 Hz +): Higher frequency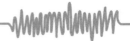

At this most subtle level, we are capable of higher level mental activity, where the brain can draw together disparate thoughts to bring deeper understanding and insight. This frequency is most active when we feel 'universal love' and expanded consciousness.

Beta (14–40 Hz): Awake and attentive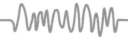

This is the most usual brain state where we are alert and conscious, functioning on the level of complex thought and engaged problem-solving. This can also include the hypervigilance of stress and anxiety. It is an energy-hungry state and the territory of inflammation and lowered immunity when not balanced with other frequencies.

Alpha (7.5–14 Hz): Resting state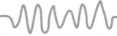

A more peaceful place, where the mind stills and we drop below our *samskaras*. We may feel greater clarity and creative insights, we can concentrate more deeply, be more present. Serotonin and endorphin-rich, this is a feel-good frequency. Desirable for reducing heightened emotional states and adrenal fatigue. Best for deep, embedded learning and mind-body integration.

Theta (4–7.5 Hz): Limbic state

The space between the conscious and the subconscious, *pratayahara*, where the senses are withdrawn. The realm of deeper meditation, where we may be able to access deep-held 'stuff' or trauma. We can be highly creative here, too; there may be powerful visualisations and profound realisations or spiritual experiences.

Delta (0.5–4 Hz): Unconscious

This is where we are beyond physical consciousness, in deep sleep or immersed in transcendental meditation. The frequency here is like a deep, slow drum. External awareness is suspended and we can heal and regenerate; physical and emotional growth is facilitated. Essential for downregulating stress – yoga *nidra* state.

FIGURE 6M. BRAINWAVES

Sound – resonance and social engagement

Sound = vibration = movement of energy. Everything in existence vibrates continuously. Sounding up into and around the heart and throat area, bringing vibration, can be deeply healing on many levels. Allowing and creating conscious sound cultivates the long, smooth exhale of breathing patterns that fully oxygenates cells.

We all have an internal resonance (*nada* – sound, tone, hidden energy) – expressed in our voice and other, less direct, ways – that has to pass through any blockages (*granthis*) in the system when being expressed audibly. By listening closely, this can give clues to their bodily locations and density, which we can loosen to aid the free flow of vibration and *prana* with sound.

Modern-day medicine uses vibrational healing to help speed up the healing rate of bones and tendinitis. Ultrasound therapies and vagus nerve stimulation are used for many mental state issues where there is an inability to self-soothe, including epilepsy and severe depression. The vagus nerve is intimately connected with the inner ear via the laryngeal nerve, so sound can be soothing. We can often inhale a little easier through the nose when creating sound. We sound on the exhale, so it immediately has an impact on the internal gaseous exchange. Sounding also generally extends the exhale, the more parasympathetic tone of the breath. It creates different vibrational frequencies throughout the body (all *koshas*), focusing the mind and enhancing awareness of the diaphragm and abdominal area.

Sounding is allowing sound to come out without the form of words or language. Expressing our simplest vowel sounds, formed before the advent of language (protolanguage) – 'oooh' and 'ahhhh', (Figure 5l) for example – frees us from needing to 'make sense'; we simply emit noise that clears the throat and our channels down to the belly. These sounds require different shapes in the palate – 'ahhhh' opens the river of the throat and frees the jaw. We can feel the vibrations reach different parts of the chest and belly. They can be used throughout *asana* practice to facilitate release and help to free the breath whenever it feels caught up above the diaphragm.

Chanting and sounding can be used with movement, *nyasa* (hand placement) or *mudra* (page 188) to increase their effectiveness. The meaning of what we sound has a direct effect on our physiology:

> The Sanskrit word *kirtana* means "narrating" or "repeating". Although it conveys a hint of praise and celebration, gods are not always involved, or sacred *mantras*... More important than the words intoned is the spirit behind them. Even chanting the phone book might be effective, as long as it is done to lose oneself in love.[38]

---

38 Simpson (2021).

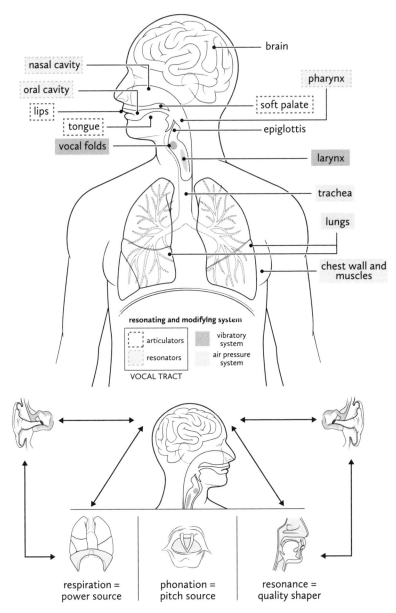

FIGURE 6N. PHYSIOLOGY OF SOUND

Religious and spiritual practices have used sound and movement for thousands of years; the healing and calming effects of prayer, chanting and devotional singing are well documented, and we can feel the resonance of coming into a group. Singing together can engender a sense of collective over the individual, enhancing community cohesion – harmonising and resonating frequency, we find where we come into synchronicity. When we sound together, we synchronise our biorhythms and retrain our breath, heart rate variability (HRV) and collective intention that helps to regulate the heart rate as a collective.

Simply putting on music, dancing, singing and letting go, without attachment to how it looks or sounds, helps to open the fifth *chakra*. Compassion from the heart below also supports our ability to express there. Singing has been linked to increased contentment and joy, as well as our emotional and physical resilience: 'singing can cause changes in neurotransmitters and hormones, including the upregulation of oxytocin, immunoglobulin A, and endorphins, which improves immune function and increases feelings of happiness'.[39]

Free and compassionate communication (from a non-judgemental, tolerant and open-minded viewpoint) supports the health relation with self and others that ripples through the whole psycho-neuro-immune system, including respiratory and immune health.

Mantra

Mantra translates as 'mind protection': *man* from *manas*, meaning 'mind', and *tra*, 'to protect' or as 'something positive', which can potentially transform. Its traditional purpose was to gain mastery over oneself. *Mantra* comes from the heart – not the mind or ego – and helps to connect to what is within. Traditionally made up of sacred, Sanskrit words from the Vedas, *mantras* are repeated with respect and held as something precious. Chanting (*mantra*), along with *pranayama* and *asana*, is considered one of the most powerful aspects of yoga. It can help engage the parasympathetic nervous system and take us out of the stress response.

Part of this is by engaging the neocortex (frontal lobes) of the brain concerned with language, offering voices other than our internal ones. *Mantra* can bring about a state of healing vibration, dissolve *granthis* and bring the mind to a peaceful, *sattvic*, state, removing that which is negative or harmful, including *avidya* (ignorance) and *dukkha* (suffering). The beat cycle used when repeating mantra affects brain frequencies (Figure 6m). Chanting slowly reduces the breath and heart rate and calms the mind, which may support those with anxiety-related and other sympathetic dominant issues, a contributing factor (or root cause) of most immune and respiratory issues.

---

39   Kang, Scholp and Jiang (2018).

'Om' or 'Aum'

Chanting is an important, subtle practice, modulating how we process our emotions:

> *Om* chanting is associated with an experience of relaxation, changes in autonomic balance and deactivation of limbic brain regions (amygdala)... Modulation of brain regions involved in emotion processing and implicated in major depressive disorder (MDD) raises a potential possibility of *OM* chanting in the treatment of MDD.[40]

Research has shown that '*Bhramari pranayama* and *Om* chanting are effective in improving pulmonary function in healthy individuals'.[41]

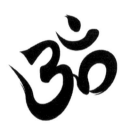

In the *Bhagavad Gita*, Lord Krishna states: 'I am the syllable *Om*... I am the sacred monosyllable... Among words, I am the monosyllable *Om*' (10.25).

'Whoever controls his mind and knowing that the souls reside in the forehead repeats the word *Om*, knowing it as representing Brahma, and thinking of Me his soul leaves the body, that person shall attain the supreme goal' (8.13).

According to Hindupedia: 'When one pronounces *Aum* correctly, all the basic sounds also echo. It is believed to be the traditional way of clearing all the impediments in the vocal cord to make one chant the hymns (*mantra*) correctly.'

FIGURE 60. '*OM*' OR '*AUM*'

Sometimes translated as 'the universal', 'everything', '*Om*' or '*Aum*' has around 22 meanings and connotations; for example: 'These three sound units consist of [the *gunas*] *sattva*, *rajas* and *tamas*... The vowel symbol "a" is the earthly realm, the vowel syllable "u" the atmosphere and the consonantal syllable "m" is the heavenly realm.'[42] In Hinduism it refers to the self within – *atman* – and ultimate divine truth – *brahman*.

Samadhi is the ultimate of the eight-limbed path laid out within Patanjali's *Yoga Sutras*, where our individual consciousness meets with the greater consciousness: 'Chanting *om* will lead us into *samadhi*.'[43] Said to be the primordial sound born with the universe, its vibration links us to the original source of creation. When we chant '*Om*', it harmonises our being with the realm of

---

40   Rao *et al.* (2018).
41   Mooventhan and Khode (2014).
42   Mallinson and Singleton (2017, *Markandeyapurana* 39.1–14).
43   Bryant (2009, *Yoga Sutra* 1.23–1.29).

oneness, a direct expression of *turiya*, which is what/who we truly are, our 'essence nature', dropping below all the layers of conditioning, the *samskaras*.

Rhyming with 'home', '*Om*' is sounded as a-a-u-u-m-(ng)-silence. The tip of the tongue is placed on the roof of the mouth to sound the last two syllables, 'm' and 'ng', which symbolise the close of the creation cycle, completing with silence, the 'empty pot' pause (*kumbhaka*), which drops us into the power of silence. The sound reverberates from the pelvic floor upward, to the crown of the head, resonating through the diaphragm and throat, via the 'instrument' of the torso.

'*Om*', the cosmic sound, is referred to as *pranava*, a word that derives from *pranu*, 'to reverberate', and ultimately from the root *nu*, 'to praise or command', but also 'to sound or shout'. It is the audible expression of the transcendental, attributeless ground of reality and infuser of *prana*: 'By opening up the back with the inhale, you are welcoming the breath as a gift, and providing space… Let the silence drape over you before inhaling again. Exhalation is an egoless state, I am not doing the *Om*, the *Om* is done through me.'[44]

Vibration and water in the body

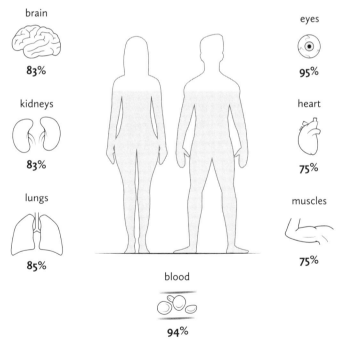

brain
83%

eyes
95%

kidneys
83%

heart
75%

lungs
85%

muscles
75%

blood
94%

FIGURE 6P. FLUIDS IN ORGANS

44   Rama Jyoti Vernon (2015).

When we consider that the body comprises 75 per cent water (with different ratios within organs, as seen in Figure 6p), and that water is sensitive to vibration, we can start to understand how theories such as Dr Masaru Emoto's Hado medicine work. This is based on experiments in which positive intention and prayer directed through water affected the formation of water crystals. Dr Emoto states:

> The theory of Hado postulates that, since all phenomena is at heart resonating energy, by changing the vibration we change the substance. Conventional science in general still does not support this notion. Yet quantum physics and in particular the "observer effect" (of Heisenberg's uncertainty principle) clearly suggests we do alter our environment.[45]

We can extrapolate from this that sound and vibrations can be used therapeutically to alter not just the fluidity and flow throughout our body, but also the very structure of the water within it.[46] A group of approximately 2000 people in Tokyo focused positive intentions toward water samples located inside an electromagnetically shielded room in California. That group was unaware of similar water samples set aside in a different location as controls. Ice crystals formed from both sets of water samples were blindly identified and photographed by an analyst, and the resulting images were blindly assessed for aesthetic appeal by 100 independent judges. Results indicated that crystals from the treated water were given higher scores for aesthetic appeal than those from the control water.[47] This lends support to the idea that vibration, sound and intention can alter the 'intrinsic vibrational pattern at the atomic level in all matter. The smallest unit of energy. Its basis is the energy of human consciousness.'[48]

Sound travels almost five times more efficiently through water, so the body conducts sound beautifully. See more in Part 3 around fluid adaptation for all of the ways that our fluid body can be affected by support of its flow, frequency and health.

Sounds in yoga

The nervous system is attuned to recognise that very high- or low-pitched sounds generally denote danger. In Indic texts, pitch is *svara*: *udatta, svarita*

---

45 Office Masaru Emoto (no date).
46 Matos *et al.* (2017).
47 Radin *et al.* (2006).
48 Office Masaru Emoto (no date).

and *anudatta* are markers that indicate tonal accents. *Langhana* ('to fast', 'to reduce', 'to diminish back to its cause') is usually soft, soothing sounds that help with elimination (letting go) and 'discharging' the exhalation, while *brahmana* sounds are more 'charging', to do with building and nourishing the inhalation.

Balam is the strength of the sound being used (see also page 278). *Nada* is said to be the sound beneath the words (like the clay is to the pot). It is internal transformation through sound and vibration: *ahata* is sound from without and *anahata* is the unstruck sound perceived by the heart *chakra*. Sounding naturally elongates the length of outbreath with vibration – *spanda* is vibration that radiates from pure consciousness, *brahman*, as well as the energy that manifests from all movement towards harmony. *Cit* or *citta* is supreme consciousness whose nature is *spanda* – a pulse, a movement, a flow.

While ancient Eastern philosophy can seem esoteric, there are clear similarities in themes that arise in modern science: 'The parallels to modern physics [with mysticism] appear not only in the Vedas of Hinduism, in the I Ching, or in the Buddhist sutras, but also in the fragments of Heraclitus, in the Sufism of Ibn Arabi, or in the teachings of the Yaqui sorcerer Don Juan.'[49]

The power of silence

In silence, the brain can relax, recalibrate, rewire and renew. That space between and after sounding is particularly powerful and potent after the vibration, for example when we listen to the fade of a singing bowl or after sounding out *mantra*, where we can tune into the resonance that follows the sound. We can feel increased capacity to understand internal and external signals and all of those within our environment, to have a greater sense of interoception/exteroception, the vibration within and outside of ourselves, where we are placed.

Often noise pollution is prevalent in our society. It can leave us feeling uneasy with silence – because we are always distracted by noise, by technology, we can feel the need to fill it, never allowing that sense of dropping down into quiet, vulnerability. Even doing yoga practice with music all the time does not give us the time to be with silence, our interoception, to really be with ourselves. Noise pollution can increase cardiac disease, depressive symptoms and cause sleep disturbance, getting in the way of our Circadian rhythms and contributing to chronic stress.[50] It can also negatively affect cognitive functioning and development in children; many children don't spend much time in silence now, which is needed when the brain is growing and neural pathways

49 Capra (2010).
50 Farooqi *et al.* (2020).

are being laid down.[51,52] This is why sympathetic dominance can lead to noise sensitivity, feelings of overload.

We are also not built for complete absence of noise; the silence referred to here is the 'deep thunderous silence' described within Zen. A hermetically sealed house is a long way from the teeming sounds of a forest, field or running water; our bodies vibrate most healthily along with the natural world we are a part of, even if so often separate from. In meditation, sounds around are part of our practice; we register a sound because it creates a vibration within us.

In yoga, *mauna* (silence) equates with peace of mind, inner quietude; this is the 'goal' of yoga, where the fluctuations of the mind are stilled (*Yoga Sutra* 1.2). Consciously quietening verbal activity – both our students' and our own! – so that attention is drawn inwards is an important part of teaching yoga, ensuring there is space between instructions for inner processing.

THE JAW AS A GATEWAY INTO SILENCE

Back to the jaw again (pages 53 and 85), to bring space around the architecture of the delicate inner ear area – and thus be able to connect with inner silence – we can direct awareness, curious and kind movement into the jaw via the whole upper body and head area; as well as that which supports it from below. Creating the space to drop beneath the 'outer chatty layers' allows us passage to meet the silence within that can often feel like the eye of the storm. This is always within us, but there is so often so much noise over the top that we can forget its presence – releasing the jaw is a gateway into a reunion with the ease, serenity, grace and acceptance within us; *samata*. As Tias Little says: 'In meditation, it is valuable to soften the muscular attachments around the jaw in order to release the delicate inner ear and connect to interior silence. Yoking to silence imparts a soothing effect on the entire brain while promoting *samata*, profound ease and serenity throughout the body. Meditation serves to bring stillness and space within the skull by imagining a third ear (like the mystical third eye) in the centre skull.'[53]

---

51 Kesar (2014).
52 Abramowicz, Kremkau and Merz (2012).
53 Little (2016).

PHYSICAL PRACTICE: BRINGING IT ALL TOGETHER – MOVEMENT WITH OPTIONAL SOUND

Sequencing

When bringing together practices from previous parts, with the optional addition of sound, we can bring conscious awareness to how we occupy the space of not doing, undoing/unravelling, smooth transitions, moving between planes and parallel posing, which all help to promote fluidity. Promoting a *sattvic* tone (page 275) regulates the nervous system (and inflammation), soothing lymphatics and supporting the microbiome – important considerations we have explored for immune and respiratory health.

Note that the sequences in this part are simply examples that also illustrate how we can incorporate sound in a simple and accessible way. You can draw in any similar sequencing from the previous parts (or others, of course) to create many permutations of sequence and theme, including:

- Grounding
- Rolling, rocking, reaching, pulsing, etc.
- Primal movements
- Starting to come off the ground
- All-fours up to lunging
- The journey to standing
- Coming back down
- Respecting the space and time of *savasana* (corpse pose).

Setting tone or intention

When planning a practice that supports the nervous system, teaching considerations include:

- Observing places where stress, tension or trauma are held, such as the jaw, eyes, throat, neck, shoulders, diaphragm, psoas, organs, hips, knees, feet…and back up to the head area.
- Holding and staying, creating containment with ease, found after

fluidity. Feeling the movement in stillness after stillness within movement.

- Setting grounding, orientation, agency.
- Shifting energy, voice, pace, strength where and when appropriate, including when a more active or stronger practice can help a student move through residues of stress in the system to be able to settle.
- Anatomical information and instructions as body-in-motion rather than reductionist facts that might take away from real-body-mind experience in the moment, for example common names for body parts, describing lines of movement or regions.
- Guiding moving in more deeply without prompting the mind's 'more is better' response – talking directly to the tissues.
- Holding focus without judgement or goal orientation – curiosity and exploration via our immediate experience in the here and now (not an idea, assumption or projection) – the phenomenological.
- Holding the space of the pause to allow processing, assimilation and integration – weaving these punctuations into the 'story'.
- Developing mindful attention – compassion and awareness (page 71).
- Breath leads, body follows, mind observes.
- Moving into patterns of protection, stress or trauma to be able to move through and resolve – respecting these boundaries of self-protection.

From here, we have the space to make more conscious and informed choices on how to respond to physical sensations, to reinforce positive and break negative feedback loops. For teachers, this means being able to give the student enough time and space to feel subtle sensations and nuances, guiding them to not get caught up in 'the story' or interpretation. Slowing down to feel and refining awareness into smaller and more subtle movements sets the scene for a more present relationship with our inner experience.

Movement with sound practice suggestions

This sequence can be done with or without the sounds suggested throughout; sounding can be as simple as 'ahh', 'ooo', 'mmm' and maybe together as 'Aum' (page 352). It could also just be adding the 'hum' or the vibration of *brahmari* breath (page 319) to practise drawing into *pratyahara*, feeling the healing qualities of the vibration in the lungs, throat, mouth (and beyond) lymphatics and tissues, promoting vagal tone (page 163).

Sound can be played with anywhere that we might synchronise breath with movement and notice the space of release with the exhalation that brings. As sound naturally elongates the out-breath, feel how there is a need to slow down the movement in response, which can also bring more awareness to its components and adaptive shifts within changing relation to gravity.

We might also simply allow such sounds of protolanguage (ancestral components of the words we use) or vowel sounds as they spontaneously arise in practice, for example an externalised expression of something moving through that is simply ready to be released. Like any part of our practice, notice where the sounding expresses a need with a quality of *sattva* (not too little, not too much). In other areas of life, a scream or a yell can be a fantastic vocal release, but within the context of a quiet, meditative practice we are attuning to the sound that resonates with introspective frequencies – that supports rather than disturbs a consistency of presence and offers deeper places of transformation.

Rather than force sound, we find the positioning of the mouth and neck (with soft jaw and eyes) to feel that the sound 'falls out' so it finds the appropriate tone, note, volume and texture for any given moment. In this way, sounding is a healing resonance rather than straining tissues – we are looking to support the throat, its microbiome, lymphatics, etc.

Here is an example of bringing sounding into movement practice with simple one-syllable sounds to build up to 'Om' ('Aum') with a moving sequence. Between each of the sounds below, include time for pause and integration, for the effects of each to be received and processed, as we might with any information: language, movement, sensation of any nature. All of the sounds engage the vagus nerve down the side of the neck to the chest (and beyond) from behind the ear, as well as a resonance into the middle ear that registers safety, so time for this to be assimilated can also be allowed within the movement.

Here the sound is part of, not separate to, the motion. Feel how the different levels change the sound resonance when we include the 'ahhh', 'ooo', 'mmm' that make up 'Aum'.

1. Prepare the space for sounding, loosening into the jaw and face, moving and breathing into the cheeks, sinuses, forehead, temples, between the eyes and muscles around and in the eye sockets.
2. Feel out the movement of a few fluid, easeful cycles of breath (inhale and exhale).

3. Sound 'ahhh' 1–3 times on the exhale, opening the mouth, jaw, throat and palate.
4. Sound 'ooo' 1–3 times on the exhale, which brings the vibration up into the tissues around the lips and mouth, maybe deepening the timbre.
5. Sound 'mmm' 1–3 times on the exhale, as in *brahmari* (page 319), taking the sound inwards, resonating into the chest and diaphragm.
6. Putting the three sounds together, continue the movement sounding '*Aum*', or move to a still place and chant three times.

These soundings can be used in any simple movement pattern, for example moving from all-fours to sound down into *balasana* (child's pose) and back up again. Feeling able to explore unlocks the creativity that helps us access the parasympathetic nervous system; repetition helps to regulate breathing. In the movements that follow, you can add in the sounds previously mentioned and as suggested in the instructions, or play with any '*Aums*', hums, *simha pranayama* (lion's breath; page 369), *bija mantra* (seed *mantra*: one-syllable sounds; page 371) and explore. Some yoga traditions bring more involved *mantra* into *asana* practice (such as *surya namaskar* (sun salutation)) to regulate the motion with the breath, and to suffuse the practice with intention and meaning; it is best to learn these directly with a teacher.

Arriving and grounding with (optional) sound

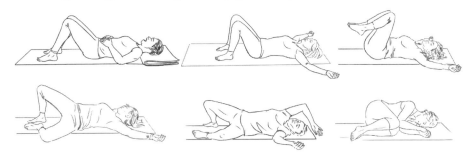

A simple sequence that takes a massaging and releasing journey through fascial nooks and crannies, while weaving in nervous system harmony. A good preparation for sound as it releases the throat and jaw, while creating fluid movement through the spine, ribs and diaphragm. Some simple sounds here

– for example, a natural and spontaneous releasing 'ahhh' or more guttural sounds helps prepare the vocal tissues and throat for the resonance to come.

1. Allow coming into CRP (page 55) for a spacious process of noticing the body, gathering sensory feedback on the ground as you come down. Hands on the belly to tune inwards; noticing any chatter in the brain, allowing the breath and natural rhythms of the body to come to the foreground of attention. Feel any swelling of the in-breath up the body that prompts a natural sigh on the exhale down towards the feet.

2. Come through pandiculations (pages 56) with any natural yawns and sounds to open down into the throat and chest from where you can bring your arms comfortably out to the side. Come into a lying spine undulation (page 58) to deepen awareness around the *jala*, throat region. Start to allow a subtle sound, like you might make if you were cleaning your glasses, space between the back teeth and around the eyes to allow a natural elongation to open up on the exhalation.

3. Draw each knee in towards the chest, massaging around the sacrum with any spontaneous movement into tissues on the back body, including the backs of the ribs and lungs.

4. Feet back to the ground, come to the Feldenkrais half-bridge roll (page 63), introducing an 'aah' sound on the exhale back to centre, signalling a decompressive quality. With this focus on release back to the midline, feel if the opening out (inhale) movement has more room to naturally open out more from the centre, for example, extending out the leg that drops to the ground and reaching across the diagonals of the torso (page 115) with the opposite arm.

5. After resting back to centre (any 'symmetrical' position), move side to side so that the movement falls just behind the breath in a softer version of the adrenal response exercise (page 118). Rather than inhale into the full 'star-shape', stay bent in the legs (feet mat-width) to roll to the side-lying foetal position on the exhale. Find a route with limbs heavy, dragging the top leg over so the movement is initiated from the belly. If comfortable, take the top arm over the head to roll to the side, fingers along the floor to open up the side ribs (or any other comfortable journey for the arm and shoulder). Keep that side-rolling movement fluid to sound as you roll to the side, allowing a natural pause at the end of the exhale so that the movement back to centre on the inhale allows a sense of 'gathering back in'.

6. The sequence ends resting on whichever side feels most intuitive, curled right in towards heart and belly on the side, breathing into the dorsal body.

Crawling to *simha pranayama* (lion's breath)

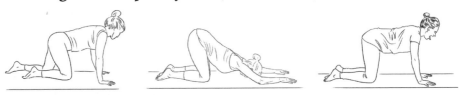

Coming to all-fours, free crawling feels out the territory – both on the ground and internally – before organising around the spine and ultimately opening that up into the throat area. This introduces resonance from the feedback on the ground; meeting spirallic movement at the centre and the vibration of strong air movement at the immune tissues of the throat and mouth.

1. Crawl back and forth, exploring the suspension of the shoulders and the hips, any and all directions – outside the confines of a mat.
2. Bring the hips above the knees (page 182), and reach the hands out – you can even extend the arms in this position, coming onto the fingertips (head up with the ears between the upper arms) and pandic-ulating (pages 56 and 290), with deep 'aahh' releases on the exhales.
3. Back to all-fours, circle the tailbone (page 128), limiting the movement in the shoulders so that the slide and glide of the viscera can be felt, waking up the belly region, loosening into the lower back. Allow that to snake up the spine so that the whole body becomes involved. Bring-ing that to stillness, notice where the head feels comfortable and least compressive in the neck and eyes.
4. Softening around the jaw, on the exhale allow the tongue to extend out in *simha pranayama* (lion's breath; page 369), looking up to the third eye, with the option to allow the breath to sound past the vocal cords with a soft, natural 'haaaa' – like a wind. Repeat three times.
5. Settle back into *balasana* (child's pose), softening around the third eye. Returning to all-fours, circle the tailbone in the opposite direction, then another three *simha pranayamas*. Come back to *balasana*, with the arms out to the side, breathing into the base of the skull and across the lower back.

Low salutation with (optional) sound

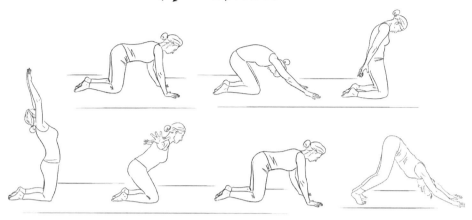

Come back into this moving meditation, to reconnect with movement that ripples upwards with the inhale of *prana* up the front spine, the dropping of *apana* down with the exhale. The mind can quieten as the movement follows the breath, and if sounding, there is more control and awareness needed in the descent back to the ground – where the out-breath is naturally elongated. You can also come to *adho mukha svanasana* (down-face dog) between each movement (or each different sounding) as an inversion to rest into the silence permeating into all *koshas*.

1. Slide the hands back to all-fours for the low *vinyasa* salutation (page 181); where the belly gathers up into the spine to come back, take the weight off the hands to reach the arms up and round to the side, sitting down as if to sit on a chair. Gather the belly to ease back down to all-fours, rippling up on the inhale and down on the exhale, three times: one with 'aaaaaaah', one 'ooooooooh', one 'mmmmmmm' on subsequent exhales on the movement down.
2. Rest in either *adho mukha svanasana* (down-face dog) or *balasana* (child's pose); feel the reverberance and resonance of the sound settle.
3. You can also add in any salutation style practice after down-face dog here – for example, stepping to lunge or the sequence on page 180.

Simple standing practice

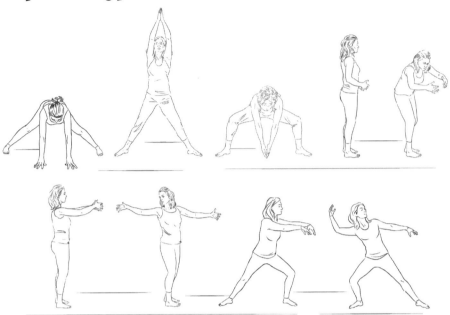

This sequence opens up the body 360 degrees, moving around the spine, improving lymphatic flow with pump and squeeze around the lungs. Standing up from the ground to feel a sense of presence, occupying your space and that around you, consider, how does the sound express differently in standing postures?

1. With the option to move freely through any primal motions from down-face dog through to *prasarita padotanasana* (wide-legged standing forward fold, page 184), come to a half-version where you can lengthen between the breastbone and pubic bone.
2. Turn the heels in and raise up into *utkata konasana* (intense angle pose) explorations 3 (page 244), playing with sounding as you exhale down the midline.
3. Settle back to *tadasana* (mountain pose), holding hands in front of your belly, fingers slightly apart, completing the circle of the pelvis. In this meditative space, we connect with the belly, and a deeper intuition of 'what is here right now'. You can come back to this reflection between each movement.
4. Raise your hands as if holding an imaginary football at about eye height or higher, as your neck feels comfortable, with arms in a circle

to keep the soft ventral space of the inner arms. Keeping your focus on the ball, rotate it – from the belly – fully in front of your body, bending your knees as you reach it down past your legs. Change direction, fully breathing as you move into the diaphragm and ribs.

5. Take the imaginary football down to chest height, inhale to reach one hand back behind you past the hip, following it with your gaze to turn from the belly. Exhale to bring it back the same way to join the other hand, then inhaling that back. Move from side-to-side, bending the knees as the hand moves past the body and retaining focus on the moving hand as you exhale back to the midline, as in previous sequences: with 'ahhh', 'ooo' and 'mmm'.

6. Coming back to *utkata konasana* (intense angle pose) explorations 2 (page 241), feel where the movement drops into a rhythm, a cadence, where the breath is supported all the way up from the feet and shifting weight side to side.

Uttanasana flow with (optional) sound

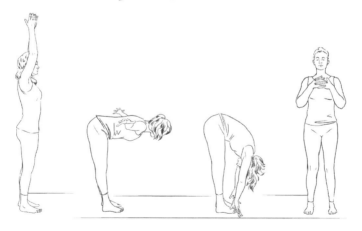

This is a simple sounding practice that explores the different frequencies felt moving through higher and lower planes, with the front body closing and then opening. Similar can be done kneeling, seated on a chair or with knees deeply bent, which may also allow those with low blood pressure or dizziness to acclimatise through the planes more easily.

1. From *tadasana* (mountain pose) inhale up and then exhale down into *uttanasana* (standing forward fold; page 236), sounding out 'aaaaaah'.

2. Bring the torso and arms back up half-way, so level with the collarbone, squeezing the back muscles to open the front body on an inhalation, another 'aaaaaaah' on the descent back into *uttanasana*.

3. Inhale to come up, raising the arms over the head, then another 'aaaaaaah' as the hands release back down to the heart.

4. Repeat the cycle 1–3 with an 'ooooooooh', then the cycle with an 'mmmmmmm' sound on each exhale moving down.

5. With the hands at the heart in *tadasana*, put those three sounds together for three '*Aums*'.

6. Settle into the silence of non-doing in *tadasana*, sensitive to the rhythm of the breath, the subtle vibration resonant in the body: 'That which is not uttered by speech that by which speech is revealed.'[54]

Supported inversion practice to *savasana* (corpse pose)

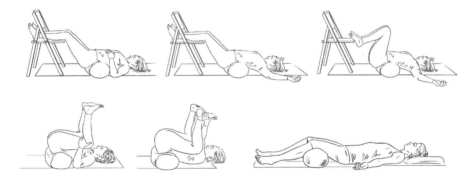

These supported inversions heighten interoception by shifting the relationship to gravity in the fascial sacs around the organs and thus create new sensation via interoceptive change. Opening the abdomen and then gathering around it, we are invited to allow any sounding before to settle deep into our unconscious realm at the belly and pelvis.

1. Coming into supported *viparati karani* (upside-down practice, page 304) feeling an easy, soft *jalandhara bandha* (throat gathering, page 336). Tune in to the natural timbre in the throat as you cultivate *ujjayi*. Feel the difference in resonance through the throat and chest with hands onto the diaphragm and out to the side, before dropping into silence.

2. Coming to supported *apanasana* (wind release pose) at the heart, even

---

54 Swami Paramananda (2013, *Kena Upanishad* 1.5).

moving into supported *ananda balasana* (happy baby pose) – wherever you can sensitively settle to feel the back of the body expanding and softening in preparation for *mantra* or *savasana* (corpse pose).

Karuna namaha, a simple *mantra* practice

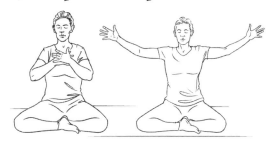

Both chanting and gesturing with an emphasis on the power of *karuna* (compassion) – brings the qualities of friendliness, generosity, non-judgement, courage and the strength of gentleness into our mind-body in a very real way. This supports the immune and respiratory systems as we switch off the threat response and move towards soothing and comfort to the self, regulating the autonomic nervous system into parasympathetic states.

1. Sit supported on a bolster, legs comfortable – rising from the front of the sit-bones, through the front spine. Cross the arms first behind the body to prepare the chest to open, lifting the sternum and the bottom of the breastbone to gather the throat, soften the eyes, moving into *jalandhara bandha* (throat gathering; page 336). Gather up the intelligence in the pelvic diaphragm into *mula bandha* (root gathering).
2. Release the arms forwards, hands back to the heart. *Karuna* means 'compassion', *namaha* 'salutations', so the chant into the heart space of *karuna namaha* is 'All hail to compassion'. First inhale to open the arms and exhale, chanting *karuna namaha,* as the hands come back to the heart three times, bringing compassion to ourselves.
3. Extend compassion outwards to others – begin with the hands on the heart, extending outwards with the *mantra* on the exhale, inhaling the hands back in to the heart. Repeat three times.
4. Settle back into the heart space, feeling the echoes of the sound within connected to the vibration of the universal.

5. After time to integrate, move into *savasana* (corpse pose). This is a very important part of our practice, where we settle into stillness of the external body, senses draw inwards and awareness becomes more subtle, a space of kind, healthy boundaries and the ability to meet others with a kind expression, all those aspects of immune and respiratory health embodied, felt in the breath.

6. Coming up from *savasana*, finish the practice with three clear '*Aums*', hands at the heart, the meeting of mind and body.

SUBTLE PRACTICES: SIMPLE SOUNDING AND *MANTRA*

Simha pranayama (lion's breath)

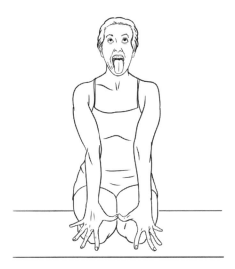

Simha pranayama is a forceful exhalation from the back of the throat, while extending the tongue from the mouth (downwards). The muscles at the front of the throat contract, and the breath passes over the back of the throat with a roaring 'haaaa' sound, creating plenty of vibration.

A 'happy' postural head placement is essential for nasal breathing: it is hard to sound easefully with the head pushed forward in an overfocusing *rajasic* place, with little space for airways and opening of the oesophagus (see 'tech neck', page 169), but *simha pranayama* can be performed in any comfortable and stable position.

It can include focus up towards the third eye (pineal gland, which regulates the hormonal system) – *bhrumadhya drishti*, 'mid-brow gazing'. This focus should be *sattvic* – neither too fierce (*rajasic*), or half-hearted, lacking in full commitment (*tamasic*).

This *pranayama* stretches the muscles and stimulates the nerves in the face, relieving tension and increasing circulation. We need softness to avoid straining the throat, so this could be done in softer ways without taking the eyes upwards if there is tension up into the forehead.

Although some practitioners like to accompany the breath with a primal sound, there is no requirement to use the vocal cord. It can be accompanied with an autogenic release, as we've seen with pandiculation (pages 56 and 290), adding in the tensing fists with the inhale to full extension of the fingers with the exhale for autonomic release.

This can be warming to prepare for *asana*, moving through tension in the throat, opening and awakening *vishuddha chakra*.

'So Hum' mantra

'So Hum' is a phrase comprised of two Sanskrit words: *So*, which translates as 'That', and *Hum* as 'I' – together making 'I Am That' (also *Sohum, Soham, So Ham, Saham*, and sometimes inverted as *Hamsah*). Many scholars of ancient Indian philosophy (Vedic) interpret 'That' as representing the Universe, and it is now widely understood that the 'So Hum' mantra symbolises the connection to universal energy that is constantly supporting and nourishing us. It falls into the same concept as 'oneness', or 'I am one with the Universe and all of creation' – an Eastern view of insight. On as simple level, it can offer feelings of larger connection, safety and unconditional support: from the *Upanishads* 'The light which is thy fairest form, I see it. I am what He is.'[55]

There are various ways to practise with 'So Hum':

- 'So Hum' words repeated many times in a cyclical structure through-out a meditation practice – both words within one breath.
- This is often chanted 108 times (counting with *mala* beads). There are many reasonings as to why that number has great spiritual significance. In the *Vedas* it is the number of planetary positions and influences that need to be harmonised or pacified – the 108 steps that the sun and moon take through heaven. These can be broken down into cycles of 27.
- Incorporating an 'Om' sound in between 'So Hum' cycles.
- Chant silently, internally, where you can also sound on the inhalation and evoke the power of silence, *mauna* (page 356) – this can be a potent focus for meditation and might be accompanied by a *nyasa* (hand placement) or *mudra*. Inhale to the thought of 'So' and exhale to the thought of 'Hum', to invite melding of individual and universal consciousness (*samadhi*).

---

55 Johnston (2020).

Bija mantra

These *mantras* have vibrational impact throughout the line of the *chakras* rising up through the *sushumna*. Each sound resonates with an element, and from there is associated with a specific *chakra*, although different elements can be chanted in different locations (for example, if more grounding is needed at the heart, we can chant '*Lam*' with a focus there). Each of the seed *bija mantras* resonates different parts of the palate starting from just behind the teeth to the top of the palate, with a relationship between the fontanelle (crown of the head), the palate and top of the heart, all resonating with how we take in food, experience and nourish ourselves on many levels.

The *bija mantras* can be chanted singly (each rhymes with 'Lang') to focus on a particular area or all (bottom-to-top) resonating up from the earth, out to the universe.

- *Lam* – earth element – base, *muladhara chakra*
- *Vam* – water element – sacral, *svadhistana chakra*
- *Ram* – fire element – solar plexus centre, *manipura chakra*
- *Yam* – wind element – heart, *anahata chakra*
- *Ham* – ether element – throat, *vishuddha chakra*
- *Om* – light element – third eye, *ajna chakra* (modern addition)
- Silence – transcends other elements/integration – crown, *sahasrara chakra* (modern addition).

Self-enquiry questions

1. How do you feel the quality of your voice and expression change with your emotional states?
2. If you ever experience sore throats, respiratory issues or immune issues when feeling run down, how does your communication change?
3. How does refined awareness of the architecture, positioning and ease needed for nasal breathing affect sounding and *mantra*?
4. How does sounding within movement and *asana* change the experience?
5. Which body or health aspects (biological, psychological or yogic/Ayurvedic) link sound with the immune and respiratory systems?

Further resources

Brené Brown (2015) *Daring Greatly: How the Courage to be Vulnerable Transforms the Way we Live, Love, Parent and Lead.* New York: Avery.

Pema Chödrön (2018) *Comfortable with Uncertainty: 108 Teachings on Cultivating Fearlessness and Compassion.* Boulder, CO: Shambhala Publications.

Deborah Dana (2021) *Anchored: How to Befriend Your Nervous System Using Polyvagal Theory.* Boulder, CO: Sounds True.

Tias Little (2016) *Yoga of the Subtle Body: A Guide to the Physical and Energetic Anatomy of Yoga.* Boulder, CO: Shambhala Publications.

Kristin Neff and Christopher Germer (2018) *The Mindful Self-Compassion Workbook: A Proven Way to Accept Yourself, Build Inner Strength, and Thrive.* New York: Guilford Press.

Russill Paul (2006) *The Yoga of Sound: Healing and Enlightenment Through the Sacred Practice of Mantra.* Novato, CA: New World Library.

References

Abramowicz, J.S., Kremkau, F.W. and Merz, E. (2012) 'Obstetrical ultrasound: Can the fetus hear the wave and feel the heat?' *Ultraschall in der Medezin 33*(3), 215–217. Available at: https://pubmed.ncbi.nlm.nih.gov/22700164 [in German].

Armour, J.A. (2003) *Neurocardiology – Anatomical and Functional Principles.* Meerssen: HeartMath Research Center, HeartMath Institute. Available at: www.heartmathbenelux.com/store/product_page.php?lang=en&id=101&product=62

Armour, J.A. (2008) 'Potential clinical relevance of the "little brain" on the mammalian heart.' *Experimental Physiology 93*(2), 165–176. Available at: https://pubmed.ncbi.nlm.nih.gov/17981929

Asokan, S., Emmadi, P. and Chamundeswari, R. (2009) 'Effect of oil pulling on plaque induced gingivitis: A randomized, controlled, triple-blind study.' *Indian Journal of Dental Research 20*(1), 47–51. Available at: https://pubmed.ncbi.nlm.nih.gov/19336860

Bellosta-Batalla, M., Ruiz-Robledillo, N., Sariñana-González, P., Capella-Solano, T., *et al.* (2017) 'Increased salivary IgA response as an indicator of immunocompetence after a mindfulness and self-compassion-based intervention.' *Mindfulness,* 5 October. Available at: https://self-compassion.org/wp-content/uploads/2018/05/Bellosta-Batalla2017.pdf

Bryant, E.F. (2009) *Yoga Sutras of Patanjali.* New York: North Point Press.

Capra, F. (2010) *The Tao of Physics: An Exploration of the Parallels between Modern Physics and Eastern Mysticism,* 5th edn. Boulder, CO: Shambhala Publications.

Del Negro, C.A., Funk, G.D. and Feldman, J.L. (2018) 'Breathing matters.' *Nature Reviews. Neuroscience 19*(6), 351–367. Available at: https://pubmed.ncbi.nlm.nih.gov/29740175

Deo, P.N. and Deshmukh, R. (2019) 'Oral microbiome: Unveiling the fundamentals.' *Journal of Oral and Maxillofacial Pathology 23*(1), 122–128. Available at: https://pubmed.ncbi.nlm.nih.gov/31110428

Emamian, M.H., Hassani, A.M. and Fateh, M. (2013) 'Respiratory tract infections and its preventive measures among Hajj pilgrims, 2010: A nested case control study.' *International Journal of Preventive Medicine 4*(9), 1030–1035. Available at: https://pubmed.ncbi.nlm.nih.gov/24130944

Farooqi, Z.U.R., Sabir, M., Latif, J., Aslam, Z., *et al.* (2020) 'Assessment of noise pollution and its effects on human health in industrial hub of Pakistan.' *Environmental Science and Pollution Research International 27*(3), 2819–2828. Available at: https://pubmed.ncbi.nlm.nih.gov/31836979

Forssmann, W.G., Nokihara, K., Gagelmann, M., Hock, D., *et al.* (1989) 'The heart is the center of a new endocrine, paracrine, and neuroendocrine system.' *Archives of Histology and Cytology 52,* 293–315. Available at: https://pubmed.ncbi.nlm.nih.gov/2530996

Goldman, B. (2017) 'Study shows how slow breathing induces tranquility.' Stanford Medicine News Center blog, 30 March. Available at: https://med.stanford.edu/news/all-news/2017/03/study-discovers-how-slow-breathing-induces-tranquility.html

HeartMath Institute (2016) *Science of the Heart: Exploring the Role of the Heart in Human Performance. An Overview of Research Conducted by the HeartMath Institute.* Volume 2. Available at: www.heartmath.org/research/science-of-the-heart/heart-brain-communication

Hoffmann, M., Kleine-Weber, H., Schroeder, S., Krüger, N., *et al.* (2020) 'SARS-CoV-2 cell entry depends on ACE2 and TMPRSS2 and is blocked by a clinically proven protease inhibitor.' *Cell 181,* 271–280.e8. Available at: https://pubmed.ncbi.nlm.nih.gov/32142651

Ishida, Y., Nakamura, F., Kanzato, H., Sawada, D., *et al.* (2005) 'Clinical effects of *Lactobacillus acidophilus* strain L-92 on perennial allergic rhinitis: A double-blind, placebo-controlled study.' *Journal of Dairy Science 88*(2), 527–533. Available at: https://pubmed.ncbi.nlm.nih.gov/15653517

Jerzynska, J., Stelmach, W., Balcerak, J., Woicka-Kolejwa, K., *et al.* (2016) 'Effect of *Lactobacillus rhamnosus* GG and vitamin D supplementation on the immunologic effectiveness of grass-specific sublingual immunotherapy in children with allergy.' *Allergy and Asthma Proceedings 37*(4), 324–334. Available at: https://pubmed.ncbi.nlm.nih.gov/27401319

Johnston, C. (2020) *Isha Upanishad and Commentary: Esoteric Classics. Eastern Studies.* Lamp of Trismegistus.

Jung, C.G. (1999) *The Psychology of Kundalini Yoga: Notes of the Seminar Given in 1932.* Princeton University Press.

Kang, K., Scholp, A. and Jiang, J.J. (2018) 'A review of the physiological effects and mechanisms of singing.' *Journal of Voice 32*(4), 390–395. Available at: https://pubmed.ncbi.nlm.nih.gov/28826978

Kesar, A.G. (2014) 'Effect of prenatal chronic noise exposure on the growth and development of body and brain of chick embryo.' *International Journal of Applied & Basic Medical Research 4*(1), 3–6. Available at: https://pubmed.ncbi.nlm.nih.gov/24600569

Lieberman, D. (2014) *The Story of the Human Body: Evolution, Health and Disease.* London: Penguin.

Lin, C.D., Tona, F. and Osto, E. (2018) 'The heart as a psychoneuroendocrine and immunoregulatory organ.' *Advances in Experimental Medicine and Biology 1065*, 225–239. Available at: https://pubmed.ncbi.nlm.nih.gov/30051388

Lin, W.Y., Fu, L.S., Lin, H.K., Shen, C.Y. and Chen, Y.J. (2014) 'Evaluation of the effect of *Lactobacillus paracasei* (HF.A00232) in children (6–13 years old) with perennial allergic rhinitis: A 12-week, double-blind, randomized, placebo-controlled study.' *Pediatrics and Neonatology 55*(3), 181–188. Available at: https://pubmed.ncbi.nlm.nih.gov/24269033

Lionetti, V., Bollini, S., Coppini, R., Gerbino, A., *et al.* (2021) 'Understanding the heart–brain axis response in COVID-19 patients: A suggestive perspective for therapeutic development.' *Pharmacological Research 168*, 105581. Available at: https://pubmed.ncbi.nlm.nih.gov/33781873

Little, T. (2016) *Yoga of the Subtle Body: A Guide to the Physical and Energetic Anatomy of Yoga.* Boulder, CO: Shambhala Publications.

Little, T. and Little, S. (no date) SATYA (Sensory Awareness Training for Yoga Attunement). [course training manual]. Accessed 2019.

Mallinson, J. and Singleton, M. (2017) *The Roots of Yoga.* London: Penguin.

Matos, L.C., Santos, S.C., Anderson, J.G., Machado, J., *et al.* (2017) 'Instrumental measurements of water and the surrounding space during a randomized blinded controlled trial of focused intention.' *Journal of Evidence-Based Complementary & Alternative Medicine 22*(4), 675–686. Available at: https://pubmed.ncbi.nlm.nih.gov/28497700

Matsuyama, S., Nagata, N., Shirato, K., Kawase, M., Takeda, M. and Taguchi, F. (2010) 'Efficient activation of the severe acute respiratory syndrome coronavirus spike protein by the transmembrane protease TMPRSS2.' *Journal of Virology 84*, 12658–12664. Available at: https://pubmed.ncbi.nlm.nih.gov/20926566

McCraty, R., Atkinson, M. and Bradley, R.T. (2004) 'Electrophysiological evidence of intuition: Part 1. The surprising role of the heart.' *Journal of Alternative and Complementary Medicine 10*(1), 133–143. Available at: https://pubmed.ncbi.nlm.nih.gov/15025887

McCraty, R., Atkinson, M., Tomasino, D. and Bradley, R.T. (2009) 'The coherent heart: Heart–brain interactions, psychophysiological coherence, and the emergence of system-wide order.' *Integral Review 5*(2), 10–115. Available at: www.heartmathbenelux.com/doc/McCratyeal_article_in_integral_review_2009.pdf

Mooventhan, A. and Khode, V. (2014) 'Effect of Bhramari pranayama and OM chanting on pulmonary function in healthy individuals: A prospective randomized control trial.' *International Journal of Yoga 7*(2), 104–110. Available at: https://pubmed.ncbi.nlm.nih.gov/25035619

Neff, K.D. (2003) 'The development and validation of a scale to measure self-compassion.' *Self and Identity 2*, 223–250. Available at: https://self-compassion.org/wp-content/uploads/publications/empirical.article.pdf

Neff, K.D. (2009) 'The role of self-compassion in development: A healthier way to relate to oneself.' *Human Development 52*(4), 211–214. Available at: https://pubmed.ncbi.nlm.nih.gov/22479080

Office Masaru Emoto (no date). Hado. Office Masaru Emoto. Accessed 31/04/2022 at: www.masaru-emoto.net/en/hado

Porges, S.W. (2017) *The Pocket Guide to the Polyvagal Theory – The Transformative Power of Feeling Safe,* Illustrated edn. New York: W.W. Norton & Company.

Radin, D., Hayssen, G., Emoto, M. and Kizu, T. (2006) 'Double-blind test of the effects of distant intention on water crystal formation.' *Explore (New York) 2*(5), 408–411. Available at: https://pubmed.ncbi.nlm. nih.gov/16979104

Rama Jyoti Vernon (2015) *Yoga: The Practice of Myth and Sacred Geometry*. Ferndown: Lotus Press.

Rao, N.P., Deshpande, G., Gangadhar, K.B., Arasappa, R., *et al.* (2018) 'Directional brain networks underlying OM chanting.' *Asian Journal of Psychiatry 37*, 20–25. Available at: https://pubmed.ncbi.nlm.nih. gov/30099280

Rein, G., Atkinson, M. and McCraty, R. (1995) 'The physiological and psychological effects of compassion and anger.' *Journal of Advancement in Medicine 8*(2), 87–105. Available at: www.heartmath.org/assets/ uploads/2015/01/compassion-and-anger.pdf

Sakai, M., Shimbo, T., Omata, K., Takahashi, Y., *et al.* (2009) 'Cost-effectiveness of gargling for the prevention of upper respiratory tract infections.' *BMC Health Services Research 8*(3), 258. Available at: https:// pubmed.ncbi.nlm.nih.gov/19087312

Satomura, K., Kitamura, T., Kawamura, T., Shimbo, T., *et al.* (2005) 'Prevention of upper respiratory tract infections by gargling: A randomized trial.' *American Journal of Preventive Medicine 29*(4), 302–307. Available at: https://pubmed.ncbi.nlm.nih.gov/16242593

Simpson, D. (2021) *The Truth of Yoga: A Comprehensive Guide to Yoga's History, Texts, Philosophy, and Practices*. New York: North Point Press.

Sungnak, W., Huang, N., Bécavin, C., Berg, M., *et al.* (2020) 'SARS-CoV-2 entry factors are highly expressed in nasal epithelial cells together with innate immune genes.' *Nature Medicine 26*, 681–687. Available at: https://pubmed.ncbi.nlm.nih.gov/32327758

Swami Muktibodhananda (1998) *Hatha Yoga Pradipika* (4th reprinted edn). India: Bihar School of Yoga.

Swami Paramananda (2013) *The Upanishads*. CreateSpace Independent Publishing Platform.

Wei, H., Wang, X., Shi, H., Shang, H., *et al.* (2012) 'Auricular acupuncture and vagal regulation.' *Evidence-Based Complementary and Alternative Medicine 2012*, 786839. Available at: https://pubmed.ncbi. nlm.nih.gov/23304215

Wilson, A.C., Mackintosh, K., Power, K. and Chan, S.W.Y. (2019) 'Effectiveness of self-compassion related therapies: A systematic review and meta-analysis.' *Mindfulness 10*, 979–995. Available at: https:// self-compassion.org/wp-content/uploads/2019/08/WilsonMackintosh2019.pdf

Yang, C.F., Kim, E.J., Callaway, E.M. and Feldman, J.L. (2020) 'Monosynaptic projections to excitatory and inhibitory preBötzinger complex neurons.' *Frontiers in Neuroanatomy 14*, 58. Available at: https:// pubmed.ncbi.nlm.nih.gov/33013329

GLOSSARY OF SANSKRIT TERMS

A

Ādhāra (adhara) Support/platform. In Hindu, the way in which *ātman (atman)* is contained in the five *kośas (koshas)*.

Amṛta (amrta) Immortal/deathless. The nectar of the *devas*, allowing them to attain higher consciousness. A synonym of soma, or ambrosia.

Anuloma With the hair/grain, natural. *Anuloma prāṇāyāma (pranayama)* is the practice of inhaling through both nostrils and exhaling alternately between right and left nostrils, using the thumb and little finger to close off the other nostril.

Apāna (apana) Air going downwards. The outwards flow of *prāṇa (prana)* from the body, eliminating waste and governing digestion and reproduction.

Āsana (asana) Sitting, sitting down, seat.

Ātma (atma) Self/body/mind.

Ātman (atman) The living entity/supreme soul/in yourself.

Āyurveda (Ayurveda) Life knowledge. The science of longevity.

B

Bandhas Lock or bind, performed to direct and regulate the flow of *prāṇa (prana)*.

Bhagavad Gītā (Bhagavad Gita) One of Hinduism's holy scriptures, a 700-verse summation of *Vedanta* dating from the second half of the first millennium BCE.

Bhastrikā (bhastrika) A rapid *prāṇāyāma (pranayama)* where the inhale and the exhale are moved quickly and deliberately by the diaphragm. A *kriya*, cleansing, practice.

Bhrāmarī (Bhramari) The Hindu goddess of black bees. *Prāṇāyāma (pranayama)* practice in which the exhale is made with the humming sound of a bee.

C

Citta Consciousness/heart/the mind/the spirit soul/the living force.

D

Dhāraṇā (dharana) Concentration of the mind. The sixth of the eight limbs in Patanjali's *Yoga Sutras*.

Dhyāna (dhyana) State of meditation where awareness is fully integrated with the object of attention. The mind is firm and stable. The seventh of Patanjali's *aṣṭānga (astanga)* path.

Dṛṣṭi (drishti) Sight/glance/gaze.

G

Granthis Doubt/a difficult knot to untie.

Guṇa (guna) In Jainism, the attributes of substance: pure (*sattva*), passionate (*rajas*) and dark (*tamas*).

H

Haṭha (Hatha) Force.

Haṭhayoga (Hatha yoga) A system of physical and mental techniques to regulate the flow of *prāṇa (prana)* and purify the inner and outer bodies. Yoga by means of force.

I

Iḍā (ida) A tubular vessel/one of the three *nāḍīs (nadis)*, channels of vital spirit, on the right side of the body. Associated with the moon and the River Ganges.

J

Jālandharabandha (Jalandhara bandha) Throat stream lock. Upwards-pulling net: 'Contracting the throat, hold the chin firmly against the chest' (*Haṭha Yoga Pradīpikā*).

Jñāna (jnana) Knowledge that is inseparable from the total experience of reality.

K

Kapālabhāti (kapalbathi) Cranium perception/knowledge/skull-shining breath. An energising *prāṇāyāma (pranayama)* that clears the lungs, nasal passages and purifies the mind. The inhale is passive and the exhale pumps the belly into the spine.

Kevala kumbhaka Absolute breath retention. Complete suspension of breath, without strain, leading to a pure state of consciousness.

Kośas (koshas) The five 'sheaths' of Vedantic philosophy, which cover *ātman (atman)*, the Self.

Kriyās (kriyas) Action, deed or effort. Yoga technique or practice to achieve a specific result.

Kumbhaka Retention of the breath after inhalation or exhalation.

Kuṇḍalinī (kundalini) Coiled snake. Divine feminine energy at the base of the spine. Spiritual liberation is believed to come from cultivating this energy through Tantric practices.

M

Manas The mind.

Mudrās (mudras) Symbolic hand or bodily gestures believed to conduct *prāṇa (prana)*, vital life energy.

Mūlabandha (Mula bandha) *Mūla (mula)* is root or base, foundation; *bandha* is bind, joining together or lock. The root lock: 'Pressing Yoni (perineum) with the heel, contract up the anus' (*Haṭha Yoga Pradīpikā*). This draws *apāna (apana)*, the downwards-moving wind in the body, forcibly up.

N

Nāḍī (nadi) The tubular stalk of any plant or tubular organ (as a vein or artery of the body), any pipe or tube. Channels of movement of *prāṇa (prana)* through the body.

Nāḍīśuddhi (Nāḍī Shodhana) (nadi shodhana) Purification of the *nāḍīs (nadis)* through alternate nostril breathing. Breathing alternately through right and left nostrils, closing off the opposite side with thumb and little finger.

O

Oṁ (Aum) Supreme personality of Godhead, the complete whole. Spiritual symbol across Indic traditions.

P

Piṅgalā (pingala) *Nāḍī (nadi)* originating from right nostril and runs parallel to *suṣumnā (susumna)*. Correlates with the Sun and the River Yamuna.

Prajñā (prajna) Wisdom. The state of understanding the true nature of phenomena.

Prāṇa (prana) The vital air/the life air/life force.

Prāṇāyāma (pranayama) *Prāṇa (prana)* is energy and *ayām (ayam)* expansion. The restraint of breath, consciously controlling of the flow of *prāṇa* through the body.

Pratyāhāra (pratyahara) Weaning away from *āhāra (ahara)*. Withdrawal of the senses, fifth limb in Patanjali's *aṣṭānga (astanga)* path.

Pūraka (puraka) Inhaling.

R

Rajas One of the three *guṇas (gunas)*. The quality of passion, dynamic activity and movement.

Rechaka (recaka) Exhaling.

S

Sahita antara kumbhaka The breath is retained when the lungs are full at the end of the inhalation.

Sahita bāhya (bahya) kumbhaka Where the breath is held after the exhalation.

Samādhi (samadhi) The eighth limb of Patanjali's *aṣṭānga (astanga)* path, achieved through intense concentration in meditation. A state of transcendent consciousness, bliss.

Samāna (samana) Equal/all alike/straight/equally adjusted.

Sāṅkhya (Sāṁkhya) (Sankhya) Classical school of Indian philosophy that views human experience as constituting *puruṣa* (consciousness) and *prakṛti* (matter).

Satkarmā (shatkarma) Bodily purifications – *netī (neti)*, *dhautī (dhauti)*, *naulī (nauli)*, *bastī (basti)*, *kapālabhatī (kapalbathi)* and *trātaka (trataka)* – to prepare for *mokṣa (moksha)* (liberation).

Sattva Goodness/steadiness/power/discretion.

Śītalī (sitali) Cooling. *Śītalī prāṇāyāma (sitali pranayama)* is a cooling breath drawn in through the tongue; the exhale is through the nose.

Sūkṣma śarīra (sukshma sarira) The subtle body.

Sūrya (surya) Sun.

Sūryabheda (suryabheda) One of the eight *kumbhakas*. Purifies the cranium.

Suṣumnā (susumna) The central *nāḍī (nadi)*, equated with the River Sarasvati. Centred *prāṇa (prana)* in *suṣumnā (susumna)* represents a clear, unwavering mind.

T

Tamas Inertia, inactivity or lethargy. One of the three *guṇas (gunas)*.

U

Udāna (udana) Soaring.

Uḍḍīyānabandha (uddiyana bandha) A *bandha* in which *prāṇa (prana)* is revitalised by drawing the belly in and up, directed towards the spine and into *suṣumnā nāḍī (susumna nadi)*.

Ujjāyī (ujjayi) Diaphramatic *prāṇāyāma (pranayama)* technique. Sometimes known as 'victorious breath', 'ocean breath' or 'whispering breath'. Inhalation and exhalation is through the nose, with a gentle drawing in of the throat on the exhale to produce a sea-like sound over the glottis.

Upaniṣad (Upanisad) Ancient Vedic scriptures, known as *Vedānta (Vedanta)*.

V

Vāyus (vayus) Currents or vital winds that move *prāṇā (prana)* around the body.

Viloma Against the hair/grain. *Prāṇāyāma (pranayama)* technique where the breath is consciously interrupted, punctuated by *kumbhaka*, to gain mastery of ventilation.

Vyāna (vyana) One of the *vāyus (vayus)*, governing the circulation of *prāṇā (prana)* through the whole body.

SUBJECT INDEX

AUTHOR INDEX

Müller-Oerlinghausen, B. 265
Munk, N. 268
Muntean, A.G. 104
Muskiet, F.A.J. 101, 156, 201
Myers, T. 115, 175

Najjar, S. 265
Nakajima, K. 265
Nakao, A. 100
National Institute of Environmental
    Health Services 221
Neff, K.D. 343
Nestor, J. 43, 45, 98
Niazi, I.K. 318
NICE 108
Nishihara, H. 211
Nutma, E. 265

Odier, D. 290
Office Masaru Emoto 354
O'Rourke, D. 132
Osto, E. 347
Owen, J. 33

Painold, A. 217
Palikaras, K. 90
Pamer, E.G. 214
Paolantonio, E.G. 44
Park, J.H. 228
Parker, L.A. 174
Parvathy, S.S. 44
Pavlov, V.A. 165
Payne, A.N. 214
Payne, P. 157
Pederson, B.K. 110
Pennisi, E. 213, 216
Persson, M. 97
Peterson, M. 85, 290
Petrie, G.N. 174
Piacentino, G. 211
Pollatos, O. 260
Porges, S.W. 83, 270, 326
Poroyko, V.A. 222
Prata, J. 213
Pruimboom, L. 101, 156, 201, 213
Purssell, E. 30

Quadt, L. 260
Queri, S. 265

Radin, D. 354

Rama Jyoti Vernon 353
Ramon, S. 106
Ramsheh, M.Y. 207
Ran, Z. 90
Rao, N.P. 352
Rein, G. 347
Rhyner, H.H. 276, 277, 293
Ricard, M. 118
Ricciotti, E. 224
Richardson, A.G. 104
Rinaman, L. 214
Rivest-Gadbois, E. 265
Rodulfo, I.J.A. 149
Roenneberg, T. 100
Rosenow, M. 268
Rothenberg, R. 283, 307, 311, 312, 313
Rowe, P.C. 147
Roxo, M.R. 161
Ruegsegger, G.N. 100
Russo, M.A. 132

Sahdra, B.K. 297
Sakai, M. 341
Salim, S. 101
Salvich, G.M. 110
Sankarâchârya 151
Santarelli, D.M. 132
Satomura, K. 340
Schadt, E.E. 104
Schleip, R. 115, 146, 172, 173, 223,
    259, 261, 262, 268, 294
Scholp, A. 351
Schöttker, B. 104
Schünemann, H.J. 39
Schwager, S. 160
ScienceDaily 197
Sedlmeier, P. 273
Segre, J.A. 199
Sehinson, C. 93
Sempowski, G.D. 92
Sen-Gupta, O. 284
Serhan, C.N. 106
Sharma, J.N. 44
Shearer, A. 18
Shen, J. 90
Shields, G.S. 297
Silverio, S. 108
Simpson, D. 18, 271, 307, 349
Singh, S. 174
Singh, U. 307
Singleton, M. 263, 310, 352
Sinha, A.N. 318